Study Guide
Medical-Surgical Nursing
Concepts & Practice
2nd Edition

D0534733

Susan C. deWit, MSN, RN, CNS, PHN
Formerly, Instructor of Nursing
El Centro College
Dallas, Texas

Candice K. Kumagai, MSN, RN
Formerly, Instructor in Clinical Nursing
University of Texas at Austin
Austin, Texas

ESL Consultants

Gail G. Boehme, BA
ESL Teaching Certification
University of California at Santa Barbara

Thomas M. Sadowski, BA, MA, GDipTESOL
Language Arts Department
Allan Hancock College
Santa Maria, California

Reviewer

Laura Bevlock Kanavy, RN, BSN, MSN
Instructor, Practical Nursing Program
Career Technology Center of Lackawanna County
Scranton, Pennsylvania

ELSEVIER
SAUNDERS

ELSEVIER

SAUNDERS

3251 Riverport Lane
St. Louis, Missouri 63043

Study Guide: Medical-Surgical Nursing
Concepts & Practice, 2nd Edition

ISBN: 978-1-4377-2211-6

Copyright © 2013, 2009 by Saunders, an imprint of Elsevier Inc.

All rights reserved. No part of this publication may be reproduced or transmitted in any form or by any means, electronic or mechanical, including photocopy, recording, or any information storage and retrieval system, without permission in writing from the publisher.

Although for mechanical reasons all pages of this publication are perforated, only those pages imprinted with an Elsevier Inc. copyright notice are intended for removal.

Notices

Knowledge and best practice in this field are constantly changing. As new research and experience broaden our understanding, changes in research methods, professional practices, or medical treatment may become necessary.

Practitioners and researchers must always rely on their own experience and knowledge in evaluating and using any information, methods, compounds, or experiments described herein. In using such information or methods they should be mindful of their own safety and the safety of others, including parties for whom they have a professional responsibility.

With respect to any drug or pharmaceutical products identified, readers are advised to check the most current information provided (i) on procedures featured or (ii) by the manufacturer of each product to be administered, to verify the recommended dose or formula, the method and duration of administration, and contraindications. It is the responsibility of practitioners, relying on their own experience and knowledge of their patients, to make diagnoses, to determine dosages and the best treatment for each individual patient, and to take all appropriate safety precautions.

To the fullest extent of the law, neither the Publisher nor the authors, contributors, or editors, assume any liability for any injury and/or damage to persons or property as a matter of products liability, negligence or otherwise, or from any use or operation of any methods, products, instructions, or ideas contained in the material herein.

Vice President: Loren Wilson
Executive Content Strategist: Teri Hines Burnham
Content Development Specialist: Tiffany Trautwein
Publishing Services Manager: Jeffrey Patterson
Senior Project Manager: Mary G. Stueck
Design Director: Karen Pauls

Working together to grow
libraries in developing countries

www.elsevier.com | www.bookaid.org | www.sabre.org

ELSEVIER   BOOK AID International   Sabre Foundation

Printed in the United States of America
Last digit is the print number: 9 8 7 6 5 4 3 2 1

To The Student

This *Study Guide* has been constructed to help you achieve the objectives of each textbook chapter and establish a solid base of knowledge in medical-surgical nursing. The exercises in this guide reinforce the material presented in the textbook and in class. Additional *Interactive Review Questions for the NCLEX® Examination* and *Interactive Exercises and Activities* are available on the Evolve website (evolve.elsevier.com/deWit/medsurg). These exercises and activities will assist you to develop solid critical thinking and priority setting skills, and some require you to call upon and synthesize previously learned information to reach an answer. Completing the exercises will help you be successful on the NCLEX® Examination.

In an effort to assist Limited English Proficient (LEP) students in mastering communication in English, a section has been included in each chapter called *Steps Toward Better Communication*. The exercises in this section are aimed at improving communication while reinforcing the content of the chapter. The exercises have been constructed so that they will be helpful to other students as well.

STUDY HINTS FOR ALL STUDENTS

- *Ask questions!* There are no bad questions. If you do not know something or are not sure, you need to find out. Other people may be wondering the same thing but may be too shy to ask. The answer could mean life or death to your patient, which certainly is more important than feeling embarrassed about asking a question.
- *Make use of chapter objectives.* At the beginning of each chapter in the textbook are objectives that you should have mastered when you finish studying that chapter. Write these objectives in your notebook, leaving a blank space after each. Fill in the answers as you find them while reading the chapter. Review to make sure your answers are correct and complete, and use these answers when you study for tests. This should also be done for separate course objectives that your instructor has listed in your class syllabus.
- *Locate and understand key terms.* At the beginning of each chapter in the textbook are key terms that you will encounter as you read the chapter. Page numbers are provided for easy reference and review, and the key terms are in bold, blue font the first time they appear in the chapter. Phonetic pronunciations are provided for terms that might be difficult to pronounce.
- *Review Key Points.* Use the Key Points at the end of each chapter in the textbook to help you review for exams.
- *Get the most from your textbook.* When reading each chapter in the textbook, look at the subject headings to learn what each section is about. Read first for the general meaning, then reread parts you did not understand. It may help to read those parts aloud. Carefully read the information given in each box and table and study each figure and its caption.
- *Follow up on difficult concepts.* While studying, put difficult concepts into your own words to see if you understand them. Check this understanding with another student or the instructor. Write these in your notebook.
- *Take useful notes.* When taking lecture notes in class, leave a large margin on the left side of each notebook page and write only on right-hand pages, leaving all left-hand pages blank. Look over your lecture notes soon after each class, while your memory is fresh. Fill in missing words, complete sentences and ideas, and underline key phrases, definitions, and concepts. At the top of each page, write the topic of that page. In the left margin, write the key word for that part of your notes. On the opposite left-hand page, write a summary or outline that combines material from both the textbook and the lecture. These can be your study notes for review.
- *Join or form a study group.* Form a study group with some other students so you can help one another. Practice speaking and reading aloud, ask questions about material you are not sure about, and work together to find answers.
- *Improve your study skills.* Good study skills are essential for achieving your goals in nursing. Time management, efficient use of study time, and a consistent approach to studying are all beneficial.

Copyright © 2013, 2009 by Saunders, an imprint of Elsevier Inc. All rights reserved.

There are various study methods for reading a textbook and for taking class notes. Some methods that have proven helpful can be found in *Saunders Student Nurse Planner: A Guide to Success in Nursing School* by Susan C. deWit. This book contains helpful information on test-taking and preparing for clinical experiences. It includes an example of a "time map" for planning study time and a blank form that you can use to formulate a personal time map.

ADDITIONAL STUDY HINTS FOR STUDENTS WHO USE ENGLISH AND A SECOND LANGUAGE (ESL)

- *Find a first-language buddy.* ESL students should find a first-language buddy—another student who is a native speaker of English and is willing to answer questions about word meanings, pronunciations, and culture. Maybe your buddy would like to learn about your language and culture. This could help in his or her nursing experience as well.
- *Expand your vocabulary.* If you find a nontechnical word you do not know (e.g., *drowsy*), try to guess its meaning from the sentence (e.g., *With electrolyte imbalance, the patient may feel fatigued and drowsy*). If you are not sure of the meaning, or if it seems particularly important, look it up in the dictionary.
- *Keep a vocabulary notebook.* Keep a small alphabetized notebook or address book in which you can write down new nontechnical words you read or hear along with their meanings and pronunciations. Write each word under its initial letter so you can find it easily, as in a dictionary. For words you do not know or for words that have a different meaning in nursing, write down how they are used and sound. Look up their meanings in a dictionary or ask your instructor or first-language buddy. Then write the different meanings or usages that you have found in your book, including the nursing meaning. Continue to add new words as you discover them. For example:

    –Primary—*Of most importance; main (e.g., the primary problem or disease); The first one; elementary (e.g., primary school)*
    –Secondary—*Of less importance; resulting from another problem or disease (e.g., a secondary symptom); The second one (e.g., secondary school ["high school" in the United States])*

PRONUNCIATION NOTES

The pronunciation of words in the *Vocabulary Building Glossary* in each chapter in this guide is shown by a simple respelling. It follows the pronunciation guide in Miller-Keane *Encyclopedia and Dictionary of Medicine, Nursing, and Allied Health, 7th edition* (Saunders, 2006):

- Long Vowels: "Long" vowels (a, e, i, o, u, y) are pronounced with the sound of the name of the letter.
    1. An unmarked vowel ending a syllable is long (*ba' be=baby*).
    2. A long vowel in a syllable ending with a consonant is marked with a long symbol or macron (̄) (*be hāv'yer*).
- Short Vowels: "Short" vowels have varying pronunciations.
    3. An unmarked vowel in a syllable ending with a consonant is short (*ab dukt' = abduct*).
    4. A short vowel at the end of a syllable is marked with a short mark or breve (̆) (*lip ĭ do' sis*). Sometimes, the vowel is followed by a silent *h* instead of using the breve (*lip ih do' sis*).
    5. Some sounds are represented by two letters:
        ah': In stressed syllables, *ah* represents the "a" sound heard in father (*fah' ther*).
        ah: In unstressed syllables, *ah* represents the "a" sound heard in sofa (*so' fah*). (It often sounds like *uh*. This sound, called a *schwa*, is represented in many dictionaries by an upside-down *e*. Many people pronounce any unaccented vowel as a schwa.)
        aw: The *aw* in paw.
        oi: The *oi* in oil.
        oo: The *oo* in food.
        ou: The *ou* in out.
    6. A stressed syllable is indicated by an accent mark (') at the end of the syllable.

Good luck!

Susan C. deWit
Candice K. Kumagai
Gail G. Boehme

Copyright © 2013, 2009 by Saunders, an imprint of Elsevier Inc. All rights reserved.

To The Instructor

The *Study Guide for Medical-Surgical Nursing: Concepts & Practice* is designed to reinforce the students' understanding of terms and concepts presented in the text. It will assist them in setting priorities, applying the nursing process, thinking critically, making good judgments and decisions, communicating therapeutically, and meeting chapter objectives. Answers are provided (for instructors only) on the Evolve website.

ORGANIZATION OF THE TEXT

Included are a wide variety of exercises, questions, and activities. Most chapters include *Terminology, Short Answer, Review Questions for the NCLEX® Examination, Critical Thinking Activities*, and a special section called *Steps Toward Better Communication* written by a specialist in English as a second language. Other sections that appear where appropriate are *Completion, Identification, Review of Structure and Function, Priority Setting*, and *Application of the Nursing Process*. Additional interactive activities and exercises are provided on the Evolve website for the textbook.

DESCRIPTION OF EXERCISES

The exercises are as follows:

- **Terminology** – Reinforce correct use of words from the chapter terms list with matching and/or fill-in-the-blank questions.
- **Short Answer** – List brief answers to reinforce knowledge and assist students to meet the chapter objectives.
- **Review Questions for the NCLEX® Examination** – Multiple choice and alternate item format questions are based on real-life situations and require knowledge, synthesis, analysis, evaluation, and application.
- **Critical Thinking Activities** – Brief scenarios and questions foster problem-solving skills in nursing care which may be practiced individually or in study groups.
- **Completion** – Reinforce chapter content with fill-in-the-blank questions.
- **Identification** – Identify appropriate steps in a process or procedure or verify normal or abnormal laboratory values.
- **Review of Structure and Function** – Re-examine anatomy and physiology of the body system pertinent to the text chapter.
- **Priority Setting** – Analyze information and make decisions to set priorities within tasks or clinical situations.
- **Application of the Nursing Process** – Apply critical thinking skills and the steps of the nursing process to real-life patient care.

STUDENTS WITH LIMITED ENGLISH PROFICIENCY

Because so many students from other countries, whose primary language is not English, are entering nursing programs in the United States and Canada, we have enlisted the aid of a specialist in English as a Second Language who has worked with many health care occupation students. She helped construct the exercises in the *Steps Toward Better Communication* within each chapter. Her letter to you follows. I hope you find this section helpful to your students with limited English proficiency.

Susan C. deWit
Candice K. Kumagai

Copyright © 2013, 2009 by Saunders, an imprint of Elsevier Inc. All rights reserved.

STEPS TOWARD BETTER COMMUNICATION

Imagine yourself back in nursing school—trying to read the texts and understand the lectures in Spanish or German. Students studying in a language that is not their native language face not only the challenge of learning the medical and physiological lessons that are required of all nursing students, but they must also decipher and use a language whose nuances and grammar are unfamiliar to them. In order to ease some of that burden, we've attempted to simplify and regularize the language of *Medical-Surgical Nursing: Concepts & Practice* and the study guide, and to explain some of the colloquial uses of English that occur.

A major part of the nursing process could be described as "knowing your patient inside and out," and one key to that knowledge is being able to accurately and sensitively communicate with the patient and colleagues. To this end, after the regular exercises, we added a section for the ESL student titled *Steps Toward Better Communication*, which offers help in pronunciation, vocabulary building, and use of grammatical issues such as verb tense, and encourages asking for help and clarification. In addition, a section on understanding cultural nuances and mannerisms helps student face real-life situations and clarify feelings. Another section offers facility in appropriately asking questions and carrying on conversations.

A note about pronunciation: we assume that the important medical terms will be used and modeled correctly by the instructor. In terms of conversation, intelligibility rather than native-like accuracy should be the goal. Correct stress is the major determining factor in how easily a person can be understood. Therefore, we chose to indicate stressed syllables in words and phrases, rather than giving phonetic pronunciations that students often find difficult to understand.

Description of Exercises

The following exercises appear in the *Steps Toward Better Communication* section as appropriate.

- **Vocabulary Building Glossary** – explains and defines idiomatic or unusual use of non-medical terms used in the chapter and indicates the stressed syllables for capitalizing them.
- **Completion Sentences** – offer opportunities to use the words presented in the Glossary, often in different context than they are used in the text, thereby offering yet another way to increase vocabulary.
- **Vocabulary Exercises** – use words from the chapter in various ways to increase ease of understanding.
- **Word Attack Skills** – deal with word segments, suffixes, prefixes, and types of words to help the student learn to decode new words and their usage.
- **Pronunciation Skills** – offer practice in pronouncing difficult terms as well as phrases and sentences, with emphasis on stress and intonation.
- **Grammar Points** – are made occasionally, especially when there is a recurring point raised by the chapter, such as the use of the past tense in taking case histories.
- **Communication Exercises** – encourage communicative interchange, writing, and dialogues that might actually be used by a practicing nurse. The value of this section is enhanced if students can be paired in first- and second-language speaker combinations, giving each the opportunity to experience the other's accent and offering the possibility for cross-cultural exchange. Answers to the Communication Exercises are provided in the TEACH Instructor Resources on the Evolve website for the text, and could be printed out for student use.
- **Cultural Point(s)** – present explanations and questions about issues and customs that may differ across the cultures represented in the class, and in the prospective patient community. They can explain the normative culture in which the individual will be working, while at the same time, acknowledge and validate an individual's cultural differences.

In preparing these materials, I have drawn on my teaching experience of practicing and aspiring health care personnel. I have found them to be dedicated and eager to improve their own lives while helping others. I have learned much from them about hard work, perseverance, humor, and what they need in order to do a better job. My colleagues in teaching English and nurses with whom I have worked have been helpful with ideas for teaching projects, indicating language areas needing to be addressed, and offering suggestions and solutions for problems. However, any omissions and errors are my own.

Copyright © 2013, 2009 by Saunders, an imprint of Elsevier Inc. All rights reserved.

I have been impressed with the similarity between learning language skills and nursing skills. Both require access to academic knowledge, but mastery occurs with hands-on practice and experience. The exercises are geared to provide this opportunity. Encourage your students to interact as often as possible. Look at each lesson with the question, "How can I structure this lesson so the students will have to generate their own language to complete the exercise?" Offer real-life challenges and tasks for speaking and communicative interaction with other students, colleagues, and patients whenever possible. An encouraging, open, and interactive classroom is the best setting for language learning and improvement. I wish you well in working with this special group of people.

Gail G. Boehme

Copyright © 2013, 2009 by Saunders, an imprint of Elsevier Inc. All rights reserved.

Illustration Credits

Chapter 18
Modified from Ignatavicius, D.D., & Workman, M.L. (2010). *Medical-Surgical Nursing: Critical Thinking for Collaborative Care* (6th ed.). Philadelphia: Saunders.

Chapter 20
From Aehlert, B. (2002). *EKGs Made Easy* (2nd ed.). St. Louis: Mosby.

Chapter 30
Modified from deWit, S.C. (2009). *Fundamental Concepts and Skills for Nursing* (3rd ed.). Philadelphia: Saunders.

Chapter 34
Modified from Lewis, S.M., Heitkemper, M.M., & Dirksen, S.R. (2011). *Medical- Surgical Nursing: Assessment and Management of Clinical Problems* (8th ed.). St. Louis: Mosby.

Chapter 35
Modified from Ignatavicius, D. D., & Workman, M. L. (2006). *Medical-Surgical Nursing: Critical Thinking for Collaborative Care* (5th ed.). Philadelphia: W.B. Saunders.

 Copyright © 2013, 2009 by Saunders, an imprint of Elsevier Inc. All rights reserved.

Contents

Copyright © 2013, 2009 by Saunders, an imprint of Elsevier Inc. All rights reserved.

Copyright © 2013, 2009 by Saunders, an imprint of Elsevier Inc. All rights reserved.

Caring for Medical-Surgical Patients

Answer Key: Textbook page references are provided as a guide for answering these questions. A complete answer key was provided to your instructor.

SHORT ANSWER

Health Care System

Directions: Provide the answers to the following questions.

1. List settings in which you might seek employment after graduation. *(3, Box 1-1)*

    a. _____

    b. _____

    c. _____

2. List three factors that contribute to the rising cost of health care. *(6)*

    a. _____

    b. _____

    c. _____

3. List at three overarching goals in the U.S. *Healthy People 2020* agenda. *(7)*

    a. _____

    b. _____

    c. _____

Nursing Functions and Responsibilities

Directions: Provide the answers to the following questions.

1. List the four functions of the LPN/LVN. *(1-4)*

    a. _____

    b. _____

    c. _____

    d. _____

Copyright © 2013, 2009 by Saunders, an imprint of Elsevier Inc. All rights reserved.

2. What are the five rights of delegation according to The National Council of State Boards of Nursing's position paper, *Delegation: Concepts and Decision-Making Process*? *(4)*

    a. _____

    b. _____

    c. _____

    d. _____

    e. _____

3. Describe three ways in which you as a nurse can actively participate in health promotion and disease prevention. *(7)*

    a. _____

    b. _____

    c. _____

4. List at least five examples of patient teaching activities performed by the LPN/LVN. *(2)*

    a. _____

    b. _____

    c. _____

    d. _____

    e. _____

COMPLETION

Directions: Fill in the blanks to complete the statements.

1. Delegation is _____ to competent unlicensed assistive personnel (UAP) the authority to perform a selected nursing task/activity in a selected patient situation that is within the job description of the LPN/LVN. *(3)*

2. _____ involves a set monthly fee charged by the provider of health care services for each member of the insurance group for a specific set of services. *(4)*

3. A(n) _____ stands up for patients' rights and intervenes in their best interests. *(3)*

4. Delegation is a(n) _____ function. *(4)*

5. You must provide unlicensed assistive personnel with the necessary _____, _____, _____, and _____ to safely carry out the delegated task/activity. *(4)*

Copyright © 2013, 2009 by Saunders, an imprint of Elsevier Inc. All rights reserved.

SHORT ANSWER

Dealing with Different Patient Behaviors

Directions: Read the clinical scenario and answer the questions that follow.

Scenario A: Mrs. Gay, age 78, has been hospitalized with a broken hip. She is very quiet, does not seem to want to be touched, and responds with "I'm just fine" when asked if she is worried about anything. *(7-9)*

1. Mrs. Gay's behavior is typical of anxiety or fear and is an expression of a need for _____ _____.

2. Write four appropriate nursing interventions to help meet Mrs. Gay's needs and modify her withdrawn behavior.

   a. _____

   b. _____

   c. _____

   d. _____

Scenario B: Mr. Parsons has had one arm amputated as a result of injuries suffered in a farming accident. He has supported his wife and three small children by working as a farmer. During his hospitalization, Mr. Parsons has become increasingly abusive and critical and has threatened to report his nurse on several occasions. *(7-9)*

1. Mr. Parsons' behavior probably indicates feelings of _____ and _____.

2. His hostile behavior is an expression of a need to _____ _____.

3. Write three appropriate nursing interventions to satisfy Mr. Parsons' needs and modify his behavior.

   a. _____

   b. _____

   c. _____

Scenario C: Ms. Stinson has become manipulative with the nursing staff. She is demanding and attempts to bargain to get out of what she is supposed to do for rehabilitation after her stroke. She insists that she get something other than the broiled fish for dinner, stating that she wants pot roast, mashed potatoes, and gravy. She announces that she will not walk in the halls anymore until she gets something "decent" to eat. *(7-9)*

1. List four nursing interventions and approaches that might help in dealing with Ms. Stinson's behavior.

   a. _____

   b. _____

   c. _____

   d. _____

Copyright © 2013, 2009 by Saunders, an imprint of Elsevier Inc. All rights reserved.

PRIORITY SETTING

Directions: Read the scenario and prioritize as appropriate.

Scenario: You are caring for five patients. They have various behavioral issues that you must address. Prioritize the order in which you will assist these patients with their needs. *(9)*

_____ a. Mrs. Bora is calling for assistance to the bathroom. She is capable of managing this for herself, but she routinely calls for assistance for many tasks that she can do for herself.

_____ b. Mr. Fogel has locked himself in the bathroom. The nursing assistant is speaking to him through the door, but he "wants some time to himself."

_____ c. Mr. Ahrens is yelling at his wife. You can hear him shout, "These nurses can't do anything right. You should have never brought me here! You are so stupid!"

_____ d. Ms. Schott wants you to immediately call her doctor. "Call him right this second, or I will make sure you get fired for incompetence!"

_____ e. Mr. McGinnis refuses to get out of bed. The nursing assistant has tried to encourage him, but he just gazes off and then starts crying.

REVIEW QUESTIONS FOR THE NCLEX® EXAMINATION

Directions: Choose the best answer(s) for the following questions.

1. The RN charge nurse delegates hanging TPN solution on a patient to the LPN/LVN. Before delegating this task, the RN should: *(Select all that apply.) (3-4)*
   1. verify that the state nurse practice act allows LPNs/LVNs to perform this procedure.
   2. question the LPN/LVN as to ability to perform the procedure.
   3. remind the LPN/LVN about the need for strict asepsis for the procedure.
   4. state when the solution should be hung.
   5. ask for a report on the patient's glucometer blood glucose level.

2. The doctor asks the LPN/LVN student to hang a unit of blood on a patient who has suddenly become very critical. The best action would be to: *(3-4)*
   1. follow the doctor's orders because of the emergency situation.
   2. refuse to do it and explain that it is outside the scope of practice.
   3. immediately get an RN to assist the physician.
   4. obtain the equipment for the doctor, but tell him that he will have to hang the blood himself.

3. The nurse must be instrumental in helping contain the cost of health care. This can be accomplished by: *(Select all that apply.) (6-7, Box 1-6)*
   1. following policies for charging for supplies used in patient care.
   2. documenting patient care for reimbursement.
   3. reusing and recycling supplies whenever possible.
   4. organizing patient care for effective and efficient use of time.
   5. decreasing patient length of stay by recommending patients leave.

4. The nurse is caring for a patient who is depressed about his health condition and he is concerned about how it will affect his ability to provide for his family. He tells the nurse, "I just don't know how my wife is going to cope if I die." What is the best response? *(8)*
   1. "You are not going to die. For goodness sakes, cheer up! Don't be so pessimistic."
   2. "What makes you think you are going to die? Your prognosis is actually quite good."
   3. "Your wife is coming to see you today and you wouldn't want her to worry about this or about you."
   4. "It sounds like you are really worried about several issues. What have you been thinking about?"

Copyright © 2013, 2009 by Saunders, an imprint of Elsevier Inc. All rights reserved.

5. The patient is constantly using the call bell and the entire nursing staff is quite frustrated and tired of this behavior. A team approach to help the patient gain independence would be to: *(8-9)*
   1. assign a different nurse every day to prevent the patient's dependency on one person.
   2. tell the patient that someone will check on him every 30 minutes if he does not use the call bell.
   3. refuse to answer the call bell if the patient uses it too much.
   4. tell the patient to do things for himself and then follow through by refusing to help him.

6. The doctor has just told the patient that she has a terminal illness. She is softly crying and the doctor instructs you to "take care of her." What would be the best immediate intervention to meet the spiritual needs of this patient? *(10)*
   1. Offer to sit with her.
   2. Offer to call the hospital clergy.
   3. Offer to call family or friends.
   4. Offer to pray for her.

7. Measures that assist in developing a therapeutic relationship might include: *(Select all that apply.)* *(8-9)*
   1. always follow through on obtaining requested information for the patient.
   2. talk encouragingly about the patient's physician.
   3. use an unhurried approach when interacting with the patient.
   4. always knock before entering the room.
   5. explain what you are going to do before performing any procedure.

8. An important part of assessment is the social assessment. An important question to ask is: *(7)*
   1. "Where did you go to school?"
   2. "What are your concerns about being away from home?"
   3. "What are your beliefs about how to stay well?"
   4. "What are your beliefs about a higher power?"

9. Medicare Part B requires a(n) _____ and does not pay for most
   _____. *(5, Box 1-3)*

CRITICAL THINKING ACTIVITIES

Scenario: You are caring for Mr. Huang, a young man who recently emigrated from a Southeast Asian country. You notice a strange bruising pattern on his back. When you question him about it, he appears to be embarrassed and just shakes his head. When you report the finding to the RN, she tells you that it may be from a culturally based home remedy known as "coin rubbing."

1. What might his nonverbal behavior mean? *(10)* _____

   _____

   _____

2. List three interventions that would help Mr. Huang to feel more relaxed and open in giving information for the data collection. *(8-9)*

   a. _____

   b. _____

   c. _____

Copyright © 2013, 2009 by Saunders, an imprint of Elsevier Inc. All rights reserved.

3. How can you increase your "cultural competence" to prepare yourself for working with coworkers and patients from a variety of different cultural backgrounds? *(9-10)*

_____

_____

STEPS TOWARD BETTER COMMUNICATION

VOCABULARY BUILDING GLOSSARY

Term	Definition
signif'icant others	important people in the life of the patient; may include family, loved ones, and close friends
collab'orative (co lab' ah ra tive)	working together
pre'mium (pree' mee um)	rate amount paid for insurance
fee'-for-service	amount paid to the doctor depending on the service given
em'pathy	understanding of another's feelings
feed'back	return information about actions or an idea
self-esteem'	one's own feelings of worth
eye contact	looking into a person's eyes while talking to him or her
compass'ion	caring
com'petence	knowing what to do and being able to do it
interact'ing	acting on each other; communicating
el'derly	polite term for people who are over age 65 years

COMPLETION

Directions: Fill in the blanks with the appropriate words from the Vocabulary Building Glossary to complete the statements.

1. The LPN/LVN, the RN, the physician, and the respiratory therapist form a(n) _____ team that provides the best and most efficient care for the patient.

2. The patient's insurance was not valid, because he forgot to pay the monthly _____.

3. The patient needed an explanation of _____ in order to understand that the insurance company would directly pay the doctor.

4. When a patient is an adult and not married, you should inquire about _____ _____ who are part of the patient's support system.

5. To evaluate the effectiveness of your patient teaching, it is important to obtain _____ from the patient.

Copyright © 2013, 2009 by Saunders, an imprint of Elsevier Inc. All rights reserved.

6. Being able to feel _____ helps you to understand the patient and to provide

    compassionate care.

VOCABULARY EXERCISE

1. The word **site** means "place." In this chapter, the places talked about are work sites, or places LVNs
    might work. On the job, you might talk about the **site** of the wound, or the **site** of the infection. Make
    two sentences using the word in the two different ways.

    _____

    _____

Two other words with the same pronunciation are **sight** (verb): to see, or sight (noun): something to see and
cite: to quote or make reference to.

2. Complete the sentences using the correct word above: **Site/sight/cite**
    a. It was quite a _____ to see Mr. Benson tangled in his oxygen tubes.

    b. This is the _____ for the new clinic.

    c. When you write your paper, be sure to _____ your sources.

    d. The original _____ of the infection is not known.

3. If medical personnel were *demeaning* and *aloof* would that be good for the patient? Why or why not?

    _____

    _____

SPECIAL VOCABULARY MEANINGS

*Directions: Each language uses words or phrases as idioms that do not translate directly, but are part of everyday
speech. Explain in your own words the meaning of the idiomatic words in the quotation marks.*

1. What does "bending the rules" mean? _____

    _____

2. Why is "skyrocketing" a good description for the cost of health care? _____

    _____

    _____

3. What is meant by "unraveling… and stitched back together" with reference to the health care system?

    _____

    _____

Copyright © 2013, 2009 by Saunders, an imprint of Elsevier Inc. All rights reserved.

4. Why would expensive and specialized medical care be called "boutique medicine"? _____

_____

_____

CLINICAL SCENARIOS

Directions: Study the following scenarios.

1. Mrs. Bazan was admitted with weight loss, abdominal pain, and a diagnosis of "rule out cancer of the colon." She underwent a colonoscopy and a bone scan. A member of her church group has come to visit and stops you in the hall to ask if Mrs. Bazan's tests show that she has cancer. You know that they did and that Mrs. Bazan has been told her diagnosis. To protect your patient's privacy and confidentiality, which of the following is the *best* response?
   a. "You will have to speak to Mrs. Bazan's doctor about that."
   b. "I really have no idea what the tests showed."
   c. "I cannot reveal the results of a patient's tests."
   d. "What did Mrs. Bazan tell you?"

2. *Communication example:* Jane is talking with a nursing assistant. "Barry, I would like you to assist Mr. Januz with his range-of-motion exercises now. Put each joint of his affected arm through the range of motion five times. If he has discomfort, stop and let me know. I will be in room 212."

   Later, Jane checks with Barry about the task delegated. "Barry, how did the range-of-motion exercises go for Mr. Januz? Did he have any discomfort? Did you encounter any problems? How many times was each joint exercised?"

3. Write out how you would delegate the following task and then describe how you would verify that the task was completed.

   Mrs. Paul needs to be dangled and then ambulated twice on your shift. Ann, the nursing assistant working with you, is capable of performing this task.

Copyright © 2013, 2009 by Saunders, an imprint of Elsevier Inc. All rights reserved.

Critical Thinking and the Nursing Process

Answer Key: Textbook page references are provided as a guide for answering these questions. A complete answer key was provided to your instructor.

IDENTIFICATION

Phases of the Nursing Process

There are five major phases or components of the nursing process: assessment, nursing diagnosis, planning, implementation, and evaluation. Four of these apply to the LPN/LVN: assessment (data collection), planning, implementation, and evaluation. *(15, 22-24, 26-27, Box 2-1)*

Directions: For each nursing action on the right, identify the name of the phase in which the action occurs.

1. _____ Noting whether the application of heat has relieved muscle pain.

2. _____ Referring the patient and family to a community support group.

3. _____ Setting a goal for prevention of damage to the skin from prolonged pressure.

4. _____ Assisting a patient to turn, cough, and breathe deeply every 2 hours after surgery.

5. _____ Changing the types of nourishing fluids offered to a patient to ones that he prefers.

6. _____ Asking how often the patient normally has a bowel movement.

7. _____ Looking at the laboratory report on a patient's chart to determine the results of a urinalysis.

8. _____ Teaching a patient to administer his own insulin.

COMPLETION

Directions: Fill in the blanks to complete the statements.

1. The nursing process is a rational way of helping nurses perform their tasks more _____
   _____. *(16-24)*

2. Graduates of practical nursing programs are expected to _____ to the development of nursing care plans. *(16-17, 24)*

3. The focus of nursing should be on _____ patient needs, _____ nursing care, and _____ the plan. *(16-17)*

Copyright © 2013, 2009 by Saunders, an imprint of Elsevier Inc. All rights reserved.

4. Ongoing _____ is a necessary and important part of the nursing process. *(27)*

5. Formulating the nursing care plan and writing outcome criteria are joint processes between the nurse and the _____. *(26)*

Assessment (Data Collection)

Directions: Answer the following questions about the process of data gathering, which occurs during the assessment phase of the nursing process.

1. A nursing history is obtained from what three sources? *(19, 22)*

   a. _____

   b. _____

   c. _____

2. An interview should be conducted in a(n) _____ and should take no longer than 20–30 minutes. *(19-20, Box 2-5)*

3. When interviewing an elderly patient, the nurse should _____ because the person probably has more health history information to relate and may speak slowly if ill. *(19)*

4. Secondary sources for interview information when the patient is incapacitated might be:

   _____, _____, _____, or _____. *(19)*

5. Cultural values that may affect a patient's care or health practices are best assessed by asking about _____. *(19, see also Chapter 1)*

6. Part of a psychological assessment is determining how a patient reacts to _____ and then determining present _____ abilities. *(19, see also Chapter 1)*

7. One way to begin a spiritual assessment is to ask if _____ is important to the patient. *(18, see also Chapter 1)*

8. Your patient weighs 165 pounds. Convert the patient's weight to kilograms: _____ kg *(see Units Conversion calculator on Evolve)*

9. Your patient states she drinks 32 ounces of fluid a day. Convert the patient's fluid intake to milliliters: _____ mL *(see Units Conversion calculator on Evolve)*

Copyright © 2013, 2009 by Saunders, an imprint of Elsevier Inc. All rights reserved.

SHORT ANSWER

LPN/LVN's Role and Use of Nursing Process

Directions: Write a short essay answer for each question.

1. During the evaluation, you find that an intervention is not effective and the patient is not meeting the goal. What is the next step? *(27)*

   _____

   _____

   _____

2. Explain why documentation of nursing care is important. (Include at least three reasons.) *(26)*

   _____

   _____

   _____

   _____

   _____

APPLICATION OF THE NURSING PROCESS

Directions: Provide the answers to the following questions.

Scenario A: The nursing diagnosis on the nursing care plan states "Pain related to surgical incision." Nursing interventions include the following: "Monitor PCA morphine effectiveness; reposition every 2 hours; provide quiet environment and rest periods; offer distraction to minimize pain." The expected outcomes state "morphine will control pain effectively; patient says pain is not interfering with rest." What would be appropriate evaluation data to determine that these expected outcomes are being met? *(18, 26-27)*

Scenario B: Your home care patient who just had a knee replacement has considerable pain in the knee. The nursing care plan has a nursing diagnosis of "Self-care deficit related to knee joint pain." Write two expected outcomes for this nursing diagnosis relevant to this patient. *(18, 26-27)*

a. _____

b. _____

Copyright © 2013, 2009 by Saunders, an imprint of Elsevier Inc. All rights reserved.

PRIORITY SETTING

Directions: Read each scenario and prioritize the needs for these patients.

Scenario A

1. Your patient has a complex health condition and as you are assessing the patient you discover several problems. You realize that priorities of care are determined by a hierarchy of needs. Which problem has the highest level of need? *(22)*
   a. Patient is vomiting and cannot retain meals.
   b. Blood pressure is elevated to 160/100 mm Hg.
   c. Respiratory rate is 32 breaths per minute.
   d. Patient has not had a bowel movement in 3 days.

Scenario B

1. Your patient is recovering from abdominal surgery. There are several important tasks that must be accomplished in the early part of the shift. It is 8:30 AM. What should be done first? *(22)*
   a. Administer the AM oral medication for type II diabetes.
   b. Have the patient turn, cough, and deep-breathe with the incentive spirometer as scheduled.
   c. Get the patient up to the chair as ordered and make the bed.
   d. Obtain the medication ordered for pain that the patient has requested.

REVIEW QUESTIONS FOR THE NCLEX® EXAMINATION

Directions: Choose the best answer(s) for the following questions.

1. The LPN/LVN contributes to the nursing care plan by: *(24)*
   1. devising the nursing diagnoses.
   2. collaborating with the RN on the nursing diagnoses.
   3. independently choosing nursing diagnoses from a list.
   4. collaborating with the patient concerning the nursing diagnoses.

2. The focus of the planning step of the nursing process is: *(15, 26)*
   1. implementing nursing interventions.
   2. collecting data to determine appropriate nursing diagnoses.
   3. determining goals and identifying expected outcomes.
   4. revising interventions according to outcomes

3. The most important part of writing expected outcomes for nursing diagnoses is to: *(26)*
   1. state the outcome so that it is measurable.
   2. include health promotion and resource management.
   3. make the outcome "short-term."
   4. base it on objective patient data.

4. Which would be considered objective data? *(Select all that apply.)* *(18)*
   1. Nausea and dizziness when rising too quickly
   2. A fecal odor on the patient's breath
   3. Skin color appears pale and is cool to touch
   4. Blood pressure is 150/90 and pulse is 112
   5. Relief 1 hour after pain medication

Copyright © 2013, 2009 by Saunders, an imprint of Elsevier Inc. All rights reserved.

5. The nurse is performing the morning assessment on a patient. There is a smell of newly mown clover noted on the patient's breath. This odor is most likely to associated with which condition(s)? *(20)*
   1. Hepatic coma
   2. Diabetic ketoacidosis
   3. Poor hygiene
   4. Chronic sinusitis

6. In order to correctly palpate the abdomen, the nurse uses which technique? *(20)*
   1. Depresses gently with the fingertips and thumb.
   2. Uses a sweeping motion with the back of the hand.
   3. Gently feels with the flat palmar surface of the hand.
   4. Warms the stethoscope bell before listening to four areas.

7. The nurse is looking at the patient's chart and other documentation to determine when the patient received the last dose of blood pressure medication. Where would be the best place to locate this information? *(22)*
   1. Physician's orders
   2. Medication reconciliation form
   3. Nurse's narrative notes
   4. Medication administration record

8. An increased number of WBCs is most likely to be associated with: *(23)*
   1. dehydration.
   2. improper diet.
   3. iron deficiency.
   4. infection.

9. The nurse knows that current vital signs are an important indication of what is happening at a given moment. In addition, vital signs should be correlated with which patient data? *(20)*
   1. Trends of the past readings
   2. Standardized normal readings
   3. The patient's ideal body weight
   4. Accuracy of the equipment

10. In the collaborative role of the LVN/LPN and RN, when developing a prioritized list of nursing diagnoses, the two nurses use _____ to determine relationships among the data. *(24)*

CRITICAL THINKING ACTIVITIES

1. You are caring for a patient with a nursing diagnosis of Impaired respiration related to anesthesia. Identify which interventions you would select for this diagnosis and briefly explain why you selected each intervention. Also, for interventions that you rejected, give your rationale in the space provided on the next page.
   a. Encourage use of the incentive spirometer every 2 hours while awake.
   b. Encourage fluids (if not contraindicated).
   c. Monitor vital signs at least once per shift.
   d. Encourage ambulation as ordered.
   e. Assist to sit in the chair for meals.
   f. Splint the surgical incision for coughing.
   g. Encourage to stretch out time between doses of narcotic pain medication.

Copyright © 2013, 2009 by Saunders, an imprint of Elsevier Inc. All rights reserved.

_____

_____

_____

_____

_____

_____

_____

_____

_____

_____

_____

_____

_____

_____

_____

STEPS TOWARD BETTER COMMUNICATION

VOCABULARY BUILDING GLOSSARY

Term	Definition
base'line data	data for reference; the beginning data against which we measure later information
cor'relate	make to match, compare points of several things
clue	a suggestion; added information or hints
da'tabase (da' tah bas)	basic information collected about the patient that is tabulated or recorded
dis'count	disregard, not pay attention to
enhance'	improve, make better, add to
entail'	includes or involves as a necessary inclusion
evalua'tion	process of judging
hi'erarchy (hi' er ark ee)	in order according to importance or rank
in'put	information from someone about facts, feelings, or attitudes
implementa'tion	the carrying out of actions
men'tate	patient's capacity to think
on'going	in progress; continuing
pru'dent	wise or careful

Copyright © 2013, 2009 by Saunders, an imprint of Elsevier Inc. All rights reserved.

COMPLETION

Directions: Fill in the blanks with the appropriate words from the Vocabulary Building Glossary above to complete the statements.

1. The patient and family should have _____ on the goals of care and the treatment plan in order to increase compliance and success.

2. You should _____ with the respiratory therapist about how the patient is to perform her respiratory exercises and how to work them into her schedule of other treatments.

3. A(n) _____ is a person with whom the patient shares closeness, intimacy, and trust in a long-term relationship.

4. When items or concepts are placed in order according to their priority, they are in a(n) _____ _____.

5. If you have a cold or cough, it is not _____ to work with patients with low resistance.

6. Don't _____ the statements the patient makes because it will give you some _____ as to how he is feeling.

7. Think of some ways you can _____ your patient's stay in the hospital.

8. Try to _____ the lab reports with what you observe with the patient.

9. Taking a good history _____ getting adequate information from the patient.

CLINICAL ACTIVITIES

Asking for Assistance

Directions: Seek assistance when something is unclear or not understood.

1. If you feel awkward auscultating the heart and lungs, ask the instructor to demonstrate the skill on your patient by saying, "Would you please show me how to auscultate my patient's lungs (or heart) properly?"

2. If you are having difficulty hearing a patient's blood pressure accurately, ask for help by saying, "I'm not certain I'm getting my patient's blood pressure accurately. Could you help me?"

Copyright © 2013, 2009 by Saunders, an imprint of Elsevier Inc. All rights reserved.

SHORT ANSWER

To assist patients with spiritual concerns, rather than saying, "Do you want...?", the patient might be more receptive if you would use a more polite form of question, such as "Would you like...?". Other polite phrases include "Might I...?", "May I...?", and "I would like to ... if that is all right with you."

Directions: In the spaces below, write polite phrases for asking a patient about reading to her, praying with her, sitting with her, calling a spiritual advisor, and calling friends. Example: "Would you like me to bring you something to read?"

1. _____

2. _____

3. _____

4. _____

5. _____

Writing Expected Outcomes

Directions: Write two expected outcomes for each of the following nursing diagnoses. Example: Patient will use PCA pump before pain becomes severe for 48 hours after surgery. (26)

1. Pain related to surgical incision.

   a. _____

   b. _____

2. Self-care deficit related to paralysis of left side.

   a. _____

   b. _____

3. Constipation related to side effects of medications.

   a. _____

   b. _____

GRAMMAR POINTS

When taking a history, you need to be sure that you and the patient are talking about the same time period.

- When you are asking about past medical history, you need to ask "Have you had...*breathing problems*...?" (chronic conditions) or "Have you **ever** had...*a stroke*...?" (a one-time happening).

- If you are asking about current symptoms, you will need to ask "Do you have...*vision or hearing problems*...?" (now).

If you do not pronounce the words carefully, or are dealing with an older person with a hearing loss or with someone who is distracted, or is a native speaker of another language, you may not receive the correct information.

Copyright © 2013, 2009 by Saunders, an imprint of Elsevier Inc. All rights reserved.

Fluids, Electrolytes, Acid-Base Balance, and Intravenous Therapy

chapter

3

Answer Key: Textbook page references are provided as a guide for answering these questions. A complete answer key was provided to your instructor.

MATCHING

Directions: Select the principle on the right that most accurately completes the statement on the left.

1. Maintaining normal composition and distribution of body fluids is essential to health because _____. *(31)*
2. The renin-angiotensin-aldosterone system causes renin _____. *(32)*
3. When there are differences in concentration of fluids in the various compartments _____. *(32)*
4. The substances in the body fluids can move in and out of capillaries and cell bodies because _____. *(32)*
5. A deficit of water in the extracellular compartment leads to cellular dehydration because _____. *(33-34)*

a. osmotic pressure will move water from the area of lesser concentration of solutes to the area of greater concentration until the compartments are of equal concentration

b. all the life processes of every cell of every organ take place in a fluid medium

c. when a semipermeable membrane separates fluids of unequal concentration, molecules of water move from the less concentrated to the more concentrated solution

d. to be released when there is decreased blood flow to the kidney

e. diffusion provides a spontaneous mixing of molecules

COMPLETION

Directions: Fill in the blanks to complete these statements about fluid and electrolyte balance.

1. Whenever sodium is retained by the body and not excreted by the kidneys, _____ is also retained. *(41)*

2. Normal transmission of nerve impulses and normal muscular activity, including that of the heart, require the presence of _____. *(43-44, Table 3-4)*

3. A potassium deficit can cause cardiac _____. *(42, 44, Table 3-4)*

4. When a patient becomes dehydrated from insufficient fluid intake, serum sodium levels _____. *(41)*

5. Four conditions that can lead to hypokalemia are improper use of _____, as well as _____, _____, and continuous _____ _____. *(42, 44, Table 3-4)*

Copyright © 2013, 2009 by Saunders, an imprint of Elsevier Inc. All rights reserved.

6. Examples of three foods high in potassium are _____, _____, and
   _____. *(44)*

7. Magnesium is important in reactions related to _____ metabolism. *(43, Table 3-4 and 45)*

8. Good sources of magnesium include _____
   _____. *(43)*

9. _____ is essential for the formation of bone. *(44-45, Table 3-4)*

10. _____ is also important as a(n) _____ to promote acid-base balance.
    (45-46)

SHORT ANSWER

Fluids and Electrolytes

Directions: Fill in the blank or supply a short answer to complete the following statements about fluid balance and intake.

1. The average intake of liquids during a 24-hour period is _____ mL. *(31, Table 3-1)*

2. A urinary output of less than _____ mL per hour indicates fluid deficit. *(31, Table 3-1)*

3. List three treatments or nursing measures that can lead to water intoxication. *(38-39)*

   a. _____

   b. _____

   c. _____

4. Name three nursing actions that can help relieve nausea and vomiting. *(35, 38)*

   a. _____

   b. _____

   c. _____

5. When a patient vomits, he loses water and which electrolytes? *(35)* _____

   _____

6. To help in the assessment of fluid volume deficit related to diarrhea, list three observations the nurse should note and record. *(38)*

   a. _____

   b. _____

   c. _____

Copyright © 2013, 2009 by Saunders, an imprint of Elsevier Inc. All rights reserved.

7. Name four nursing measures useful for treating fluid volume deficit related to diarrhea. *(38)*

    a. _____

    b. _____

    c. _____

    d. _____

8. Name two causes of fluid volume deficit in the elderly patient undergoing gastric suction. *(37)*

    a. _____

    b. _____

9. List three nursing actions that should be included in the care plan of a patient with generalized edema. *(39-40)*

    a. _____

    b. _____

    c. _____

10. List three common nursing diagnoses for patients with problems of vomiting, diarrhea, or draining wounds. *(34-38)*

    a. _____

    b. _____

    c. _____

SHORT ANSWER

Signs and Symptoms of Fluid and Electrolyte Imbalance

1. A 78-year-old patient is admitted with hyponatremia. What signs and symptoms of this problem would you expect to find in this patient? _____ _____ *(41-42, Table 3-4)*

2. A patient with cardiac problems enters the hospital with diarrhea. He is hypokalemic. What signs and symptoms are of hypokalemia are expected? Why is this condition so dangerous? _____ _____ *(42, 44, Table 3-4)*

Copyright © 2013, 2009 by Saunders, an imprint of Elsevier Inc. All rights reserved.

TABLE ACTIVITY

Fluid Deficits

Directions: Complete the following table which compares the three major conditions related to fluid deficits. (34-38)

	Vomiting	Diarrhea	Draining Wounds
Clinical manifestations to be documented			
Possible causes			
Nursing interventions			
Medical management			

Copyright © 2013, 2009 by Saunders, an imprint of Elsevier Inc. All rights reserved.

IDENTIFICATION

Intravenous Therapies

Directions: For each type of intravenous therapy on the left, identify and list all interventions on the right that apply.

1. _____ Total parenteral nutrition (TPN) *(50-51, 56-57)*

2. _____ Intravenous therapy *(50-52)*

3. _____ Blood transfusion *(51)*

a. Two nurses must check and verify the bag label with the patient's ID band and information.

b. Started at no more than 60–80 mL per hour.

c. Take baseline vital signs including temperature before starting.

d. Monitor the site, flow rate, and how patient is tolerating the infusion hourly.

e. Monitor blood sugar frequently during the first week.

f. Monitor the elderly patient carefully for signs of fluid overload.

g. Stop the infusion if the patient becomes short of breath.

h. Always use an IV infusion pump to administer it.

i. Slowly decrease the rate of infusion before stopping it.

j. Take vital signs every hour while administering it.

CALCULATIONS

Directions: Calculate the correct flow rates for the following orders and situations. (53)

1. Ordered: 1000 mL D_5RL over 8 hours
   Administration set delivers 20 gtts/mL
   How many drops per minute should be administered? _____

2. Ordered: 500 mL $D_{10}W$ at 150 mL/hour
   Administration set delivers 20 gtts/mL
   How many drops per minute should be administered? _____

3. Your patient had an IV count of 325 mL at the beginning of your shift. You infused two piggybacks during the shift; the first was 125 mL and the second was 50 mL. You hung a new 1000 mL bag of fluid at 1:00 PM. The IV count at the end of your shift was 800 mL.
   What was the total IV intake for the shift? _____

Copyright © 2013, 2009 by Saunders, an imprint of Elsevier Inc. All rights reserved.

PRIORITY SETTING

You are assigned to care for the following patients:
  a. Ms. Toms, age 76, who has nausea, vomiting, and dehydration.
  b. Mr. Wilson, age 68, who had surgery and is receiving a transfusion of packed red cells.
  c. Mr. Whitts, age 36, who has pancreatitis and is receiving TPN.

1. After you receive report, which patient would you visit and check first? _____

You have a nursing assistant assigned to help you with your patients. You need vital signs on all three patients at 8:00 AM.

2. Which patient would you assign to the nursing assistant for measuring vital signs? _____

3. You need to do an initial shift assessment on each of the three patients. Which one would you assess first? _____

IDENTIFICATION

Blood Gas Analysis

Directions: Under each laboratory value given below, add ↓ if the value is below normal, ◊ if normal, and ↑ if above normal. Then decide whether the data set indicates metabolic acidosis, respiratory acidosis, metabolic alkalosis, or respiratory alkalosis. (47-50)

Example:	pH	pCO_2	HCO_3
	7.32	44 mm Hg	21 mEq/L
	↓	◊	↓

Indicates metabolic acidosis

1.	pH	pCO_2	HCO_3
	7.33	50 mm Hg	26 mEq/L

Indicates _____

2.	pH	pCO_2	HCO_3
	7.48	32 mm Hg	25 mEq/L

Indicates _____

3.	pH	pCO_2	HCO_3
	7.50	45 mm Hg	28 mEq/L

Indicates _____

Copyright © 2013, 2009 by Saunders, an imprint of Elsevier Inc. All rights reserved.

REVIEW QUESTIONS FOR THE NCLEX® EXAMINATION

Directions: Choose the best answer(s) for the following questions.

1. Factors in the formation of edema may include: (*Select all that apply.*) *(39-40)*
   1. drinking too much water in hot weather.
   2. a diet leading to protein deficiency.
   3. obstruction of lymphatic circulation.
   4. burns causing capillary permeability.
   5. infusion of 4 L of normal saline.

2. The patient with hypercalcemia may exhibit: (*Select all that apply.*) *(43, 44, Table 3-4)*
   1. nausea.
   2. stupor.
   3. abdominal pain.
   4. polyuria.
   5. parasthesias.

3. Safe administration of intravenous fluids includes: *(51-53)*
   1. shaking the bag to mix the solution thoroughly.
   2. checking the infusion rate every 30–60 minutes.
   3. weighing the patient daily.
   4. checking electrolyte levels before hanging a new bag of IV solution.

4. The data indicating effectiveness of interventions for an elderly patient with a fluid volume deficit are: (*Select all that apply.*) *(34-38)*
   1. weight gain of 2 pounds.
   2. successful infusion of 3000 mL of normal saline.
   3. patient can answer questions without confusion.
   4. moist mucous membranes in the mouth.
   5. drinking 8 ounces every 2 hours

5. Nursing actions for a patient receiving intravenous fluids should include: (*Select all that apply.*) *(51-53)*
   1. re-dress the IV insertion site each shift.
   2. stabilize the cannula in the vein to prevent trauma to the surrounding tissues.
   3. set the intravenous fluid to run at the prescribed rate of flow.
   4. speed up the flow rate of intravenous fluids when necessary to catch up on fluids that have not been administered at the prescribed rate.
   5. observe and record the patient's response to the administration of fluids.
   6. maintain strict asepsis when changing the intravenous tubing and bag.

6. When a patient shows signs of a transfusion reaction, the nurse must: *(51, see also Chapter 17)*
   1. increase the rate of flow of the saline via the "Y" tubing.
   2. take the vital signs and wait 15 minutes, then take them again.
   3. slow down the rate of flow and notify the physician.
   4. stop the transfusion, notify the physician, and keep the intravenous line open with normal saline.

7. Calculation: Find the correct number of drops per minute for the following order: 500 mL D5½NS IV q 8 hrs. Available: Microdrip tubing. _____ *(53-55)*

Copyright © 2013, 2009 by Saunders, an imprint of Elsevier Inc. All rights reserved.

8. Place an "X" on the diagram below where a central line would most likely be inserted for the administration of TPN. *(56)*

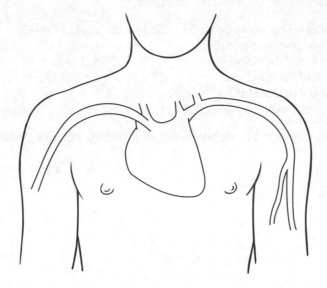

9. Metabolic acidosis is more likely to occur in a person who: *(48)*
   1. is unable to metabolize carbohydrates normally or who ingests few or no carbohydrates.
   2. is unable to metabolize fats normally.
   3. suffers from kidney failure with excessive reabsorption of bicarbonate from the urine.
   4. has diarrhea with excessive loss of bicarbonates in the feces.

10. Nursing measures recommended to prevent central line infection include: *(Select all that apply.)* *(56)*
    1. cleansing the insertion site with chlorhexidine solution for dressing changes.
    2. performing hand hygiene whenever changing fluids or performing dressing changes.
    3. daily review of the need for the central line.
    4. changing the dressing every 3 days.
    5. using barrier precautions when changing the dressing.

CRITICAL THINKING ACTIVITIES

Scenario: Intestinal Surgery

Your patient is a 68-year-old female who had intestinal surgery 4 days ago. She is NPO, has a nasogastric tube set to intermittent suction, an intravenous line with D5½NS at 125 mL/hr. Physical assessment data includes: Alert and oriented but groggy, diaphoretic, fine crackles in the lower lobes of both lungs, moving all extremities, and complaining of abdominal pain and a dry mouth. Bowel sounds are hypoactive, no BM since surgery, and is voiding dark amber urine without difficulty. Urine sp. gr. is 1.030. NG output in last 2 hours is 200 mL of dark green secretions. Vital signs: T 101.2° F, P 92, BP 128/78. Intake last 24 hours: 2480 mL, output was 2010 mL. Laboratory values: K+ 3.1 mEq/L, Na+ 140 mEq/L, Cl- 91 mEq/L.

1. What other assessment data should you acquire related to her fluid status? *(33-50)*

Copyright © 2013, 2009 by Saunders, an imprint of Elsevier Inc. All rights reserved.

2. Do the assessment findings indicate a fluid deficit or fluid excess problem? Explain using the assessment data. *(33-40)*

3. What is her electrolyte status? Does she have any electrolyte abnormalities? If so, which one(s)? Give your rationale for your answers. *(40-45)*

Scenario: Pneumonia

Your patient is a 76-year-old male who was just admitted with pneumonia. He is anorexic and has a temperature of 102.4° F, P 98, R 26 and shallow, BP 138/64. He is diaphoretic. Lung sounds reveal decreased breath sounds in bases with rhonchi in upper lobes. He is somewhat confused.

1. What assessments would you make regarding fluid and electrolyte status? *(57-58)*

2. What might be causing the patient's confusion? *(48, 57, Table 3-4)*

3. Would you expect that the patient would have an acid-base imbalance? If so, what would it probably be? *(Table 3-4)*

STEPS TOWARD BETTER COMMUNICATION

VOCABULARY BUILDING GLOSSARY

Term	Definition
syno'via (sin o' vee ah)	secreting membrane found in joints
a'queous (a' kwee us) hu'mor	transparent fluid between the lens of the eye and the cornea
paren'teral (pah ren' ter al)	by subcutaneous, intramuscular, intravenous, or method other than by mouth into the gastrointestinal tract
cru'cial (kru'shul)	of extreme importance
diaphore'sis (di ah for ee'sis)	excessive perspiration, a great deal of sweating
clam'my	cool and damp
sprue	disorder causing lack of nutrient absorption from the intestine
per'meable (per'mee a bul)	permitting passage of a substance (a property of membranes)
vis'cous (vis' kus)	thick, like honey (a property of fluids)

Copyright © 2013, 2009 by Saunders, an imprint of Elsevier Inc. All rights reserved.

VOCABULARY EXERCISE

Table of prefixes to remember:

Prefix	Meaning	Examples
extra-	outside	extracellular
hyper-	more	hypertonic hyperglycemic
hypo-	less	hypotonic hypoglycemic
inter-	between among	internal interstitial intervention
intra-	within	intracellular intravascular intravenous
iso-	same, equal	isotonic isometric
trans-	through, across	transcellular transfusion transport

COMPLETION

Directions: Fill in the blanks with the correct terms from the glossary list.

1. _____ fluid is located in the joints and acts as a lubricant for the joints.

2. Fluid balance is _____ to the well-being of an elderly person.

3. The patient with a high fever often experiences _____.

4. Normal saline intravenous solution is _____.

5. A 10% dextrose intravenous solution is _____.

6. An intravenous infusion places fluid in the _____ space.

7. The patient who is experiencing shock has skin that feels _____.

8. Enteral feeding solutions are more _____ than intravenous solutions.

9. Patients who have _____ often experience considerable diarrhea.

10. A membrane must be _____ for diffusion to take place across it.

Copyright © 2013, 2009 by Saunders, an imprint of Elsevier Inc. All rights reserved.

COMMUNICATION EXERCISE

Patient Teaching

A. *Directions: A nurse is instructing a patient about input and output. Note their interaction.*

Nurse: "Mrs. T., the doctor wants us to measure everything you drink. This sheet will be here for you to write down the amount each time you drink something."

Mrs. T.: "How will I know how much I drank?"

Nurse: "See how this cup is marked with lines indicating the amount of fluid?"

Mrs. T.: "Oh, yes, I do see that now."

Nurse: "Now tell me what you will do."

Mrs. T.: "I need to look to see how much fluid is in the cup and then how much is left when I have had a drink. Do I subtract to determine the exact amount I drank?"

Nurse: "Yes, that's correct. If you have trouble, just call me and I'll help you. Let's try it now. The cup has 120 mL in it. Take a drink. Good. Now it has 60 mL left. So if we subtract 60 from 120, we find that you drank 60 mL. Let's write that down."

Mrs. T.: "It doesn't seem too complicated. Leave the paper and pencil next to the cup to remind me to write the amount down each time I drink, please."

Nurse: "Of course, Mrs. T. Also, I need to measure your urine output. So whenever you use the toilet, be certain that the little white "hat" is sitting in it. Call me when you have finished and I will measure and record it. Try to drop any toilet paper into the toilet behind the hat so it doesn't alter the measurement."

Mrs. T.: "O.K., I'll try."

B. *You have a patient who cannot tolerate dairy products; they cause diarrhea. What can you teach this patient about planning a diet that contains sufficient calcium?*

_____

_____

_____

Copyright © 2013, 2009 by Saunders, an imprint of Elsevier Inc. All rights reserved.

Care of Preoperative and Intraoperative Surgical Patients

chapter

4

Answer Key: Textbook page references are provided as a guide for answering these questions. A complete answer key was provided to your instructor.

COMPLETION

Preoperative Care

Directions: Fill in the blank with the correct word(s) to complete the sentences.

1. A colostomy procedure indicates that the patient's colon would be _____ _____. **(64)**

2. The surgeon should be alerted if a patient's temperature is _____. **(64)**

3. The elderly patient is more prone to fluid and electrolyte imbalances during and after surgery because she is more likely to have _____ _____ _____. **(64)**

4. Before surgery, it is important to know if the patient has any _____ and if he is taking _____. **(64-65)**

5. Obese people are at higher risk with surgery because fat contains fewer blood vessels, causing _____ and a greater threat of _____. **(67)**

6. The malnourished patient is also at risk because _____ is needed to replace blood cells and serum lost during surgery. **(67)**

7. Patients are encouraged to quit smoking before surgery because smoking has a negative effect on _____ and _____. **(67)**

8. A patient who is allergic to _____ is at high risk of exposure during surgery. **(65)**

9. Poorly controlled diabetes leads to postoperative complications such as _____ and _____. **(67)**

10. _____ and _____ should be discontinued _____ days before surgery. **(65)**

Copyright © 2013, 2009 by Saunders, an imprint of Elsevier Inc. All rights reserved.

PRIORITY SETTING

Directions: You have finished receiving report and are ready to begin patient care. You are assigned a preoperative surgery patient who is scheduled for surgery at 8:30 AM. How would you prioritize your actions? Number the actions listed below in the order (from 1 to 8) in which you would perform them. **(64-74)**

_____   a.   Complete the preoperative checklist.

_____   b.   Check to see that the patient's signature is on the surgical consent form.

_____   c.   Check that all diagnostic test results are back and determine if there are any abnormal lab values.

_____   d.   Have the patient shower, if possible.

_____   e.   Remind the patient to remain NPO and not to swallow any fluids or food.

_____   f.   Have the patient remove any metal hairpins and jewelry and all underclothes, leaving on only a clean hospital gown.

_____   g.   Start the presurgical nurse's notes in the chart which will be finished when the transport person comes for the patient.

_____   h.   Explain to the family where the surgical waiting room is and how to get there.

MATCHING

Surgical Risk Factors and Their Effects on Recovery

Mr. J. is admitted to the same-day surgery unit for repair of an inguinal hernia. He is 48 years old, has diabetes mellitus for which he takes insulin, is 140 pounds overweight, and smokes one and a half packs of cigarettes a day. He has smoked since age 15 and has chronic bronchitis with a productive cough.

Directions: Match each of Mr. J.'s surgical risk factors with the effect it can have on his recovery from surgery. Note that there may be more than one effect for each risk factor. **(67)**

1. _____   Diabetes mellitus

2. _____   Smoking and chronic bronchitis

3. _____   Obesity

a.   Slower healing and risk of infection because adipose tissue has fewer blood vessels

b.   Decreased lung expansion due to chronic lung disease

c.   Decreased lung expansion due to upward pressure of enlarged abdomen against thorax

d.   Wide variations in blood glucose levels

e.   Potential for wound dehiscence because of added stress on sutures

f.   Accumulations of secretions in air passages

g.   Infection related to less phagocytic action against microorganisms

h.   Reduced level of functional hemoglobin

i.   Abnormal clot formation and obstruction of blood vessels

Copyright © 2013, 2009 by Saunders, an imprint of Elsevier Inc. All rights reserved.

COMPLETION

Directions: Fill in the blank with the correct word(s) to complete the statements.

1. The function of the _____ is important in the surgical patient because this is where anesthetic agents are metabolized. *(66)*

2. The _____ nurse is responsible for opening sterile supplies during surgery. *(75-76)*

3. Surgery is a risk for the elderly patient because _____ formation is greater the older the patient. *(67)*

4. In addition to physiological preparation, most surgical patients have a need for _____ support. *(65-66)*

5. As the patient leaves for surgery, family members should be informed about which three things? *(72)*

   a. _____

   b. _____

   c. _____

6. When a patient asks why he can't have anything to eat or drink for 8 hours prior to surgery, how should the nurse respond? *(70)* _____

   _____

APPLICATION OF THE NURSING PROCESS

Scenario: Mrs. Sutton, age 38, is to undergo a simple mastectomy for early breast cancer. She will have general anesthesia. She has recently remarried and is concerned about her husband's feelings regarding her surgery.

1. List the nursing diagnoses that would be appropriate for Mrs. Sutton in the preoperative period. *(64-72)*

   _____

   _____

   _____

2. State an outcome objective for each of the above nursing diagnoses. *(64-72)*_____

   _____

   _____

   _____

3. List interventions that you would perform when the transport person comes to take Mrs. Sutton to surgery. *(72)*

   _____

   _____

   _____

Copyright © 2013, 2009 by Saunders, an imprint of Elsevier Inc. All rights reserved.

4. How would you evaluate the preoperative care given to Mrs. Sutton? *(74)* _____

_____

_____

_____

_____

SHORT ANSWER

Intraoperative Care

Directions: Provide a brief answer to each question.

1. Describe autologous blood collection and reinfusion. *(64)* _____

_____

_____

2. What are the advantages of regional anesthesia? *(76)* _____

_____

3. List four procedures for which local anesthesia is used. *(76-77)*

    a. _____

    b. _____

    c. _____

    d. _____

4. Name three measures that are used to prevent the possibility of surgical infection in the operating suite? *(75-76)*

    a. _____

    b. _____

    c. _____

5. Identify the various measures that are used to prevent "wrong patient, wrong site" surgery from occurring. *(72, 74)*

_____

_____

_____

_____

6. No matter what type of anesthesia is used, the goals of anesthesia should be kept in mind. They are: *(75)*

    a. _____

    b. _____

    c. _____

Copyright © 2013, 2009 by Saunders, an imprint of Elsevier Inc. All rights reserved.

7. Potential complications of surgery include the following. Describe an intervention to monitor and/or prevent their occurrence. *(77-78)*

   a. Infection: _____

   _____

   b. Fluid volume imbalance: _____

   _____

   c. Hypothermia/hyperthermia: _____

   _____

   d. Injury: _____

   _____

REVIEW QUESTIONS FOR THE NCLEX® EXAMINATION

Directions: Choose the best answer(s) for the following questions.

1. The patient who is a heavy smoker is at increased risk of complications after surgery with general anesthesia because: *(66-67)*
   1. blood pressure swings may occur when nicotine is withdrawn.
   2. respiratory muscles are weakened, making coughing difficult.
   3. nicotine withdrawal causes considerable nervousness.
   4. irritated lung tissues produce more secretions from inhaled anesthesia.

2. The patient who has liver disease is at increased risk from surgery because: *(Select all that apply.)* *(66)*
   1. good liver function is needed to metabolize drugs and anesthetics.
   2. the liver helps cleanse the blood of microorganisms.
   3. blood pressure swings are likely when liver function is poor.
   4. clotting times may be affected causing the patient to bleed excessively.
   5. the liver stores extra blood that can be released if the patient becomes hypovolemic.

3. Skin preparation is performed prior to surgery to: *(Select all that apply.)* *(70)*
   1. provide a better visual field for the surgeon.
   2. sterilize the skin.
   3. help prevent wound contamination.
   4. facilitate postoperative dressing changes.
   5. reduce the number of microorganisms at the surgical site.

4. The patient is scheduled for an exploratory laparotomy for an abdominal mass. The preoperative laboratory results are: *(66)*
   CBC: Hgb= 14.5 g, RBC 5.1, WBC 8600
   UA: sp. gr. 10.25, glucose negative, ketones negative, WBCs 57 per low power field, casts 10.
   Which test finding would you report to the surgeon? _____

5. Which point(s) should be covered before a patient signs a surgical consent form? *(Select all that apply.)* *(68)*
   1. The correct name of the procedure to be performed
   2. The names and credentials of all surgical assistants
   3. The potential complications that may occur from the surgery
   4. The length of time the patient will be in the PACU
   5. The benefits of the surgery
   6. Verification that the patient is mentally competent and not coerced into signing the form

Copyright © 2013, 2009 by Saunders, an imprint of Elsevier Inc. All rights reserved.

6. Functions of the scrub nurse include: *(Select all that apply)* **(75)**
   1. assisting with ties of surgical team's gowns.
   2. preparing the instrument table.
   3. labeling and handling surgical specimens.
   4. assisting with transfer of the patient to the operating table.
   5. handing instruments and supplies to the OR team during surgery.
   6. maintaining sterility within the sterile operating field during surgery.

7. Procedural sedation is used for many surgeries. It consists of: **(76)**
   1. a nerve block combined with oral sedation.
   2. local or regional anesthesia and IV sedation.
   3. inhalation of short-acting anesthetic.
   4. intravenous anesthesia and sedation.

CRITICAL THINKING ACTIVITY

Scenario: Mrs. Holt is scheduled for a colectomy for diverticulosis after many episodes of diverticulitis. She has been feeling much better since she finished the antibiotics for the last episode. You have the preoperative checklist in hand and are preparing her for surgery. She tells you that she has decided she doesn't want the surgery after all, because she is feeling so much better. **(66-67)**

1. What do you do? Describe the specific steps you would take in this situation.

2. How would you document this event in her medical record?

STEPS TOWARD BETTER COMMUNICATION

VOCABULARY BUILDING GLOSSARY

Term	Definition
laparoscopic (lap a ro skop' ik)	seen or performed though a laparoscope, an instrument for direct visualization into the peritoneal body cavity
invasive (in vay' siv)	involving a puncture or incision of the skin
hemodilution (hee' mo di loo' shun)	increase of the fluid content of the blood which decreases its concentration
coercion (co er' shun)	using force or threats to make a person do something

Copyright © 2013, 2009 by Saunders, an imprint of Elsevier Inc. All rights reserved.

COMPLETION

Fill in the blank in the following sentences with the correct word from the glossary.

1. Administering too much intravenous fluid may cause _____.

2. Telling a patient that she will surely die without the surgery would be _____ in order to get the patient to sign the surgical consent form.

3. Even laparoscopic surgery is _____.

4. Gallbladder surgery is often a(n) _____ procedure these days.

GRAMMAR POINTS

Verb Forms—Future Tense

The nurse prepares the patient for surgery by performing preoperative teaching. Instructions to the patient are given using the future tense, such as "You will…" or "you should…", or "The nurse is going to…". For the following set of orders, write out the instruction or explanation you would give to the patient as part of the preoperative teaching.

1. NPO after midnight:_____

    _____

2. Report at 0600 to outpatient surgery unit: _____

    _____

3. Surgical prep:_____

    _____

4. Restoril 30 mg p.o. H.S.:_____

    _____

Directions: Other instructions you would give to the patient might include the following. Fill in the blanks with the proper verb forms.

5. "The nurse _____ you to cough and deep-breathe every 2 hours."

6. "Turning _____ required every 2 hours after surgery."

7. "You will need _____ for pain medication and should do so before the pain becomes severe."

8. "Your valuable belongings _____ locked up in the business office or given to your husband."

9. "You _____ your necklace prior to surgery."

10. "The side rails _____ raised after you have been given your preoperative medications."

Copyright © 2013, 2009 by Saunders, an imprint of Elsevier Inc. All rights reserved.

CULTURAL POINTS

What special items might you need to think about if you are preparing an older patient for surgery?

_____

_____

_____

What information would you give him or her about the items? Write out how you would state that information.

_____

_____

_____

Copyright © 2013, 2009 by Saunders, an imprint of Elsevier Inc. All rights reserved.

Care of Postoperative Surgical Patients

Answer Key: Textbook page references are provided as a guide for answering these questions. A complete answer key was provided to your instructor.

TABLE ACTIVITY

Anesthesia Implications

Directions: Complete the following table which compares the nursing implications of various types of anesthesia. **(81)**

Type of Anesthesia	Postoperative Nursing Implications
Inhalation (general anesthesia)	
Intravenous drugs (procedural sedation)	
Regional or topical	

SHORT ANSWER

PACU Care

Directions: Provide the answers to the following questions in the blank spaces provided.

1. The correct way to open the airway of a patient who is still unconscious after surgery with general anesthesia is to: _____

    _____ . *(81-82)*

Copyright © 2013, 2009 by Saunders, an imprint of Elsevier Inc. All rights reserved.

2. Oxygen is administered in the PACU to the patient who has undergone general anesthesia for two reasons, which are: *(81)*

    a. _____

    b. _____

3. Discharge criteria from the PACU is based on a scoring system that includes assessment of:

    _____

    _____ *(82)*

Postoperative Care

Directions: Answer the following questions in the spaces provided.

1. General anesthesia causes some atelectasis. The nurse must encourage deep-breathing and coughing to re-expand the lung alveoli because:

    _____

    _____ *(84)*

2. List five nursing responsibilities regarding the care of active surgical drains. *(90)*

    a. _____

    b. _____

    c. _____

    d. _____

    e. _____

3. Signs that circulation is adequate distal to the surgical site are _____

    _____ . *(85)*

4. If there is no written order for dressing changes, what should be done? *(90)*_____

    _____

5. What should be recorded on the patient's chart when a dressing is changed and drainage noted? *(90)*

    _____

    _____

6. What signs and symptoms indicate an infected surgical wound? *(90)*_____

    _____

7. What is the correct procedure for the immediate care of a patient who experiences wound dehiscence and evisceration? *(91)*

    _____

    _____

Copyright © 2013, 2009 by Saunders, an imprint of Elsevier Inc. All rights reserved.

COMPLETION

Directions: Fill in the blanks to complete the statements.

1. Besides checking the rate of respirations, it is important to check both the _____

   and _____. *(83-84)*

2. Besides medicating for pain, measures to promote comfort in the immediate postoperative period in-

   clude providing _____ and medicating as needed for _____. *(87-88)*

3. The three initial classic signs of shock resulting from hypovolemia due to hemorrhage are

   _____. *(93)*

4. In addition to those above, describe other physical changes that occur with the progression of shock. *(93)*

   a. Pulse: _____

   b. Blood pressure:_____

   c. Respirations: _____

   d. Skin: _____

   e. Level of consciousness: _____

5. Another complication to which the elderly patient is more susceptible is overhydration. Signs that
   would make the nurse suspect overhydration include: *(92, Table 5-2)*

   _____

   _____

6. A postoperative patient is complaining of shortness of breath and chest pain; he is very anxious and has

   a cough, rapid pulse, and rapid respirations. These could indicate the complication of _____

   _____. *(92, Table 5-2)*

APPLICATION OF THE NURSING PROCESS

Scenario: Mr. Takanaki, age 72, has undergone a colectomy. He did well through surgery and in the recovery room. He has an IV with D_5NS hanging, an NG tube set to low suction, and a urinary catheter. He has a history of arthritis and chronic bronchitis. He is usually an "active senior," playing golf several times each week and tending his garden. He is breathing shallowly when you assess him and is complaining of pain at 7 out of 10 on the pain scale.

1. Choose the top four nursing diagnoses that would appropriate for Mr. Takanaki during this postoperative period. *(83-84)*

   _____

   _____

   _____

   _____

Copyright © 2013, 2009 by Saunders, an imprint of Elsevier Inc. All rights reserved.

2. Write at least one expected outcome for each of the above nursing diagnoses. *(84)*

    a. _____

    b. _____

    c. _____

    d. _____

3. What nursing interventions should be included on the plan of care to monitor for pulmonary problems? *(84-91)*

    _____

    _____

    _____

4. What adjunct measures could you use along with pain medication to treat this patient's pain? *(87-88)*

    _____

    _____

5. What measures would you institute to promote good oxygenation and circulation? *(84-85)*

    _____

    _____

    _____

    _____

    _____

6. What evaluation criteria would tell you that the patient is breathing effectively? *(84)*

    _____

    _____

7. What evaluation criteria would tell you that the patient's pain is adequately controlled? *(87-88)*

    _____

    _____

Copyright © 2013, 2009 by Saunders, an imprint of Elsevier Inc. All rights reserved.

PRIORITY SETTING

You are assigned to care for Mr. Takanaki who is just returning from surgery. He has had a colectomy. You receive report from the PACU nurse and settle the patient in the bed. Number the actions listed below in the order (from 1 to 12) in which you would perform them. *(81-83)*

_____ a. Inspect the surgical dressing.

_____ b. Check all tubes and drains for patency.

_____ c. Take the vital signs.

_____ d. Adjust the IV drip rate to the ordered flow rate.

_____ e. Inquire about the patient's pain level.

_____ f. Ask the patient to take four deep breaths.

_____ g. Hook the NG tube to the suction.

_____ h. Document the postoperative assessment.

_____ i. Verify that the correct IV solution is hanging.

_____ j. Provide an additional warmed blanket.

_____ k. Allow the family to visit.

_____ l. Auscultate the heart and lungs.

REVIEW QUESTIONS FOR THE NCLEX® EXAMINATION

Directions: Choose the best answer(s) for the following questions.

1. If a surgical patient develops malignant hyperthermia, which sign(s) would the nurse expect? (*Select all that apply.*) *(92-93, Table 5-2)*
   1. Shortness of breath
   2. Dark, cola-colored urine
   3. Hypotension and tachypnea
   4. Widened pulse pressure
   5. Cardiac arrhythmia

2. The patient most likely to have pulmonary complications after surgery is the one who has had a(n): *(84)*
   1. appendectomy.
   2. hysterectomy.
   3. tonsillectomy.
   4. cholecystectomy.

3. Adynamic ileus can occur after anesthesia and abdominal surgery. Signs and symptoms found on assessment include: *(87, 92 Table 5-2)*
   1. high-pitched, frequent bowel sounds in all four quadrants.
   2. diarrhea, cramping, and high-pitched bowel sounds.
   3. absence of bowel sounds in upper quadrants.
   4. abdominal distention, pain, no passage of feces or flatus, and no bowel sounds.

4. Coughing after surgery is evaluated not only by the amount of airflow produced by the cough but also by: *(84)*
   1. the loudness of the sound made.
   2. the number of coughs produced at one time.
   3. the degree of inspiration prior to the cough.
   4. whether secretions are moved up and out of the bronchial tree.

Copyright © 2013, 2009 by Saunders, an imprint of Elsevier Inc. All rights reserved.

5. Surgery may cause psychological problems. The nurse should assess for signs of ineffective coping such as: *(94)*
   1. excessive pain.
   2. withdrawn behavior.
   3. constant complaining.
   4. demanding behavior.

6. A non-infected surgical wound should be cleaned with _____. *(91)*

7. The plan of care for the immediate postoperative period should include which safety measure? *(84)*
   1. Keeping an emesis basin within the patient's reach
   2. Positioning the patient on her side until she is alert to prevent aspiration
   3. Talking to the patient and reorienting her frequently
   4. Covering the patient with warmed blankets to decrease chilling

8. Other safety measures for the postoperative patient include: *(Select all that apply.) (81-83)*
   1. cautioning the patient not to get out of bed without assistance while receiving narcotic analgesics.
   2. answering the patient's call light promptly.
   3. assessing the patient for bladder distention every 8 hours.
   4. monitoring fluid intake and output closely.
   5. assessing urine output every 2 hours.
   6. assessing vital sign trends.

9. The order reads: Infuse D_5RL 1000 mL over 6 hours. The IV tubing delivers 10 drops per mL. The drop rate should be _____ gtts/minute.

10. When assisting the patient to arise from the bed postoperatively, you would have him *first: (82, 85)*
    1. push up from the bed with his elbows.
    2. turn toward the side of the bed from which he is going to exit it.
    3. bend the knees and plant the feet flat on the mattress.
    4. grab the top side rail and push up to a sitting position.

CRITICAL THINKING ACTIVITY

Scenario: Mr. T. has just returned to his room from the PACU. He has had a colectomy performed. He is receiving IV fluids and antibiotics.

1. On the third postoperative day, he has abdominal distention. He is not passing flatus and no bowel sounds are detected. What complication of surgery might he be experiencing? *(87, 92 Table 5-2)*

   _____

2. An NG tube is inserted and attached to suction. He is placed on NPO status. The last shift assessment found that he is tachycardic, has decreased urine output, poor skin turgor, and his blood pressure has dropped 20 points. What would you suspect is the problem? *(86, 92, Table 5-2)*

   _____

3. Mr. T. improves and is ready for discharge. He will continue oral antibiotics at home. What instructions should he be given? *(94, 96-97)*

   _____

   _____

   _____

Copyright © 2013, 2009 by Saunders, an imprint of Elsevier Inc. All rights reserved.

STEPS TOWARD BETTER COMMUNICATION

VOCABULARY BUILDING GLOSSARY

Term	Definition
allay' (ah lay')	to calm, to place at rest
induce' (in doos')	to bring on by outside means
grog'gy	unsteady or shaky with an unclear mind
numb (num)	lack of sensation; no feeling
kink'ed (kinkt)	bent sharply so as to block the flow inside
malaise' (mah layz')	general feeling of bodily discomfort

COMPLETION

Directions: Fill in the blanks in the following sentences with the correct word from the glossary above.

1. Mrs. P. is awake from anesthesia, but is still very _____.

2. The nurse must carefully check each tube and drain after turning a patient to be certain that no tube is

   _____.

3. After spinal anesthesia, the patient's legs are _____ for a few hours.

4. Mr. R.'s wound was healing nicely, but he is suffering from _____.

5. Certain drugs can sometimes _____ anaphylactic shock.

GRAMMAR POINTS

As a nurse, you will be giving postoperative discharge instructions to your patients. Some instructions are about things the patient *should* do (ought to do, are strongly advised); others are about things that she *should not* do. Certain things *must* be done (are necessary to do, cannot be avoided) to prevent complications; other things *must not* be done or they may interfere with recovery. Insert the correct instruction before each statement.

You should   You should not   You must   You must not

1. _____ walk for 5–10 minutes three times a day.

2. _____ inspect the incision for signs of redness or drainage every day.

3. _____ scratch the incision if it starts to itch.

4. _____ lift anything heavier than 5 pounds for at least 4 weeks.

5. _____ call the physician if your temperature rises to 100.2° F (38.0° C).

Copyright © 2013, 2009 by Saunders, an imprint of Elsevier Inc. All rights reserved.

COMMUNICATION EXERCISE

Dialogue Example

Joan, an LVN, is getting Mr. Cox out of bed to sit in the chair for the second time since his surgery yesterday. Note how Joan interacts with Mr. Cox.

Joan: "Mr. Cox, it is time to get you up to sit in the chair for about 20 minutes now. I'll help you sit on the side of the bed and put on your robe."

Mr. Cox: "Do I have to get up now? I just finished breakfast."

Joan: "Yes, your doctor left orders for you to be up in the chair after breakfast."

Mr. Cox: "You won't leave me there too long, will you?"

Joan: "No, I'll be back in about 20 minutes to help you back into bed."

Mr. Cox: "OK."

Joan: "Place your left hand on the side rail and turn toward me." (She raises the head of the bed slightly and helps Mr. Cox to turn on his side and swing his feet over the side of the bed into a sitting position. She helps him put his arms into his robe while he is seated.)

Mr. Cox: "Whee, I feel just a little dizzy."

Joan: "Just sit here for a moment until the dizziness passes."

Mr. Cox: "OK. I feel better now."

Joan: "Let me put your slippers on your feet and then I'll help you to stand up. Place your hands on my shoulders and stand on the count of three." (Joan helps Mr. Cox to stand by supporting him while he rises.)

Mr. Cox: "I made it."

Joan: "That was very good. Now we'll walk over to the chair and turn so that you are ready to sit down."

Mr. Cox: "I don't want to miss the seat when I sit down."

Joan: "Move back so the chair is touching the back of your legs. Place your right hand on the arm of the chair and slowly lower yourself into the chair." (Mr. Cox does this successfully.) "That was great. Would you like a blanket over your legs to keep you warm?"

Mr. Cox: "No, I'm warm enough. That wasn't as hard as it was yesterday. Thank you."

Joan: "OK. It is 9:10 now, so I'll be back at 9:30."

Copyright © 2013, 2009 by Saunders, an imprint of Elsevier Inc. All rights reserved.

Infection Prevention and Control

chapter

6

Answer Key: Textbook page references are provided as a guide for answering these questions. A complete answer key was provided to your instructor.

COMPLETION

Directions: Fill in the blanks to complete the statements.

1. All streptococci and staphylococci are gram-_____ organisms. *(115)*

2. Pinworms are most commonly found in children and cause significant itching in the _____ area. *(103)*

3. Insufficient hand hygiene by medical staff and other people in contact with patients is a major cause of _____ infections. *(108, 114)*

4. *Chlamydia* is typically transmitted via _____ contact. *(103)*

5. Pathogens are transmitted by three routes: _____, _____, and _____. *(101)*

SHORT ANSWER

Causes and Symptoms of Infection

Scenario: You are caring for patients on a general medical-surgical unit. Currently, there are several post-operative patients; therefore, you are vigilant for signs and symptoms of infection in these patients. You also have an elderly patient who is fairly immobile, so you are aware of the need to assess her for signs of pneumonia.

Directions: Provide the answers to the following questions.

1. List four specific signs and symptoms that suggest presence of a respiratory infection. *(107)*

    a. _____

    b. _____

    c. _____

    d. _____

Copyright © 2013, 2009 by Saunders, an imprint of Elsevier Inc. All rights reserved.

2. What are five local signs and symptoms of inflammation? *(107)*

   a. _____

   b. _____

   c. _____

   d. _____

   e. _____

3. Identify seven signs and symptoms of systemic or generalized infection. *(107)*

   a. _____

   b. _____

   c. _____

   d. _____

   e. _____

   f. _____

   g. _____

Nursing Interventions for Patients with Infections

Directions: Provide the answers to the following questions.

1. List three nursing interventions that can be used to reduce high fevers. *(104)*

   a. _____

   b. _____

   c. _____

2. What are three teaching points to help patients avoid spreading respiratory infections to others? *(108-110)*

   a. _____

   b. _____

   c. _____

3. List five things that you should do to help prevent health care–associated infections. *(111-114, Table 6-8)*

   a. _____

   b. _____

   c. _____

   d. _____

   e. _____

Copyright © 2013, 2009 by Saunders, an imprint of Elsevier Inc. All rights reserved.

TABLE ACTIVITY

Directions: Complete the following table by supplying appropriate information in each column. Some of the blocks have been filled in for you. (110, Table 6-5)

Category-Specific Isolation Precautions (Expanded Precautions)

Isolation Category	Private Room	Masks	Gowns	Gloves	Common Diseases Placed into Isolation Category
Airborne Infection Isolation	Always; door to room must be kept closed at all times		No, unless draining wounds		Pulmonary or laryngeal tuberculosis, or draining tuberculous skin lesions; smallpox, viral hemorrhagic fever, severe acute respiratory syndrome (SARS); measles; varicella, disseminated zoster
Contact Precautions				Always; if patients are cohorted, staff must perform hand hygiene and change PPE *between* patients	
Droplet Precautions		Wear a surgical mask when entering room; patient should wear mask during transport and observe cough etiquette			

PRIORITY SETTING

Scenario: You are caring for a patient who was admitted for a leg infection. She needs IV antibiotic medication. She is unsure, but she believes that it will be the first time that she will receive this medication.

Directions: Prioritize the steps below for safe administration. (118-119, Table 6-9)

_____ a. Check the order and know why the patient is to receive an antimicrobial drug.

_____ b. Check that the dosage of the antimicrobial drug is appropriate for the patient.

_____ c. Verify allergies with the patient before administering an antimicrobial drug.

_____ d. Obtain cultures prior to administering the antimicrobial agent.

_____ e. Check to see if serum drug levels or cultures have been ordered.

_____ f. Monitor patient for signs of allergic reaction, such as rash, hives, itching, drug fever, swelling of the mucous membranes, difficulty breathing, or anaphylaxis.

Copyright © 2013, 2009 by Saunders, an imprint of Elsevier Inc. All rights reserved.

SHORT ANSWER

Sepsis

Scenario: You are working in an extended-care facility. Mr. Amberski is an elderly patient who is generally alert, cheerful, and conversant. Today, you immediately notice a marked change in his behavior and he appears very ill. You are aware that he has had some urinary symptoms (i.e., frequency and urgency) over the past two days.

Directions: Answer the following questions about sepsis.

1. List four signs and symptoms of sepsis. *(115-116)*

    a. _____

    b. _____

    c. _____

    d. _____

2. How might these symptoms differ in an elderly person? *(115-116)* _____

    _____

APPLICATION OF THE NURSING PROCESS

Care of the Patient at Risk for Infection

Directions: Write a short-term and a long-term goal and 4–6 interventions and an example of an evaluation statement for the short-term goal.

Mr. Jones is a 70-year-old gentleman residing in an extended-care facility. He has chronic poor circulation to his lower extremities; the skin just above the ankles has a brownish discoloration and is very leathery. He complains of itching and frequently scratches his legs; there are some very faint superficial scratches noted on the right ankle.

Nursing Diagnosis: Risk for infection related to poor circulation and skin ulceration

Goals/Expected Outcomes	Nursing Interventions	Evaluation

Copyright © 2013, 2009 by Saunders, an imprint of Elsevier Inc. All rights reserved.

REVIEW QUESTIONS FOR THE NCLEX® EXAMINATION

Directions: Choose the correct answer(s) for the following questions.

1. When a nurse assesses the patient for signs of local infection, which sign(s) or symptom(s) would indicate a local infection? *(Select all that apply.)* **(107)**
    1. Redness of skin and adjacent tissues
    2. Swelling at the site and surrounding tissues
    3. Pain at the site and surrounding tissues
    4. Limited function of the involved part
    5. Decreased peripheral pulses

2. The patient requires Expanded Precautions because of a draining wound positive for MRSA. The patient must go to the radiology department for diagnostic testing. What should the nurse do? **(109)**
    1. Call the physician and ask if the testing is really needed.
    2. Reschedule the test for after the MRSA is resolved.
    3. Put a mask on the patient just prior to transport.
    4. Call the radiology department and report presence of MRSA.

3. A patient has a staphylococcal infection that developed in an abdominal wound. The dressing must be changed once each shift. The patient is underweight, suffering from malnutrition, and has a fever. Which nursing action(s) is (are) essential? *(Select all that apply.)* **(104, 116-117)**
    1. Assess bowel and urine elimination regularly.
    2. Monitor temperature and promptly report abnormal readings.
    3. Encourage the patient to eat well-balanced, nutritious meals.
    4. Strictly adhere to precautions to avoid spreading infection.
    5. Plan active exercise to promote mobility.

4. A medication likely to be prescribed to combat a staphylococcal infection is: **(120, Table 6-10)**
    1. acetaminophen (Tylenol).
    2. trimethoprim-sulfamethoxasole (Septra).
    3. ketoconazole (Nizoral).
    4. penicillin V (Pen-Vee K).

5. A patient has a hacking cough, a runny nose, and painful swallowing because of a sore throat. He is diagnosed with a streptococcal infection of the throat. The nurse should use gloves for which type of activity? **(116)**
    1. Taking a radial pulse.
    2. Obtaining a throat swab culture and sensitivity.
    3. Delivering the throat culture tube to the lab.
    4. Reviewing the culture results.

6. Which patient(s) are most likely to have depression of the immune system? *(Select all that apply.)* **(104-106)**
    1. Patient who takes antibiotics for a urinary tract infection
    2. Patient who drinks excessive alcohol
    3. Patient who has chronic renal failure
    4. Patient who has been on corticosteroids for a long time
    5. Patient who is overweight for height
    6. Patient who is employed in a long-term care facility

7. To help a patient recover from a throat infection, what should he be advised to do? **(116-118)**
    1. Continue his normal workout routine but to get plenty of rest at night.
    2. Drink 8 ounces of liquid every hour while he is awake.
    3. When the sore throat stops, discontinue prescribed medications.
    4. Take an antipyretic with meals or a snack.

Copyright © 2013, 2009 by Saunders, an imprint of Elsevier Inc. All rights reserved.

8. The patient comes to the clinic for a chief complaint of burning with urination and urinary urgency. Based on her complaints, what additional assessment data would be most appropriate to obtain *first*? *(116-118)*
   1. Assess her genitalia for signs of inflammation.
   2. Check her chart for a history of kidney problems.
   3. Check her temperature to assess for a fever.
   4. Ask her about drug and food allergies.

9. While waiting to see the physician for urinary symptoms, the patient tells the nurse that she has to go to the bathroom to urinate. The nurse should: *(116)*
   1. ask her to delay urination until after the physician has examined her.
   2. instruct her to obtain a clean-catch midstream urine specimen.
   3. get an order for a Foley catheterization to relieve her urinary urgency.
   4. allow her to void freely and wait for the physician's orders.

10. The nurse observes a new nursing assistant using a mask, a gown, foot covers, and gloves for every patient that she is assigned to. What should the nurse do *first*? *(109)*
    1. Check the assignment sheet to see what kinds of patients the assistant is assigned to.
    2. Ask the charge nurse to intervene because the assistant is wasting supplies.
    3. Assess the assistant's understanding of Standard and Expanded Precautions.
    4. Allow her to continue to work because her actions prevent health care–associated infection.

11. Alcohol-based hand sanitizer is frequently adequate; however, when caring for patients with infections, which types of pathogens require strict soap-and-water hand hygiene? (*Select all that apply.*) *(114)*
    1. *Clostridium difficile*
    2. *Staphylococcus aureus*
    3. *Candida albicans*
    4. *Pseudomonas aeruginosa*
    5. *Klebsiella pneumoniae*

12. Which action(s) would the nurse take to reduce the risk of health care–associated infections for patients who are at risk? (*Select all that apply.*) *(114)*
    1. Position the patient in a supine position for comfort.
    2. Offer and assist with frequent oral hygiene.
    3. Obtain an order for indwelling catheter for incontinent patients.
    4. Encourage patients to cough and deep-breathe.
    5. Advocate for removal of nasogastric feeding tubes as soon possible.
    6. Alert physician to culture and sensitivity reports for appropriate antibiotic use.

13. The patient is being treated for a *Staphylococcus aureus* skin infection. The nurse sees an order for ketoconazole. What should the nurse do *first*? *(116, 120, Table 6-10)*
    1. Give the medication as ordered and observe for side effects.
    2. Call the physician and question the order.
    3. Call the pharmacy and ask why the drug was ordered.
    4. Check laboratory results to verify presence of a fungal infection.

14. A mother reports giving her child ½ teaspoon of liquid children's fever reducer. How many milliliters (mL) did she give? _____ *(see Units Conversion calculator on Evolve)*

15. Physician orders 600 mg of acetaminophen. Pharmacy delivers a 3-ounce bottle of acetaminophen 325 mg/10.15 mL. How many mL should be given? _____ *(see Units Conversion calculator on Evolve)*

Copyright © 2013, 2009 by Saunders, an imprint of Elsevier Inc. All rights reserved.

CRITICAL THINKING ACTIVITIES

Scenario A: You observe that a new nursing assistant has a cough and runny nose. She is assigned to care for a patient with neutropenic precautions. You realize that she may be unfamiliar with this type of isolation, or that she may not know how to deal with the situation. *(109-115)*

1.   What should you do? _____

   _____

   _____

Scenario B: You see a laboratory technician drawing blood from a patient. He is not wearing gloves, stating, "I don't need gloves." He appears to be competent and is quickly able to draw the blood without apparent contact with body fluids. *(109-115)*

1.   Explore how you would handle this situation. _____

   _____

   _____

   _____

   _____

STEPS TOWARD BETTER COMMUNICATION

VOCABULARY BUILDING GLOSSARY

The following words from Chapter 6 have the long **a** sound, as in *name*. Perhaps you can find others.

Term	Definition
surveil'lance (ser vay'lenz)	continuous watching for something
malaise'(mah layz')	feeling of illness
-phage (fahj)	eating, swallowing
mac'rophage (mak' row fahj)	large phagocytic cell
phagocyto'sis (fag ow sytow' sis)	surrounding of microorganism by phagocytes
asep'tic	free from bacteria
asep'sis	method to prevent infection, keep bacteria-free

PRONUNCIATION SKILLS

The long **a** sound can be spelled in a number of ways.

Spelling	Examples
a	latent, anal, patient, dangerous, table, dilation, incubation
a–e	invade, isolate, palpate, dilate, lactate, incubate, drape, -phage, make, mistake (silent "e" at end)
ai	brain, pain, malaise, daily, wait, straight
ay	day, say, stay, May
ea	great, break, steak
ei	vein, weigh, nucleic, eight
ey	they, obey

Copyright © 2013, 2009 by Saunders, an imprint of Elsevier Inc. All rights reserved.

MATCHING

Directions: Match the following terms with their correct definitions.

1.	_____ Asepsis	a.	General feeling of illness, not well
2.	_____ Malaise	b.	Containing pus
3.	_____ Exudate	c.	Watching for
4.	_____ Purulent	d.	Keeping free from bacteria
5.	_____ Surveillance	e.	Discharge that is composed of tissue, fluid, and dead cells

PRONUNCIATION SKILLS

*Directions: In the following sentences, underline the letters in the words that have the long **a** sound.*

1. Draping the patient on the table before a procedure protects the patient's privacy and modesty. It helps to maintain aseptic conditions.

2. Ms. Clay has fever and malaise and her wound has green exudate.

3. Mrs. James is not having any pain, but she has gained more than eighteen pounds in weight.

COMMUNICATION EXERCISES

Directions: Write out what you would say for the following situations.

1. Mrs. Compton is admitted for a hysterectomy but has a boil in the axilla. How would you explain the importance of hand hygiene and using clean towels and washcloths to bathe when she goes home?

   _____

   _____

   _____

   _____

   _____

   _____

2. You have a patient with a large infected wound on his shin. How would you explain to him how infection is spread and the precautions that must be taken in caring for him and changing his dressings?

   _____

   _____

   _____

   _____

   _____

   _____

   _____

Copyright © 2013, 2009 by Saunders, an imprint of Elsevier Inc. All rights reserved.

Care of Patients with Pain

Answer Key: Textbook page references are provided as a guide for answering these questions. A complete answer key was provided to your instructor.

TABLE ACTIVITY

Common Terms to Help Patients Describe Their Pain

Directions: Fill in the table with some common terms to help your patient describe pain. (130, Table 7-3)

Degree of pain (from least to most severe)	
Quality of pain	
Frequency of pain	

COMPLETION

Directions: Fill in the blanks to complete the statements.

1. The body produces _____, which can attach to pain receptors and block the pain sensation. *(125)*

2. Sinus infection pain reflected in the upper molars is termed _____ pain. *(130)*

3. Rest _____ pain tolerance and improves response to analgesia. *(127, 138)*

4. One "rule" to keep in mind is that massage should *not* be used on areas _____ _____. *(139)*

5. A dressing change or an uncomfortable procedure can be made less painful if you ask the patient questions and _____ his attention during the procedure. *(138-139)*

Copyright © 2013, 2009 by Saunders, an imprint of Elsevier Inc. All rights reserved.

6. Repositioning is an important measure in _____ pain, especially in the elderly. *(140-141)*

7. Examples of narcotic analgesics are _____, _____, and

   _____. *(135)*

8. A measure of the effectiveness of control of chronic pain is how well the patient can accomplish

   _____. *(128)*

SHORT ANSWER

Pain and Pain Management

Directions: Read the scenario and answer the questions that follow.

Scenario: You have been asked to assist the nurse manager to develop an in-service for the nursing staff about pain and pain management. He has asked you to collect some relevant information that can be reviewed with the staff and to make a handout that compares acute and chronic pain.

1. What are five facts that dispel false perceptions about pain? *(126-128, 130-134, Table 7-4)*

   a. _____

   b. _____

   c. _____

   d. _____

   e. _____

2. List four nonphysical factors that affect pain tolerance. *(126-131)*

   a. _____

   b. _____

   c. _____

   d. _____

3. List at least six nonpharmacologic approaches that can be used as adjuncts to medication. *(138-140)*

   a. _____

   b. _____

   c. _____

   d. _____

   e. _____

   f. _____

4. Briefly explain how imagery and meditation can assist with pain control. *(139)* _____

   _____

   _____

Copyright © 2013, 2009 by Saunders, an imprint of Elsevier Inc. All rights reserved.

TABLE ACTIVITY

Acute Versus Chronic Pain

Directions: Fill in the table to compare features of acute and chronic pain. **(127-128, Table 7-2)**

Pain	Acute	Chronic
Duration		
Prognosis for relief		
Cause		
Psychosocial effects		
Effect of therapy		

APPLICATION OF THE NURSING PROCESS

Caring for a Patient with Acute Pain

Directions: Provide the answer to the following questions.

Mr. Jung sustained injuries in a tour bus accident and was transferred 2 days ago from the ICU to the general medical-surgical unit. He has a broken arm, rib fractures, and soft tissue trauma on both legs. Mr. Jung has a difficult time verbalizing his pain to the nursing staff and frequently declines medication. He is quiet and withdrawn and often appears very uncomfortable.

1. List at least six physiologic clues that upon assessment might indicate Mr. Jung is experiencing pain. *(127-129)*

   a. _____

   b. _____

   c. _____

   d. _____

   e. _____

   f. _____

Copyright © 2013, 2009 by Saunders, an imprint of Elsevier Inc. All rights reserved.

2. List at least five behaviors you might observe that indicate that Mr. Jung may be having pain. *(127-129)*

   a. _____

   b. _____

   c. _____

   d. _____

   e. _____

3. You are reinforcing teaching points to help Mr. Poroj understand pain management. *(Select all that apply.)* *(133-134)*
   a. Medication is more effective if taken before pain is too severe.
   b. Taking medication regularly helps control the pain.
   c. Pain actually interferes with wound healing.
   d. Patient addiction to narcotics is usually less than 1%.
   e. Pain tolerance does not vary greatly from one person to the next.

4. List five areas that should be covered in documentation about pain and measures taken for the treatment of pain. *(132-133, 137, Box 7-1)*

   a. _____

   b. _____

   c. _____

   d. _____

   e. _____

PRIORITY SETTING

Directions: Read the scenarios and prioritize tasks and patients' needs appropriately.

Scenario A: You are caring for Mr. Rojas. He sustained a broken ankle with severe soft tissue swelling and many abrasions in a motorcycle accident. He was admitted and has an external fixation procedure for the ankle fracture. He received IV morphine before the procedure, procedural sedation, and a nerve block for the fixation. The current order is for morphine by PCA pump. Prioritize the following nursing responsibilities that are related to giving analgesic medications. Ibuprofen 800 mg is ordered for his many abrasions and muscle pain.

_____ a. Verify PCA pump settings with order.

_____ b. Reinforce teaching about medications.

_____ c. Use nonpharmacologic measures such as elevation or ice packs.

_____ d. Report to the physician when measures are not effective.

_____ e. Assess the patient's pain.

_____ f. Check the medication record for last dose of ibuprofen.

Copyright © 2013, 2009 by Saunders, an imprint of Elsevier Inc. All rights reserved.

Scenario B: You are caring for several patients on a busy medical-surgical unit. While you are aware that all patients expect and deserve to receive timely and adequate relief of their pain, you also recognize the need to organize and prioritize your actions. Based on your knowledge of pain and pathophysiology, prioritize the order in which you will attend to the analgesic needs of these patients.

_____   a. Mr. Jasper is 2 days postoperative for a hernia repair. He complains of pain 8/10 in the lower abdominal area.

_____   b. Mrs. Quentin reports pain in the left neck and jaw which radiates down to the back.

_____   c. Mr. Davoudi reports severe pain that started 10 minutes ago, in the area distal to his lower extremity cast.

_____   d. Mr. Ramirez is a diabetic who has continuous neuropathic pain in his lower legs.

REVIEW QUESTIONS FOR THE NCLEX® EXAMINATION

Directions: Choose the best answer(s) for the following questions.

1. The patient is experiencing pain in a limb after amputation. What type of pain is this patient experiencing? *(126)*
   1. Chronic pain
   2. Phantom pain
   3. Referred pain
   4. Nociceptive pain

2. The nurse understands that the choice of a pain scale to use for a patient depends on the: *(129-130)*
   1. pain scales available on the unit.
   2. age and physical and cognitive ability of the patient.
   3. nurse's preference for a pain scale.
   4. World Health Organization's recommendation.

3. Which pain scale would be appropriate for a patient who is cognitively impaired? *(129-130)*
   1. Visual scale
   2. Color scale
   3. Pieces of pain scale
   4. Behavioral pain scale

4. Gabapentin (Neurontin) is given to relieve which type of pain? *(136)*
   1. Acute pain
   2. Chronic pain
   3. Neuropathic pain
   4. Nociceptive pain

5. A patient is undergoing rehabilitative therapy. When would be the best time to give analgesic medication? *(133-135)*
   1. Give PRN medications every 4–6 hours.
   2. Give early in the morning before performing ADLs.
   3. Give on a schedule to minimize pain during therapy sessions.
   4. Give whenever the pain is greater than 4/10.

Copyright © 2013, 2009 by Saunders, an imprint of Elsevier Inc. All rights reserved.

6. The patient is unable to verbalize pain. Which patient behavior is the best indicator that pain medication is successfully addressing the patient's pain? *(129-131)*
   1. Patient sleeps unless aroused by nurse.
   2. Patient watches TV without grimacing.
   3. Patient actively participates in physical therapy.
   4. Patient smiles at friends and family when they visit.

7. The nurse gives the patient a 4-mg IM dose of morphine at 10:00 AM. When should the nurse next evaluate the effectiveness of the pain control medication? *(137)*
   1. 10:15 AM
   2. 10:45 AM
   3. 11:00 AM
   4. 2: 00 PM

8. When evaluating the effectiveness of pain medication, in addition to assessing physical body language, the nurse should rely on: *(132, 137)*
   1. the length of time between requests for pain medication.
   2. how sedated the patient becomes after receiving the medication.
   3. whether the patient experiences nausea from the medication.
   4. what the patient says about his pain relief.

9. Packs or compresses for heat therapy are usually left in place for _____. *(Fill in the blank.)* *(138)*

10. Intramuscular analgesic injections are not recommended for the elderly because: *(137)*
    1. kidney function is decreased and the drug is excreted more slowly.
    2. circulation is sluggish and the medication is not picked up quickly.
    3. skin and tissue are more fragile and bruising is likely.
    4. muscle and fat tissue are diminished which may affect bioavailability.

CRITICAL THINKING ACTIVITIES

Scenario: Mrs. Cole, age 54, is admitted to the hospital for a laparoscopic cholecystectomy. She has a history of chronic gallbladder disease with episodes of pain, nausea, and vomiting. During her initial assessment upon admission, you learn that Mrs. Cole has had rheumatoid arthritis of the knees and hips for about 15 years.

1. Which statement most accurately applies to Mrs. Cole's problem of arthritis pain?
   a. If she does not mention having pain due to her arthritis, it is because she has gotten used to it over the years and it no longer bothers her much.
   b. Unless some degeneration of the joints is shown by x-rays, there is little reason to believe that a person has pain with arthritis.
   c. The use of moist heat in the morning upon arising can diminish pain with movement.
   d. Aspirin, a non-narcotic analgesic, and hot packs applied to her knees help relieve Mrs. Cole's pain at home and could be continued in the hospital.

2. If Mrs. Cole states that she often feels pain under her right shoulder blade when her gallbladder "acts up," you can assume that Mrs. Cole:
   a. probably also has an undiagnosed heart condition.
   b. is feeling referred pain.
   c. is confused about where her pain really is.
   d. is pretending to have pain that does not really exist.

Copyright © 2013, 2009 by Saunders, an imprint of Elsevier Inc. All rights reserved.

3. The admitting physician has not ordered anything for relief of Mrs. Cole's arthritic pain. In this circumstance, the best nursing action would be to:
   a. explain to Mrs. Cole that whatever she receives for pain after surgery will probably relieve the pain she has in her knees and hips.
   b. ignore the omission of orders because Mrs. Cole's arthritic pain is not as important as her gallbladder disorder.
   c. ask Mrs. Cole what measures she uses at home for relief of her arthritic pain, record the information, institute nursing measures, and ask her physician to order the analgesic she uses.
   d. tell Mrs. Cole nothing can be done about her painful joints because her physician did not write an order for any relief measures.

4. On the evening after her surgery, Mrs. Cole has a long visit with her daughter. During that time, you look in on Mrs. Cole and she seems to be comfortable and happy. After her daughter leaves, Mrs. Cole asks for something for pain. Mrs. Cole's behavior probably indicates that:
   a. she does not have as much real pain as she says she has.
   b. she is afraid to complain in her daughter's presence.
   c. her daughter brought some medication from home to relieve her mother's pain.
   d. her daughter's visit effectively distracted Mrs. Cole and diverted her attention from her pain.

STEPS TOWARD BETTER COMMUNICATION

VOCABULARY BUILDING GLOSSARY

Term	Definition
com pounds'	(verb) increases or adds to; makes worse
creep'ing	moving slowly and with difficulty
frail	having delicate health; weak; easily breakable
grim'ace	tense facial expression indicating pain
im'agery	mental pictures
indic'ative	suggesting; pointing out; revealing
place'bo	a substance given as medication that contains no actual medication
keep a "stiff upper lip"	bear something without an outward show of emotion or body change (slang); to endure without complaint
tol'erance	point in drug therapy where the drug no longer works

COMPLETION

Directions: Fill in the blanks with the appropriate words from the Vocabulary Building Glossary above.

1. The use of _____ helps patients relax and take a short "mental vacation."

2. The patient was experiencing back pain and was _____ across the room to the bathroom.

3. When the nurse turned the patient onto his left side, his _____ indicated that he was experiencing pain.

4. Fatigue _____ the problem of pain and makes it more difficult to cope with.

Copyright © 2013, 2009 by Saunders, an imprint of Elsevier Inc. All rights reserved.

5. The 88-year-old lady had lost 7 pounds and appeared very _____.

6. Some patients respond well to a(n) _____ in place of a narcotic analgesic.

7. Mr. Thomas presented a(n) _____, not even flinching when the doctor bent his knee after surgery.

8. When a patient frequently complains of pain much sooner than usual after a dose of pain medication, either something is making the pain worse or the patient is developing _____ to the pain medication.

9. When a pain medication is no longer effective for the patient, it is _____ of the need for a change in the medication order.

MATCHING

Directions: Match the abbreviations with their correct terms.

1. _____   OTC   a. Transcutaneous electrical nerve stimulation

2. _____   PCA   b. Over-the-counter

3. _____   TENS   c. Patient-controlled analgesia

TERMINOLOGY

Evaluating Pain

Directions: Rank (from 1 to 9) the following words for degrees of pain from the least to the worst.

_____   moderate

_____   minimal

_____   extremely severe

_____   exquisite

_____   mild

_____   very severe

_____   absent

_____   fairly severe

_____   severe

Copyright © 2013, 2009 by Saunders, an imprint of Elsevier Inc. All rights reserved.

MATCHING

Directions: Match the terms indicating the quality of pain on the right with the correct category headings on the left (each category will have more than one term).

1. _____ Heat
2. _____ Knife
3. _____ Stretching
4. _____ Vibrating
5. _____ Pressure

a. Burning
b. Pulsating
c. Dull
d. Twisting
e. Tearing
f. Throbbing
g. Biting
h. Searing
i. Stabbing
j. Crushing
k. Tingling
l. Pulling
m. Sharp

COMMUNICATION EXERCISES

Directions: Read the following scenarios and answer the related questions.

1. Your patient's ordered medication is not controlling the pain for more than 1 hour. You need to call the doctor and ask for the order to be changed. Write out what you would say during the phone call. (Remember you will need to know the current vital signs.) _____

   _____

   _____

   _____

   _____

2. You have given your patient an injection of morphine for pain. An hour later, you notice that the patient's respirations have dropped to 10 per minute. You must notify the charge nurse of the patient's condition. Write out how you would tell the charge nurse this information. _____

   _____

   _____

   _____

   _____

   _____

Copyright © 2013, 2009 by Saunders, an imprint of Elsevier Inc. All rights reserved.

Care of Patients with Cancer

Answer Key: Textbook page references are provided as a guide for answering these questions. A complete answer key was provided to your instructor.

COMPLETION

Directions: Fill in the blanks to complete the statements.

1. Malignant cells grow in a(n) _____ manner compared to normal cells. *(144)*

2. A(n) _____ is a tumor composed of fibrous tissue. *(146)*

3. Malignant growths are divided into four main types: _____,
_____, _____, and _____. *(146)*

4. TNM staging system identifies cancers by how much the malignancy has spread and includes three basic parts: *T* for _____, *N* for _____, and *M* for _____
_____. *(146-147)*

5. _____, _____, air and water pollution, and certain
_____ found in food packaging are all considered to be carcinogens. *(147-149)*

6. There are three traditional modes of therapy for malignancies: _____,
_____, and _____. *(158-165)*

7. Many antineoplastic drugs are _____, which can cause tissue damage and severe local injury if they escape from the vein into which they are administered. *(163)*

8. Suppression of the _____ is the major reason that doses of chemotherapy must be limited. *(168)*

9. A leiofibroma contains both _____ cells and _____
_____. *(146)*

10. Radiation therapy of the abdomen or lower back often produces_____, _____,
and _____ starting 7–10 days after the beginning of treatment. *(162, Table 8-3)*

11. The doctor orders Roxenol 20 mg PO q 4 h for pain. The pharmacy delivers a 90-mL bottle of Roxenol 10 mg/mL. How many mL should be given? _____

Copyright © 2013, 2009 by Saunders, an imprint of Elsevier Inc. All rights reserved.

MATCHING

Risk Factors for Cancer

Directions: Match each high-risk factor on the left with its associated site of malignancy on the right. **(147, Table 8-1)**

1. _____   Diet heavy in pickled or salted foods
2. _____   Frequent sex in early teens
3. _____   Early menarche; late menopause
4. _____   Estrogen therapy
5. _____   Over age 65; African-American
6. _____   Heavy smoker; asbestos exposure
7. _____   Use of smokeless tobacco

a. Stomach
b. Prostate
c. Uterine and endometrial
d. Breast
e. Uterus and cervix
f. Lung
g. Mouth

SHORT ANSWER

Interventions for the Side Effects of Chemotherapy

Directions: Read the clinical scenario and answer the questions that follow.

Scenario: You are caring for a patient who is receiving chemotherapy. List at least five nursing activities (assessments or interventions) to include in the care plan of the patient experiencing the common problems related to cancer or the toxic side effects of chemotherapy.

1. Common problem: diarrhea *(164, 167)*

   a. _____

   b. _____

   c. _____

   d. _____

   e. _____

2. Toxic effect: thrombocytopenia *(168)*

   a. _____

   b. _____

   c. _____

   d. _____

   e. _____

3. Toxic effect: mucositis *(166-167)*

   a. _____

   b. _____

   c. _____

   d. _____

   e. _____

Copyright © 2013, 2009 by Saunders, an imprint of Elsevier Inc. All rights reserved.

4. Toxic effect: immunosuppression *(168)*

   a. _____

   b. _____

   c. _____

   d. _____

   e. _____

APPLICATION OF THE NURSING PROCESS

Caring for a Patient with Non-Hodgkin's Lymphoma

Directions: Provide the answer to the following questions.

Mrs. Junic is diagnosed with non-Hodgkin's lymphoma. She is receiving combination chemotherapy and radiation. She is trying to be brave and "not bother the nurses or worry her family," but you walk in and find that she is crying. She admits to nausea, vomiting, and diarrhea, but she states, "I know that is just part of the therapy, so I am trying to deal with it."

1. List at least four things to assess related to Mrs. Junic's vomiting and diarrhea. *(167)*

   a. _____

   _____

   b. _____

   _____

   c. _____

   _____

   d. _____

   _____

2. Which nursing diagnosis is a priority for Mrs. Junic? *(167)*
   a. Alteration in nutrition (less than body needs), risk for, related to nausea, vomiting, and diarrhea
   b. Diarrhea related to effects of cancer treatment
   c. Knowledge deficit related to drugs and side effects
   d. Ineffective individual coping related to side effects of treatment

3. List six nonpharmacologic interventions for nausea. *(167)*

   a. _____

   b. _____

   c. _____

   d. _____

   e. _____

   f. _____

Copyright © 2013, 2009 by Saunders, an imprint of Elsevier Inc. All rights reserved.

4. List at least five resources that a cancer patient and his or her family might use to help them cope with the problems associated with malignancy. *(171, 175)*

   a. _____

   b. _____

   c. _____

   d. _____

   e. _____

5. Which statement by Mrs. Junic indicates that she understands how to deal with the side effects of chemotherapy? *(157, 171)*
   a. "All drugs, including chemotherapy drugs, have side effects."
   b. "I should report side effects; they could be an adverse response to therapy."
   c. "After I learn to recognize the side effects, I can cope independently."
   d. "A few side effects are okay as long as they don't interfere with activities of daily living."

PRIORITY SETTING

Directions: Read the following scenario and prioritize as appropriate.

Scenario: You are assigned to care for five patients on an oncology unit. You have just received report from the night shift nurse. Prioritize the order in which you will attend to the needs of these patients.

   _____   a. Ms. Hobbs needs her AM dose of Megace.

   _____   b. Mrs. Hiroshi needs assistance with eating breakfast.

   _____   c. Mr. Lopez' laboratory report shows a platelet count of 20,000/mm^3.

   _____   d. Mr. Nehru is asking for a PRN pain medication.

   _____   e. Ms. Jaiswal wants information about cancer support groups.

REVIEW QUESTIONS FOR THE NCLEX® EXAMINATION

Directions: Choose the best answer(s) for the following questions.

1. When assessing the effect of anorexia on maintaining ideal body weight, a significant loss of weight would be: *(166)*
   1. 1 pound per month.
   2. 0.5 pound per week.
   3. 2 pounds per month.
   4. 2 pounds or more per week.

2. The nurse directs the nursing assistant in safety measures to be used while caring for a patient undergoing radiation therapy with a sealed implant. Which would be appropriate to include? *(161-162, Figure 8-6)*
   1. Use ordinary Standard Precautions, but nothing else is required.
   2. Limit total time in patient's room to 60 minutes/8-hour shift.
   3. Wear a radiation detection badge to detect the amount of radiation exposure.
   4. Wear a lead apron to decrease exposure to radiation.

Copyright © 2013, 2009 by Saunders, an imprint of Elsevier Inc. All rights reserved.

3. When providing care for a patient undergoing internal radiation, you would: *(161, Box 8-5)*
    1. wear a lead apron when at the bedside.
    2. quickly and efficiently provide hands-on care.
    3. stay out of the patient's room as much as possible.
    4. ask a family member to feed the patient.

4. When evaluating the patient's response to chemotherapy, which assessment finding is the greatest immediate concern? *(168)*
    1. Constipation and straining
    2. Bleeding after brushing teeth
    3. Alopecia or change in hair color
    4. Fatigue and irritability

5. The patient is newly diagnosed with cancer and faces enormous stress. Which response by the nurse would be the most useful in helping the patient cope? *(172)*
    1. "The doctor will give you all the information you need to know."
    2. "Tell me what the doctor told you and maybe I can help to clarify things."
    3. "Try to read or watch television. Just keep your mind busy."
    4. "Don't worry about chemotherapy, my aunt had it and she did just fine."

6. When assessing for the side effect of bone marrow depression from chemotherapy, the nurse would: *(Select all that apply.) (168)*
    1. check the CBC lab results.
    2. assess for easy bruising.
    3. assess for signs of infection.
    4. check for hearing loss.

7. Alopecia resulting from chemotherapy is: *(169)*
    1. temporary.
    2. irreversible.
    3. treatable.
    4. preventable.

8. The nurse gives the patient a booster PCA dose of morphine 2 mg. The nurse would assess the response to the medication in: *(169-170)*
    1. 15 minutes.
    2. 20 minutes.
    3. 30 minutes.
    4. 60 minutes.

9. Which statement by the family indicates an understanding of palliative care? *(172)*
    1. "We want him to be comfortable, so oral medications are preferred."
    2. "We should encourage water and other nourishment as much as possible."
    3. "He'll feel short of breath and we'll hear the "death rattle."
    4. "He'll continue with his cancer treatments if they don't cause side effects."

10. The patient is having diarrhea secondary to radiation therapy of the pelvic area. Which statement by the patient indicates a need for additional teaching about the diarrhea? *(167)*
    1. "I will cleanse the rectal area and apply petroleum jelly."
    2. "I will report an increase in the number and frequency of bowel movements."
    3. "I will avoid eating foods such as bananas and cheese."
    4. "I may need to have my electrolytes checked if the diarrhea is severe."

Copyright © 2013, 2009 by Saunders, an imprint of Elsevier Inc. All rights reserved.

11. *Promoters* are substances that: *(148)*
    1. help prevent cancer cells from invading other cells.
    2. cause cancer cells to grow faster.
    3. help cancer cells metastasize to other areas.
    4. enhance the effect of chemotherapy drugs.

12. All cancers are caused by _____ that malfunction and cause overgrowth of cells. *(149)*

CRITICAL THINKING ACTIVITIES

Scenario: Mr. Long is scheduled to begin receiving external radiation therapy to his chin and neck for cancer of the mandible.

1. Select all of the correct teaching points to share with Mr. Long about his therapy. *(159-160)*
   a. Local skin irritation may not appear immediately, but may appear later.
   b. The treatment will be delivered in divided doses over many days.
   c. He must avoid contact with others to avoid exposing them to radiation.
   d. Written instructions are provided to help manage the expected side effects.
   e. Skin damage will be permanent, but the area will be very small.

2. Which of these side effects is most likely to occur as a result of radiation to the neck? *(162, Table 8-3)*
   a. Thrombocytopenia
   b. Loss of taste
   c. Alopecia
   d. Leukopenia

3. Choose measures that would be included in the care plan for Mr. Long. *(Select all that apply.)* *(159-160)*
   a. Increase fluid intake
   b. Artificial saliva to be used as needed
   c. Minimal brushing of teeth to reduce irritation
   d. Avoid spicy food and alcohol
   e. Limit protein intake

4. To minimize damage to the skin exposed to radiation, Mr. Long should be instructed to do which of the following? *(160)*
   a. Wear a tight-fitting scarf around his neck to protect it from sunlight.
   b. Wash the skin gently with mild soap, tepid water, and a soft washcloth.
   c. Avoid applying any lotions or powders unless prescribed by physician.
   d. Examine the condition of his skin weekly and report any blistering.

5. Mr. Long becomes unusually angry and demanding after his third treatment. You recognize that: *(160)*
   a. he had a bad experience with the radiation therapy team.
   b. anger is one of the normal stages in the grieving process.
   c. the physician should be notified to prescribe an anxiolytic drug.
   d. confusion and personality changes are side effects of therapy.

6. In helping Mr. Long to deal with his anger, choose the most therapeutic response. *(160)*
   a. "Everything will be okay, Mr. Long. Let me sit with you for awhile."
   b. "You don't seem like your usual self. Tell me what happened."
   c. "Those treatments are really tiring. Just rest for awhile."
   d. "I can see that you are upset. Why are you acting this way?"

Copyright © 2013, 2009 by Saunders, an imprint of Elsevier Inc. All rights reserved.

STEPS TOWARD BETTER COMMUNICATION

VOCABULARY BUILDING GLOSSARY

Term	Definition
ad'juvant	serving to help or assist; used in addition to (another treatment)
be'nign	not malignant; gentle or kind
carcin'ogen	substance that tends to produce a cancer
depletes'	uses up; seriously decreases the supply
immunocom'petent	able to develop immunity
in si'tu	contained within the original site
intrin'sic	naturally belonging to or within something
malig'nant	uncontrolled growth that is harmful and may cause death
metas'tasis	spread of cancer cells to other parts of the body
oc'cult	hidden; not readily detectable
transforma'tion	change in nature, character, or appearance
ves'icant	agent that causes severe irritation and can cause blisters

WORD ATTACK SKILLS

Combining Forms: Prefixes

adeno-	gland
carcino-	cancer
melano-	black
fibro-	fiber; refers to connective tissue
leio-	smooth muscle
leuko-	white blood cell; white
lipo-	fat; lipid
lympho-	lymphocyte (clear tissue fluid)
osteo-	bone
radio-	radiant energy waves such as in radiation therapy

Combining Forms: Suffix

-oma	tumor

Word Families

metas'tasis	(noun) invasive spread of tumor cells
metas'tasize	(verb) to spread throughout the body
metasta'tic	(adjective) capable of spreading throughout the body
carcino'ma	(noun) malignant tumor of epithelial tissue
carcin'ogen	(noun) agent that may cause cancer
carcinogen'ic	(adjective) capable of causing cancer

Copyright © 2013, 2009 by Saunders, an imprint of Elsevier Inc. All rights reserved.

PRONUNCIATION SKILLS

Directions: Look at the accent mark on each of the following words and practice their pronunciations.

mes en chy' mal (*ch* sounds like "k")   prog no' sis

ma lig' nant   car cin no' ma   (kar sin no ma)

per i to ne' al   car cin' o gens   (kar sin o jens)

car cin o gen' ic (car sin o jen ik)   de oxy ribo nu cle' ic   (dee oxy rybow noo klay ic)

mi cro scop' ic ally (*ically* sounds like "ikly")

COMPLETION

Directions: Fill in the blanks with the appropriate words from the Vocabulary Building Glossary to complete the statements.

1. Chemotherapy drugs that are highly irritating are administered into a vein that has a high blood flow; such drugs may cause blisters and are termed _____.

2. A tumor whose cells reproduce in an uncontrolled, nonstructured pattern is called a(n) _____ tumor.

3. If a malignant tumor occurs in the gastrointestinal tract, the only early symptom may be _____ bleeding.

4. When certain body cells are exposed to a(n) _____ repeatedly over time, the cells may undergo malignant changes.

5. When chemotherapy or radiation is effective on a solid tumor, the cells in the tumor undergo a(n) _____ and the tumor shrinks or stops growing.

6. A brain tumor may be _____ and still be life-threatening.

7. The excessive malignant growth of a tumor places a strain on the body and _____ nutritional stores.

8. The use of tamoxifen is a(n) _____ therapy added to surgery, radiation, and/or chemotherapy for breast cancer.

9. A normal, healthy body has the _____ ability to fight and kill beginning cancer cells.

10. Poor nutrition, exposure to toxic substances, chronic illness, and long periods of excessive stress make the body less _____ and may contribute to the growth of cancer.

11. When found _____, cervical cancer has a very good cure rate.

12. Breast cancer, as well as many other types of cancer, tends to _____ to other parts of the body if not caught and treated early.

Copyright © 2013, 2009 by Saunders, an imprint of Elsevier Inc. All rights reserved.

Types of Tissues

Directions: From what type of tissue does each of the following tumors arise? **(146)**

1. Adenocarcinoma: _____

2. Leiomyoma: _____

3. Lymphoma: _____

4. Melanoma: _____

5. Osteosarcoma: _____

6. Fibroma: _____

COMMUNICATION EXERCISE

Mr. Tomm, age 72, has metastatic prostate cancer. He is to undergo radiation therapy. Practice what you would say in the remainder of the dialogue.

Nurse: "Good morning, Mr. Tomm. How do you feel this morning?"

Mr. Tomm: "Pretty good, I guess. I woke up a lot last night."

Nurse: "Were you worrying about this morning's radiation treatment?"

Mr. Tomm: "I am a bit anxious, yes."

(Continue with statements by both the nurse and Mr. Tomm.)

Copyright © 2013, 2009 by Saunders, an imprint of Elsevier Inc. All rights reserved.

Chronic Illness and Rehabilitation

Answer Key: Textbook page references are provided as a guide for answering these questions. A complete answer key was provided to your instructor.

SHORT ANSWER

Chronic Illness and Immobility

1. Five chronic diseases or conditions that require extra care or rehabilitation are: *(178, Box 9-1)*

   a. _____

   b. _____

   c. _____

   d. _____

   e. _____

2. Four goals of care in a long-term care facility are: *(183)*

   1. _____

   2. _____

   3. _____

   4. _____

3. The patient with a chronic illness often feels _____. *(178)*

4. The patient must develop new _____ mechanisms in order to effectively deal with the changes the illness or situation has brought. *(178)*

5. Restorative programs focus on _____ and _____ . *(183)*

6. Prevention of problems of immobility begins when a patient first becomes _____
   _____. *(178)*

7. Early effects of immobility include: *(178)*

   _____

   _____

   _____

Copyright © 2013, 2009 by Saunders, an imprint of Elsevier Inc. All rights reserved.

8. The elderly are more susceptible to the complications of immobility. It is especially important to monitor an elderly immobile patient for signs of: *(179-182, Table 9-1)*

    a. _____

    b. _____

    c. _____

    d. _____

    e. _____

TABLE ACTIVITY

Directions: Complete the following table with the measures used to prevent complications within the particular body system. *(179, Table 9-1)*

Body System	Measures to Prevent Complications
Musculoskeletal	
Gastrointestinal	
Cardiovascular	
Neurologic	
Renal/urinary	
Respiratory	
Integumentary	

Copyright © 2013, 2009 by Saunders, an imprint of Elsevier Inc. All rights reserved.

COMPLETION

Directions: Fill in the blanks to complete the statements.

1. When working with a rehabilitation patient, the nurse must recognize that the patient is the _____ team. *(188)*

2. The rehabilitation team often consists of the physician, nurse, vocational counselor, and the _____, _____, _____, and _____ therapists. *(188)*

3. The basis of the philosophy of rehabilitation nursing is recognition of _____ _____. *(189)*

4. Safety restraints may only be used if they _____ or are needed for _____. *(185, Box 9-7)*

5. The first step in the prevention of falls is recognition of which _____ _____. *(183)*

6. The second step in the prevention of falls is recognition of _____ _____ that could precipitate a fall. *(183)*

7. Encouraging elderly residents of long-term care facilities to _____ to pick up something and _____ to dry the feet to help prevent dizziness or loss of balance and a fall. *(Box 9-5)*

8. The resident immobilized with a security device must be checked at least every _____ to ensure the body is in good alignment and that there are no problems. *(185)*

9. To help relieve or prevent venous stasis in the immobile patient, encourage _____ _____ every 2 hours. *(179, 185, Table 9-1)*

10. Sensory deficits such as impaired _____ or _____ may add to a patient's confusion and anxiety at night. *(186)*

11. Residents who are taking diuretics must be constantly monitored for _____ _____, which might cause confusion. *(183)*

12. A major psychosocial issue for the greatly immobilized patient is _____ _____ due to inability to socialize. *(187)*

13. The goal of home care is to keep the patient _____ and enable her to _____. *(191)*

14. In the long-term care facility, the core caregivers are _____ and they should be treated respectfully. *(183)*

Copyright © 2013, 2009 by Saunders, an imprint of Elsevier Inc. All rights reserved.

REVIEW QUESTIONS FOR THE NCLEX® EXAMINATION

Directions: Choose the best answer(s) for the following questions.

1. A patient who has suffered burns over 35% of the body has a nursing diagnosis of Impaired tissue integrity. The best expected outcome for this patient would be: *(188, 190)*
    1. patient will regain mobility within 3 months.
    2. patient's skin will heal with grafting as needed within 3 months.
    3. patient's pain will be well-controlled within one week.
    4. patient will consume enough calories for tissue regeneration.

2. Within the long-term care environment, the LPN/LVN usually functions in the capacity of: *(179)*
    1. supervisor of the facility.
    2. admission nurse with Medicare paperwork duties.
    3. basic caregiver.
    4. charge nurse guiding the care team.

3. The goals of care for the long-term or extended-care facility are to: *(Select all that apply.)* *(183)*
    1. provide a safe environment.
    2. promote individual independence.
    3. instruct in new hobbies.
    4. supply sufficient fluids for hydration.
    5. allow maintenance of autonomy.
    6. assist to maintain or attain as much function as possible.

4. Restorative care programs are beneficial in preventing falls. A restorative program focuses on: *(183)*
    1. restoring skin integrity.
    2. muscle strengthening.
    3. maintaining functionality.
    4. disability prevention.
    5. ambulation.

5. When working with a rehabilitation patient, the nurse's function is to assist her to achieve an optimal state of health as: *(188)*
    1   agreed upon by the health care team.
    2. defined by the physician.
    3. defined by the patient.
    4. defined by the nurse and physical therapist.

6. An appropriate expected outcome for the nursing diagnosis of Impaired physical mobility for the resident who is right-handed and who has right-sided hemiparesis from a stroke is: *(180-182, 191)*
    1. bedrest will be maintained at all times.
    2. resident will begin crutch walking within 4 weeks.
    3. resident will comb hair and brush teeth by the end of 4 weeks.
    4. resident will show no signs of infection at time of discharge.

7. When assigning a task to an unlicensed assistive person, as the charge nurse, you must: *(180-183)*
    1. be sure it is acceptable to the resident for the person to perform the task.
    2. ask the unlicensed person if he or she knows how to perform the task.
    3. be certain that competence in performing the task has been documented for the unlicensed person.
    4. test the unlicensed person for competence.

Copyright © 2013, 2009 by Saunders, an imprint of Elsevier Inc. All rights reserved.

8. A nursing intervention that can help prevent ambulatory residents from falling on the way to the bathroom is to: *(180-182, 191)*
   1. clear the path to the bathroom.
   2. instruct the patient not to get up without assistance.
   3. place the patient's slippers within reach at the bedside.
   4. place the call bell within reach.

9. Physical and chemical restraints may be ordered and applied only when the patient: *(184-185, Box 9-7)*
   1. pulls the tubes out repeatedly.
   2. refuses to stay where he belongs.
   3. keeps interrupting the activities of others.
   4. is a danger to himself or others.

10. When working with a confused resident on dressing, it is best to gain cooperation by: *(185-186)*
   1. providing a variety of choices of what to do when.
   2. limiting choices and the need to make decisions.
   3. decreasing sensory input as much as possible.
   4. keeping the resident engaged in activities during the day.

CRITICAL THINKING ACTIVITIES

Scenario A: J.T., age 22, was in a motorcycle accident. He fractured his left leg, cervical spine (nondisplaced), and sustained a head injury. He is in the rehabilitation institute for rehabilitative care. He is in halo traction, has a leg brace, and is alert, but has some cognitive problems such as aphasia and memory loss.

1. What services would you expect to be included in J.T.'s care? *(187-191)*

2. What specific interventions should be on his interdisciplinary care plan related to his skin? *(180-182, 187-191)*

3. What measures would be on the plan to preserve and promote mobility? *(180-182, 187-191)*

Scenario B: Ms. O.P., age 78, suffered a cerebrovascular accident (CVA, stroke). She has left-sided hemiparesis and is undergoing rehabilitation in the long-term care facility. She had been living at home alone. She is beginning to show improvement in use of her extremities.

1. What do you think would be the overall goals for this resident? *(179-187)*

2. What therapies would have the highest priority? *(179-187)*

Copyright © 2013, 2009 by Saunders, an imprint of Elsevier Inc. All rights reserved.

3. What physical concerns should be addressed within her care plan? *(179-187)*

STEPS TOWARD BETTER COMMUNICATION

VOCABULARY BUILDING GLOSSARY

Term	Definition
ascertain' (as er tayn')	(verb) make certain or sure
co'ping (ko'ping)	(verb) dealing with difficulties and problems and attempting to overcome them; managing difficulties
op'ti'mal	ideal; the highest; the best, as in *the best treatment*
peo'ple skills	social abilities that help a person get along well with other people
sub'op'ti'mal	less than ideal
sundowning	(noun) when a person becomes confused as the sun goes down

COMPLETION

Directions: Fill in the blanks with the appropriate words from the Vocabulary Building Glossary.

1. The nurse and social worker work with the patient to improve his _____ skills.

2. Mr. Jones exhibited _____ by becoming very agitated during the evening shift.

3. Sometimes the nurse must _____ what is preventing the patient from making progress toward his goals.

4. Mr. Otong achieved a(n) _____ recovery from his stroke as he can walk quite well.

5. To work well on a rehabilitation team, the nurse must develop very good _____.

6. Mrs. Krause has not regained use of her arm after her stroke and her recovery is considered _____.

Copyright © 2013, 2009 by Saunders, an imprint of Elsevier Inc. All rights reserved.

PRONUNCIATION SKILLS

The consonant blend **th** in English is difficult for many people, especially since it has two different sounds. To make the **th** sound, such as in "**th**ank you" and "**th**ree," put your tongue between your front teeth and blow out air between your tongue and top teeth; slide your tongue back, scraping the top of your tongue against your upper teeth. Practice. Practice the following words:

ar**th**ritis	**th**anks
ba**th**	**th**igh
bir**th**day	**th**in
brea**th**	**th**irst
mon**th**	**th**ree
mou**th**	**th**umb
tee**th**	**Th**ursday

To make the voiced <u>**th**</u> sound, such as in "<u>**th**</u>ere" and "<u>**th**</u>ey," make the **th** sound but use your voice; try not to slide your tongue backwards—let it vibrate against your upper teeth. Compare the following:

Noun	**Verb**
bath	ba<u>the</u>
teeth	tee<u>the</u>
breath	brea<u>the</u>

Notice that the silent **e** makes the preceding vowel sounds long. Practice the following words having voiced <u>**th**</u> sounds:

ba<u>the</u>	<u>th</u>ere
brea<u>the</u>	<u>th</u>ese
o<u>th</u>er	<u>th</u>ey
<u>th</u>an	<u>th</u>is
<u>th</u>at	<u>th</u>ose
<u>th</u>e	toge<u>th</u>er

COMMUNICATION EXERCISES

1. Read the following communication. Circle every **th** sound, and put a line under every *voiced* <u>**th**</u> sound.

    The therapist will come to see you on Thursday. We will come together. I hope your arthritis is better by then. Take your bath and brush your teeth before we come. These are the breathing exercises that you need to practice. They will help you feel better. Thanks for being such a good sport.

Copyright © 2013, 2009 by Saunders, an imprint of Elsevier Inc. All rights reserved.

2. You are working in a long-term care facility. Write out what you would say when you ask another nurse to cover your assigned patients while you are at lunch.

_____

_____

_____

_____

_____

_____

Copyright © 2013, 2009 by Saunders, an imprint of Elsevier Inc. All rights reserved.

Student Name_____ Date_____

The Immune and Lymphatic Systems

Answer Key: Textbook page references are provided as a guide for answering these questions. A complete answer key was provided to your instructor.

COMPLETION

Review of Anatomy and Physiology

Directions: Fill in the blanks to complete the statements.

1. _____ patches help defend against ingested pathogens. *(196)*

2. _____ are immunoglobulins that identify and neutralize foreign objects. *(200)*

3. The _____ is the first barrier encountered by pathogens. *(198)*

4. The neutrophils and macrophages of the hematologic system assist the immune system by _____ when an antigen is encountered. *(196)*

5. When the body produces an immune response to a "self" cell or tissue, this causes a(n) _____ disorder. *(202-203)*

Labeling

Anatomy of the Organs of the Immune System

Directions: Label the following structures on the diagram of the body. (196)

tonsils
lymph nodes
thymus gland
spleen
bone marrow
gut-associated lymphoid tissue

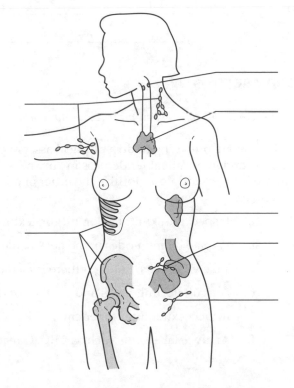

Copyright © 2013, 2009 by Saunders, an imprint of Elsevier Inc. All rights reserved.

Caring for a Patient with an Immune Disorder

Directions: Read the clinical scenario and answer the questions that follow.

Scenario: You are caring for Mr. Watson. He has an immunodeficient condition. The doctor orders transmission-based isolation precautions (protective). Mr. Watson appears very apprehensive when you first meet him and he tells you that he is not sure why he is isolated, or what to expect, or what he should be doing to help himself. *(212, see also Chapter 17)*

1. Explain the purpose of isolation to Mr. Watson: _____

    _____ .

2. Share three goals of nursing care with Mr. Watson to help him understand the plan of care.

    a. _____

    b. _____

    c. _____

3. Describe some of the psychological implications for patients who have isolation precautions.

    _____

    _____

    _____

4. Name three important teaching points for Mr. Watson to help him understand things he can do to prevent infection after being discharged from the hospital.

    a. _____

    b. _____

    c. _____

PRIORITY SETTING

Directions: Read the scenario and prioritize as appropriate.

Scenario: You are preparing to do a physical assessment on Mr. Stevens. He reports having some generalized fatigue and intermittent tenderness in "my neck, just underneath my ears." He was referred to the clinic for a immunologic workup. Prioritize the order of the elements below that are part of the physical assessment. *(206-209)*

_____ a. Inspect the skin for color, turgor, texture, and presence of lesions.

_____ b. Palpate lymph nodes in the neck to identify enlargement or tenderness.

_____ c. Take vital signs, noting if there is an increase in temperature or pulse rate.

_____ d. Auscultate lung fields and assess work of breathing.

_____ e. Inspect extremities for edema.

_____ f. Analyze lab results such as CBC, C-reactive protein, and antibody screening tests.

Copyright © 2013, 2009 by Saunders, an imprint of Elsevier Inc. All rights reserved.

APPLICATION OF THE NURSING PROCESS

Caring for a Patient with an Allergic Reaction

Directions: Provide the answer to the following questions.

Scenario: Ms. Roman comes to the clinic for a rash after eating peanuts several days ago. She also reports, "This has never happened to me before and this really itches! Is this going to happen to me again?"

1. While you are examining Ms. Roman's skin, what assessments and observations are you making? *(206)*

   _____

   _____

   _____

2. Write a patient-centered goal for the following diagnosis: Risk for impaired skin integrity secondary to irritation and scratching. *(210, Table 10-4)*

   _____

3. List five interventions to use for Ms. Roman's Risk for impaired skin integrity. *(210, Table 10-4)*

   a. _____

   b. _____

   c. _____

   d. _____

   e. _____

4. Which statement(s) indicate(s) that Ms. Roman has understood the patient education regarding allergy testing? *(Select all that apply.) (209)*
   a. A scratch test may be done by dropping extracts of allergens into scratches made on the skin.
   b. Intradermal injection of allergens will cause an anaphylactic reaction.
   c. Patches containing allergens can reduce peanut allergies.
   d. Inflammation and itching identify those allergens that provoke the immune system.
   e. Allergy testing is not necessary, because her immune reaction was typical for peanut allergies.

REVIEW QUESTIONS FOR THE NCLEX® EXAMINATION

Directions: Choose the best answer(s) for the following questions.

1. What is necessary for the immune system to function properly? *(200)*
   1. Detection of the absence of a foreign agent when it leaves body cells.
   2. Exacerbation of the process of inflammation.
   3. Inhibition of phagocytosis and the membrane-attack complex.
   4. Memory of a particular foreign agent if it appears in the body a second time.

2. Having a case of chickenpox provides a person with which type of immunity? *(203)*
   1. Passive artificial immunity
   2. Active naturally acquired immunity
   3. Active artificially acquired immunity
   4. Natural (innate) immunity

Copyright © 2013, 2009 by Saunders, an imprint of Elsevier Inc. All rights reserved.

3. The patient sustains trauma to the right lower extremity. In order to reduce the pain and edema associated with the inflammatory response, which action would the nurse perform *first*? *(198)*
   1. Obtain an order for an antiinflammatory medication.
   2. Assess the distal pulses and sensation to touch.
   3. Elevate the right lower extremity.
   4. Immobilize the leg with a splint.

4. What is the purpose of giving "booster doses" of an immunizing agent, such as tetanus toxoid? *(204)*
   1. Provides an immediate supply of antibody when a person is in danger of contracting the disease.
   2. Provides active immunity for a short period until any danger of the person developing the disease is past.
   3. Stimulates the memory of plasma cells and thereby stimulates synthesis of greater quantities of antibody.
   4. Boosts the synthesis of antibodies by sensitizing the immune cells for the first time.

5. The physician has ordered an annual influenza vaccination and a tetanus booster for an elderly patient living in a long-term care facility. The patient refuses to cooperate. What is the best response? *(204)*
   1. "I'll be really quick and gentle, because I know you don't like shots."
   2. "It's okay to refuse. We can wait and talk to your doctor about this."
   3. "Everyone in the facility is getting the vaccines, including all the staff."
   4. "I'd like to understand your point of view, so let's talk about your decision."

6. The patient has a fever. Which task(s) would be appropriate to assign to the nursing assistant? *(Select all that apply.) (209-211)*
   1. Help the patient remove excess clothing.
   2. Ask the patient about fever and chills.
   3. Obtain an antipyretic from the medication room.
   4. Take the temperature with an oral thermometer.
   5. Talk to the patient about over-the-counter fever reducers.
   6. Get the patient a popsicle.

7. The nurse is reviewing a patient's laboratory values. Which laboratory value indicates that the patient is having the desired response to antibiotic therapy? *(207-209, Table 10-3)*
   1. White blood cell (WBC) count of 11,000/mm^3
   2. Red blood cell count of 5.4 million/mm^3
   3. Platelet count of 150,000 mm^3
   4. Culture results show sensitivity to antibiotic

8. A nursing student is assisting the nurse to perform cooling measures for a patient with a high fever. The nurse would intervene if the student took which action? *(209-211)*
   1. Removed excess blankets from the patient
   2. Obtained a basin of cold water for sponging
   3. Offered the patient cool oral fluids
   4. Checked the physician's order for an antipyretic

9. The nurse is caring for several patients who have returned from diagnostic testing related to an immune disorder. Which patient needs to have the legs elevated following the procedure? *(207-209, Table 10-3)*
   1. Patient had a spleen sonogram.
   2. Patient had testing for C-reactive protein.
   3. Patient had a lymphangiogram.
   4. Patient had a lymph node biopsy.

Copyright © 2013, 2009 by Saunders, an imprint of Elsevier Inc. All rights reserved.

10. The nurse is working in a clinic that provides immunization service to the community. Which action would the nurse take to address possible adverse hypersensitivity reactions to immunizing agents? (*Select all that apply.*) **(205)**
    1. Advocate that all patients should have scratch testing prior to immunization.
    2. Administer vaccines only if patients have previously been immunized.
    3. Ask all patients about history of allergies and allergic reactions prior to immunization.
    4. Ensure the emergency equipment and rescue medications are easily accessible.
    5. Advise all patients to remain in the clinic for 15-20 minutes after receiving an injection.

CRITICAL THINKING ACTIVITIES

Scenario A: You are working with a new nursing assistant and you have asked her to carefully monitor vital signs for a patient with a fever. She appears eager and willing to help you. **(209-211)**

1. What specific directions should you give to the nursing assistant about this task?_____

    _____

    _____

    _____

    _____

    _____

STEPS TOWARD BETTER COMMUNICATON

VOCABULARY BUILDING GLOSSARY

Term	Definition
bad'ger	harass, annoy, or pester, bother frequently
con sti tu' tion	a person's overall health or disposition (also structure or organization); general body strength
im mu no glob' ulin	protein that functions as an antibody
jog	nudge as a reminder (also run at a slower pace)
mi' grate	move around
neu' tral ize	make safe or to reduce the effect
pre dis pose'	to be inclined toward, to have a tendency toward
sur veil' lance (ser va'lenz)	watch regularly or monitor

COMPLETION

Directions: Fill in the blanks with the appropriate words from the Vocabulary Building Glossary to complete the statements.

1. There are five classes of _____ (Ig): IgA, IgD, IgE, IgG, and IgM.

2. Antivenins that contain antibodies may _____ snake venom.

Copyright © 2013, 2009 by Saunders, an imprint of Elsevier Inc. All rights reserved.

3. Living in close proximity to others (i.e., homeless shelters, long-term care facilities) may

    _____ an individual to infectious disease.

4. Advise your patient that although he may have a naturally strong _____, adequate

    nutrition, immunizations, and healthy lifestyle habits will help to prevent immune disorders.

5. The Centers for Disease Control performs _____ for infectious disease, such as West

    Nile virus.

6. When supervising nursing assistants, give instructions and feedback about performance, but do not

    _____ them about minor mistakes.

7. Cancer cells can _____ to different locations in the body.

8. Taking a review course will help to _____ your memory before you take the test for

    licensure.

WORD ATTACK SKILLS

Prefixes and Suffixes

A *prefix* is attached to the beginning of a word or a word root to change the meaning. A vowel is used when
needed to connect the prefix to the word.

a-, an-	no, not, without, absence of
anti-	against, opposing
auto-	self, by itself
hyper-	excessive, more than normal; higher than needed
hypo-	decreased, less than normal; lower than needed
immun/o-	provide immunity
in-	not; (or into)
lymph/o-	lymph, lymphatic
lys/o-	destruction

A *suffix* is attached to the end of a word or root to change the meaning or the way the word is used.

-cyte	cell
-penia	deficiency of
-genic	produced by

COMPLETION

Directions: Complete the sentences with the correct prefix or suffix.

1. If sterile technique is not used for Foley catheter insertion, the patient may develop an **iatro-**_____

    infection.

Copyright © 2013, 2009 by Saunders, an imprint of Elsevier Inc. All rights reserved.

2. Lupus erythematosus is an example of a(n) _____ **-immune** disorder.

3. In a person with a normally functioning immune system, the presence of an antigen in the body will cause formation of a(n) _____ **-body.**

4. Patients with **neutro-**_____ are very susceptible to infection.

Word Families

Actor	Action	Process	Result
pro tec' tor	pro tect'	pro tec ' tion	
med' ia tor	me d' iate	me dia' tion	
re ac' tor	re act'	re ac' tion	
al' ler gen			al' ler gy

Singular and Plural Forms

Singular	**Plural**
serum	sera
diagnosis	diagnoses
phenomenon	phenomena
criterion	criteria

PRONUNCIATION SKILLS

The following words have the long <u>e</u> sound (underlined), as in the word "he." Notice the sound can be written with e, ee, ea, ei, i, or y.

m<u>e</u> 'd<u>i</u> ate
di ag no's<u>es</u>
pro c<u>e</u> 'dure
r<u>e</u>' nal
se cr<u>e</u>' tions
tech n<u>i</u>que'
f<u>e</u>'ver
d<u>ee</u>p br<u>ea</u>th'ing
d<u>e</u> cr<u>ea</u>se'/in cr<u>ea</u>se'

Directions: Underline the letters in the words that make the long e sound.

1. Please use standard precautions for handling body secretions.

2. Her fever has increased, but she is breathing deeply.

3. Does he know the procedure for keeping the needles clean?

Copyright © 2013, 2009 by Saunders, an imprint of Elsevier Inc. All rights reserved.

GRAMMAR POINTS

Active Versus Passive

Immunizations can be active or passive, and the English language can be active or passive, too. In acquired immunity, a person can either actively produce his own antibody or passively receive antibodies that have been produced by another person or animal. In English, when the subject of a sentence or clause does the action, the sentence or clause is called *active*.

Examples: *The housekeeper cleans the room.*
A nurse takes vital signs several times a day.
People produce their own antibodies.

The housekeeper, the nurse, and people do the action, so these are active sentences.

Passive sentences or clauses are used when it is not known who does the action or it is less important who or what does the action.

Examples: *The bed is made.*
Vital signs are taken in the morning and evening.

The bed and vital signs do no action (some other agent does it), so these are passive sentences.

Scientific writing often uses the passive form because there may not be an actor, or there may be no action, only a state of being. However, it is preferable to use active voice whenever possible.

Examples: *Allergies are divided into three major groups.*
Antibodies are found in the serum of blood.

Who or what divides or finds is not important.

If the agent of the action must be included, a "by" or "through" phrase is usually used to tell who or what does the acting.

Examples: *Temperatures and blood pressures are taken <u>by a nurse</u>.*
The bed is made <u>by the housekeeping staff</u>.
Antibodies are produced <u>by the plasma cells</u>.
Trends can been seen <u>by taking vital signs</u> on a regular schedule.
Vaccination became accepted <u>through the efforts of Edward Jenner</u>.
AIDS is caused <u>by transmission of HIV</u>.
Edema is characterized <u>by tight, shiny skin</u>.

The action is not done by the subjects of these passive sentences, but rather by the nouns in the underlined phrases.

A *passive verb* is formed by using the verb "to be" in any form (am/is/are, was/were, have/has been, will/would be, and so on) followed by a past participle. The *past participle* of a regular verb is its *-ed* form, such as *divided, prepared,* and *used*. Other past participles are irregular, such as *found, taken, seen, made,* and *known*.

Copyright © 2013, 2009 by Saunders, an imprint of Elsevier Inc. All rights reserved.

Care of Patients with HIV/AIDS

chapter

11

Answer Key: Textbook page references are provided as a guide for answering these questions. A complete answer key was provided to your instructor.

TERMINOLOGY

Directions: Match the term on the left with the correct definition, function, or statement on the right.

1. _____ Disseminated
2. _____ Immunocompetence
3. _____ Sentinel infections
4. _____ Wasting syndrome
5. _____ Opportunistic infection
6. _____ Barrier protection
7. _____ Diagnosis of AIDS
8. _____ T helper cells
9. _____ HAART
10. _____ Coccidiomycosis

a. Infection caused by normal body flora *(217, 221)*
b. Opportunistic infections that indicate immunosuppression *(219)*
c. Fungus found in soil *(223)*
d. Widespread *(223)*
e. Latex, polyurethane or deproteinized latex condoms *(218)*
f. Highly active antiretroviral therapy *(220)*
g. T cells that have the protein CD4 on their surface *(217)*
h. HIV+ with CD4 T-lymphocyte count less than 200 cells/μL *(217)*
i. Immune system stimulates physiologic responses for protection *(215)*
j. 10% weight loss with at least 30 days of diarrhea or weakness with fever *(229)*

SENTENCE COMPLETION

1. The largest proportion of new cases (53%) of HIV was found in _____ _____. *(217)*

2. HIV is a(n) _____ that integrates itself into the genetic material of the host cell. *(217)*

3. An unsafe practice is to be the _____ partner in anal or vaginal intercourse without using some form of _____ such as a latex condom. *(218)*

4. The first sign of cytomegalovirus in the eye is _____. *(222)*

5. In HIV-infected individuals, _____ usually manifest as white patches on the surface of the tongue and buccal mucosa. *(224)*

Copyright © 2013, 2009 by Saunders, an imprint of Elsevier Inc. All rights reserved.

SHORT ANSWERS

HIV/AIDS

You are working in a HIV/AIDS clinic that provides testing, information, referrals, and outpatient care. The clinic also takes an active role in the community to provide health information seminars and to be a resource for families.

Directions: Write brief answers for the following questions.

1. List at least five of the initial symptoms of AIDS. *(219)*

   a. _____

   b. _____

   c. _____

   d. _____

   e. _____

2. Identify four modes of transmission for HIV. *(217-218)*

   a. _____

   b. _____

   c. _____

   d. _____

3. Describe in your own words the diagnostic testing for HIV. *(219-220)* _____

   _____

   _____

   _____

   _____

   _____

   _____

   _____

4. Identify at least four teaching points for persons who are HIV positive. *(218-220)*

   a. _____

   _____

   b. _____

   _____

Copyright © 2013, 2009 by Saunders, an imprint of Elsevier Inc. All rights reserved.

c. _____

_____

d. _____

_____

5. List four important things to assess for a patient with AIDS-related dementia. *(225)*

a. _____

b. _____

c. _____

d. _____

REVIEW QUESTIONS FOR THE NCLEX® EXAMINATION

Directions: Choose the best answer(s) for the following questions.

1. Opportunistic infections occur when: *(217, 221)*
   1. the body is weakened or the immune system is suppressed.
   2. heavy exposure to tuberculosis occurs.
   3. another infection is already present in the body.
   4. antiviral therapy has affected the immune system.

2. What is a common sign of Kaposi's sarcoma? *(225)*
   1. A lung infection
   2. A central nervous system infection
   3. Blisters on the skin
   4. A "bruise" or large area of plaque on the skin

3. Which statement by an elderly patient indicates a need for additional patient teaching about risk for HIV? *(218)*
   1. "Condoms are not needed because pregnancy is not an issue."
   2. "There is a decline in functioning of the immune system for elderly people."
   3. "I may have to remind my health care provider to ask about sexual health."
   4. "Skin and mucous membranes are more fragile in the elderly person."

4. A patient is diagnosed with herpes zoster. What is the drug of choice for herpes? *(222)*
   1. Acyclovir (Zovirax)
   2. Foscavir (Foscarnet)
   3. Valganciclovir (Valcyte)
   4. Cidofovir (Vistide)

5. Why is additional intravenous normal saline administered when giving cidofovir (Vistide) and foscarnet (Foscavir)? *(222)*
   1. To counteract the nephrotoxic effects
   2. To prevent hepatotoxic effects
   3. To decrease irritation to the veins
   4. To flush the medication from the IV line

Copyright © 2013, 2009 by Saunders, an imprint of Elsevier Inc. All rights reserved.

6. The patient comes to the clinic for a physical examination and HIV testing. He tells the nurse that he thinks he may have been recently exposed to HIV. Which assessment item(s) should be included at this point? *(Select all that apply.)* **(225-226)**
   1. Sexual history
   2. IV drug use
   3. Current medications
   4. Vital signs
   5. Presence of anasarca
   6. Change of mental status

7. The doctor orders several diagnostic tests including an HIV test for a patient. What is appropriate information to give to the patient? **(219-220)**
   1. He can use an FDA-approved home test for HIV which is adequate and confidential.
   2. He will first have an enzyme-linked immunospecific assay (ELISA).
   3. He will have the Western Blot test as the first initial screening for HIV.
   4. He must fast after midnight and return in the early AM for specimen collection.

8. The patient should be advised that if the first HIV test is negative, a second test must be conducted. When should the second HIV test be conducted? **(219-220)**
   1. 1–3 months later
   2. 4–6 months later
   3. 6–12 months later
   4. 3–6 weeks later

9. The patient becomes upset when he is told that there is a waiting period between the first HIV and the second HIV test. "I can't believe that you won't give me a simple straight answer!" The best response is: **(219-220)**
   1. "Try to calm down and I'll have the doctor give you more information."
   2. "I can see you are upset, but there is nothing I can do about it."
   3. "This is really frustrating. Let's talk about what you should do in the interim."
   4. "Just wait for the test results. I'm sure that everything will be okay."

10. The nurse hears in report that a patient with AIDS also has thrush. What intervention would the nurse plan to use during the shift? **(224)**
    1. Restock the supplies for contact isolation.
    2. Offer the patient ice pops or chilled applesauce.
    3. Check to make sure there is an order for folic acid.
    4. Ensure that the patient has a patent IV for antibiotics.

CRITICAL THINKING ACTIVITIES

Scenario A: You are taking a patient history on a young woman who admits to having sex with several young men whom she knows and describes as good friends. The woman states that, "I'm pretty sure that none of us have HIV."

1. What kinds of questions should you ask? **(225-226)**

2. What are the CDC recommendations for HIV testing? **(219-220)**

3. If this young woman declines a screening test for HIV, what are your responsibilities? **(219)**

Copyright © 2013, 2009 by Saunders, an imprint of Elsevier Inc. All rights reserved.

Scenario B: The physician orders postmedication IV hydration for a patient. The current maintenance IV is infusing at 125 mL/hour per pump. The order is to increase the IV fluid to 200 mL/hour X 3 hours then resume previously ordered rate. It is now 8:00 AM.

1. What volume should the patient have received at the end of 3 hours? _____ .

2. At 8:00 AM, you should set the pump to deliver how many mL/hour? _____ .

3. At 11:00 AM, you should reset the pump to deliver how many mL/hour? _____ .

STEPS TOWARD BETTER COMMUNICATION

VOCABULARY BUILDING GLOSSARY

Term	Definition
CDC	Centers for Disease Control
gay	homosexual (male or female)
myth (mith)	traditional belief or ancient story
opportunis' tic	to use an opportunity; (medical field) a microorganism that normally does not cause disease but may do so when the immune response is impaired

PRONUNCIATION AND MEANING

When you encounter long medical words, try breaking them down into smaller parts. This will help you with their meanings.

Example: antiretroviral = anti (against) + retro (backward) + viral (relating to a virus)

It will also help you to pronounce the words correctly.

Examples:

cryptococcosis	krip' tow kok o' sis
disseminate	di sim' in ate
immunosuppression	im' you no sa pre' shun
cytomegalovirus	si' tow meg' ah low vi' rus

COMPLETION

Directions: Fill in the blanks in the sentences with the correct terms from the Vocabulary Building Glossary.

1. In someone with a suppressed immune system, an infection caused by an organism that normally would not cause infection is called a(n) _____ infection.

2. There have been many cases of AIDS transmitted from partner to partner among the _____ population in this country.

Copyright © 2013, 2009 by Saunders, an imprint of Elsevier Inc. All rights reserved.

3. Guidelines for infection control are compiled and published by the _____

_____.

4. Difficulty breathing in the AIDS patient may be the _____ of an opportunistic infection affecting the lungs.

5. The belief that elderly adults are unlikely to contract AIDS is a(n) _____.

TERMINOLOGY

Directions: Name the organ or structure to which each condition below is related. (Hint: each word contains a part that means a specific organ or structure.)

1. Retinitis: _____

2. Meningitis: _____

3. Encephalopathy: _____

4. Nephrotoxicity: _____

5. Mucocutaneous: _____

6. Neuralgia:_____

7. Neutropenia: _____

MATCHING

Directions: Match the acronym (abbreviated term) on the left with what it stands for (meaning) on the right. **(215, 217, 219-223, see also Chapter 6)**

1.	_____	HIV	a.	Personal protective equipment
2.	_____	HAART	b.	Cytomegalovirus
3.	_____	CDC	c.	Acquired immune deficiency syndrome
4.	_____	HSV	d.	Centers for Disease Control
5.	_____	NRTI	e.	*Mycobacterium avium* complex
6.	_____	AIDS	f.	*Herpes simplex* virus
7.	_____	CMV	g.	Opportunistic infection
8.	_____	MAC	h.	Nucleoside reverse transcriptase inhibitor
9.	_____	PPE	i.	*Varicella-zoster* virus
10.	_____	VZV	j.	Highly active antiretroviral therapy
11.	_____	OI	k.	Human immunodeficiency virus
12.	_____	ELISA	l.	Enzyme-linked immunospecific assay

Copyright © 2013, 2009 by Saunders, an imprint of Elsevier Inc. All rights reserved.

Care of Patients with Immune and Lymphatic Disorders

chapter

12

Answer Key: Textbook page references are provided as a guide for answering these questions. A complete answer key was provided to your instructor.

TERMINOLOGY

Directions: Match the term on the left with the correct definition, function, or statement on the right.

1. _____ Anaphylaxis
2. _____ Angioedema
3. _____ Erythema
4. _____ Urticaria
5. _____ Immune deficiency
6. _____ Allergy
7. _____ Autoimmune disorder
8. _____ Lymphoma
9. _____ Lymphedema
10. _____ Fibromyalgia

a. Leaves the body unable to resist foreign microbes or toxins *(234)*

b. Abnormal response to certain substances *(236)*

c. Hives *(241)*

d. Patchy congestion of capillaries of the skin with blood *(245)*

e. Extreme allergic reaction that is life-threatening *(236)*

f. 18 tender points *(253-254)*

g. Lymphatic cancer that primarily starts in the lymphocytes *(249)*

h. Swelling beneath the skin *(241)*

i. Large amounts of fluid accumulate, causing swelling *(253)*

j. Immune system reacting against the body's own cells *(234, 243)*

Copyright © 2013, 2009 by Saunders, an imprint of Elsevier Inc. All rights reserved.

TABLE ACTIVITY

Directions: On the table below, list the effects that could occur with exposure to different allergens. **(237, Table 12-2)**

Four Broad Categories of Allergens

Category	Method of Exposure	Triggers	Effects
Contactants	Direct contact with mucosa/skin/tissue	Dust, wool fabrics, detergents, soaps, lotions, cosmetics, plants such as poison ivy, dyes, metals in jewelry, latex	
Ingestants	Swallowed	Food: citrus fruits, tomatoes, strawberries, cow's milk, wheat, eggs, dairy products, seafood, chocolate, nuts, monosodium glutamate (MSG), other preservatives, and artificial food coloring Drugs: aspirin, barbiturates, anticonvulsants, antimicrobials, but any drug may cause an allergic reaction	
Inhalants	Entry through nose or mouth	Dust, molds, pollen, fragrances, animal dander, insect feces, and some chemicals	
Injectables	Via needle; i.e., hypodermic, intramuscular, intravenous Animal or snake bites, insect stings	Medications, vaccines, animal saliva, snake or insect venoms	

APPLICATION OF THE NURSING PROCESS

Disorders of Inappropriate Immune Response

Directions: Read the scenario and write brief answers for the following questions.

Scenario: Janice Euway suspects that she may have allergies to environmental allergens. She reports runny nose, sneezing, and watery eyes that seem to be unassociated with a fever or cold.

1. Identify five factors that should be assessed in collecting data and taking a history from Ms. Euway. **(236-237)**

    a. _____

    b. _____

    c. _____

    d. _____

    e. _____

Copyright © 2013, 2009 by Saunders, an imprint of Elsevier Inc. All rights reserved.

2. Which nursing diagnosis is the priority for Ms. Euway today? *(240)*
   a. Knowledge deficit related to self-care
   b. Risk for ineffective breathing related to systemic reaction to allergens
   c. Anxiety related to new health condition
   d. Altered nutrition related to food restrictions

3. List four drug classifications that are used to alleviate systemic reactions to allergens. *(239, Table 12-3)*

   a. _____

   b. _____

   c. _____

   d. _____

4. The doctor suggests that she initially try an over-the-counter medication. List five common side effects of medication such as diphenhydramine (Benadryl). *(239, Table 12-3)*

   a. _____

   b. _____

   c. _____

   d. _____

5. List six suggestions that will help Ms. Euway control environmental allergens. *(240)*

   a. _____

   b. _____

   c. _____

   d. _____

   e. _____

   f. _____

PRIORITY SETTING

Directions: Read the scenario and prioritize nursing actions as appropriate.

Scenario: You are working in a smaller clinic and you hear one of the x-ray technicians calling for help. The patient is having an anaphylactic reaction to IV contrast dye and the radiologist asks you to help. The patient has a patent IV line and the emergency equipment is in the room. Prioritize these five measures used to treat anaphylaxis.

_____ a. Provide psychological support

_____ b. Administer oxygen

_____ c. Establish a patent airway

_____ d. Administer antihistamine (diphenhydramine hydrochloride, Benadryl)

_____ e. Administer aqueous epinephrine

Copyright © 2013, 2009 by Saunders, an imprint of Elsevier Inc. All rights reserved.

REVIEW QUESTIONS FOR THE NCLEX® EXAMINATION

Directions: Choose the best answer(s) for the following questions.

1. Which group of drugs commonly tends to cause allergies in many people? *(241)*
   1. Antihypertensives, diuretics, and antiarrhythmics
   2. Aspirin, barbiturates, anticonvulsants, and antibiotics
   3. Vitamin and mineral supplements and electrolyte replacements
   4. Antibiotics, antianginals, sedatives, and antipsychotics

2. The patient has a medical diagnosis of fibromyalgia and a nursing diagnosis of Acute pain. Which medication is most likely to be prescribed for this patient? *(254)*
   1. Morphine
   2. Ibuprofen
   3. Fluoxetine
   4. Azathioprine

3. Which problems are related to the use of antihistamines in aging males? *(238)*
   1. Hesitancy and urinary retention
   2. Orthostatic hypotension and dizziness
   3. Angina and cardiac arrhythmias
   4. Depression and general malaise

4. A patient was recently diagnosed with systemic lupus erythematosus. Which sign(s) and symptom(s) would the nurse expect to find documented in this patient's medical record? *(Select all that apply.)* *(246-247)*
   1. Painful or swollen joints
   2. Red rash usually on the face
   3. Fatigue and weakness
   4. Nausea, vomiting, and diarrhea
   5. Unexplained fever
   6. Sensitivity to the sun

5. Which medications are likely to be prescribed for a patient with systemic lupus erythematosus? *(247)*
   1. NSAIDs and prednisone
   2. Doxorubicin (Adriamycin) and vincristine (Oncovin)
   3. Isoniazid (INH) and rifampin (Rifadin)
   4. Lamivudine (Combivir) and ethambutol (Myambutol)

6. The nurse is giving skin care instructions to a patient with systemic lupus erythematosus. Which set of instructions is appropriate? *(247)*
   1. Use alcohol-based skin care products for the antibacterial action.
   2. Avoid use of cosmetics, moisturizers, and soaps.
   3. Wear long pants, a long-sleeved shirt, and a hat when in the sun.
   4. Apply over-the-counter hydrocortisone cream as needed.

7. During the routine physical, the nurse notices that a patient has some swollen lymph glands. On further questioning, the patient admits to pain in the lymph nodes after bouts of excessive drinking. This is significant to report because this type of pain is diagnostic for: *(249-250)*
   1. Hodgkin's.
   2. non-Hodgkin's.
   3. lymphedema.
   4. fibromyalgia.

Copyright © 2013, 2009 by Saunders, an imprint of Elsevier Inc. All rights reserved.

8. The physician recommends that a patient be scheduled for a diagnostic test to detect presence of Reed-Sternberg cells in the tissues to rule out lymphatic cancer. Which diagnostic test will detect these cells? *(243)*
   1. Computed tomography
   2. Biopsy of the lymph nodes
   3. Biopsy of the bone marrow
   4. Positron emission tomography

9. The patient begins to cry. "I am really scared. Am I going to die of cancer? Why is this happening to me?" What is the best response? *(253)*
   1. "Let me get your wife and the two of you can have some privacy."
   2. "You should not be using your energy to be worried right now. You should wait until the doctor verifies the diagnosis."
   3. "I'd be scared too. My aunt had cancer and I know just how you feel."
   4. "I can tell you're scared and I don't know why this is happening, but we are here to give you support and information."

10. The patient asks the nurse to explain some of the differences between Hodgkin's and non-Hodgkin's. What information about Hodgkin's is correct? *(249-253)*
    1. Hodgkin's is more widespread through the lymphatic tissues.
    2. Hodgkin's is less widespread through the lymphatic tissues.
    3. Hodgkin's identified as B cell and T cell lymphoma.
    4. Hodgkin's has a lower survival rate and a worse prognosis.

CRITICAL THINKING ACTIVITIES

Scenario A

1. You are working in walk-in clinic. The physician orders an antibiotic injection for a patient. You give the medication as ordered. Almost immediately after receiving the medication, the patient tells you, "I feel kind of funny. Maybe a little short of breath. Is that normal?" What should you do? *(243)*

   _____

   _____

   _____

   _____

   _____

   _____

2. List four signs and symptoms that may indicate an anaphylactic reaction. *(241-242)*

   a. _____

   b. _____

   c. _____

   d. _____

Copyright © 2013, 2009 by Saunders, an imprint of Elsevier Inc. All rights reserved.

STEPS TOWARD BETTER COMMUNICATION

VOCABULARY BUILDING GLOSSARY

Term	Definition
iatrogenic	a side effect caused by medical treatment
relapse	reappearance of cancer cells; also a return to a former state
remission	disease is under control
syndrome	group of symptoms associated with a condition
reject	to refuse to accept
immunosuppression	inhibit the normal immune system response

COMPLETION

Directions: Complete the sentences using the correct term.

1. After the patient completed treatment for cancer, there was a(n) _____of symptoms.

2. The patient's prolonged usage of steroids resulted in _____ effects.

3. Goodpasture's _____ affects lungs and the kidneys.

4. I was following a very healthy diet, but I had a(n) _____ into the bad habit of eating too many sweets.

5. Her application for nursing school was _____ because her grades were too low.

6. _____ can be therapeutic for transplant patients.

PRONUNCIATION OF DIFFICULT TERMS

Directions: Practice pronouncing the following words.

Term	Pronunciation
anaphylaxis	(ă-nă-fă-LĂK-sĭs)
cellular immunity	(SĔL-ū-lăr ĭ-MŪ-nĭ-tē)
environment	(ĕn-VĪ-rŏn-mĕnt)
erythema	(ĕr-ĭ-THĒ-mă)
insufficiency	(ĭn-să-FĬSH-ăn-sē)
lymphedema	(lĭm-fĕ-DĒ-mă)

Copyright © 2013, 2009 by Saunders, an imprint of Elsevier Inc. All rights reserved.

WORD ATTACK SKILLS

In this chapter, you learned how the immune system protects the body and how failure of the immune system manifests as different types of disease and disorders. *Immuno-* is a combining form that is frequently used in this chapter.

Directions: Below are several terms that begin with "immuno-." Can you remember other words from Chapter 12 that also used the combining form "immuno-"?

immunodeficiency (ĭm-ū-nō-dě-FĬSH-ĕn-sē)

immunocompromised (ĭm-ū-nō-KŎM-pro-mīzd)

immunocompetence (ĭm-ū-nō-KŎM-pě-těns)

immunotherapy (ĭm-ū-nō-THĚR-ǎ-pē)

Copyright © 2013, 2009 by Saunders, an imprint of Elsevier Inc. All rights reserved.

The Respiratory System

chapter

13

Answer Key: Textbook page references are provided as a guide for answering these questions. A complete answer key was provided to your instructor.

REVIEW OF ANATOMY AND PHYSIOLOGY

Terminology

Directions: Match the term on the left with the correct statement, function, or definition on the right.

1. _____ Bronchioles *(258)*
2. _____ Pleural cavity *(258)*
3. _____ Cilia *(257-259)*
4. _____ Compliance *(259)*
5. _____ Cough reflex *(259)*
6. _____ Alveoli *(259)*
7. _____ Oxyhemoglobin *(260)*
8. _____ Inspiration and expiration *(259)*
9. _____ Elastance *(260, Box 13-1)*
10. _____ Total lung capacity *(264, 268, Table 13-3)*

a. Tiny air sacs
b. Carry air to alveoli
c. Hairlike projections that trap and help expel inhaled foreign particles
d. Elasticity of the lungs
e. Carries majority of the oxygen to the cells of the body
f. When depressed, secretions are retained and pneumonia may occur
g. Pressure within is less than that of outside atmosphere
h. Controlled by movement of diaphragm and muscles in chest wall
i. Extent to which lungs can return to their original position after being barely stretched
j. Amount of air or gas lung can hold at end of maximal inspiration

Completion

Directions: Fill in the blank(s) to complete the following sentences.

1. _____ decreases surface tension on the alveolar wall, allowing it to _____ more easily with _____ and preventing alveolar collapse upon _____. *(259)*

2. Two conditions that can interfere with oxygen and carbon dioxide exchange are _____ surfactant and interstitial _____. *(259)*

3. Respiratory gases are carried mostly in the bloodstream by the _____. *(259-260)*

4. A large percentage of carbon dioxide is transported in the blood plasma in the form of _____ ions. *(260)*

Copyright © 2013, 2009 by Saunders, an imprint of Elsevier Inc. All rights reserved.

5. Carbon dioxide combines with _____ within the red blood cell, forming _____. *(260)*

SHORT ANSWER

Age-Related Changes Affecting the Respiratory System

Directions: Provide a short answer to the following questions. (260)

1. Why are the elderly more susceptible to respiratory infections?_____

   _____

2. Why is the potential for aspiration greater in the elderly person? _____

   _____

   _____

3. What is the significance to the respiratory system of the 50% decrease in total body water after age 70?

   _____

   _____

4. What alveolar changes affect respiration in the elderly person?_____

   _____

   _____

5. How could osteoporosis impact respiratory function?_____

   _____

   _____

TERMINOLOGY

Assessment

Directions: Match the terms on the left with the statements on the right that best describe them. (There may be more than one answer for each.)

1. _____ Assessment of mouth and pharynx *(264)*

2. _____ Indirect laryngoscopy *(267, Table 13-3)*

3. _____ Thoracentesis *(267, Table 13-3)*

4. _____ Capnography *(265, Table 13-3)*

5. _____ Throat culture *(268)*

a. Simple removal of polyps can be done during this procedure.
b. Endoscope is passed to visualize interior of larynx.
c. Patient is NPO until gag reflex returns.
d. Uses a nasal cannula and a finger probe.
e. Usually performed to confirm infection with streptococcus.
f. To remove pleural fluid, instill medication, or obtain fluid for diagnostic studies.
g. Examiner uses warm laryngeal mirror, head mirror, and light source.
h. Examiner uses tongue blade and light source.
i. Biopsy can be taken during examination.
j. Food and liquids withheld 6–8 hours before procedure.

Copyright © 2013, 2009 by Saunders, an imprint of Elsevier Inc. All rights reserved.

SHORT ANSWER

Directions: Provide a short answer to the following questions.

1. Why is obtaining a history of smoking and alcohol intake pertinent to a respiratory assessment? *(262)*

   _____

   _____

2. What can skin color tell you that is pertinent to a respiratory assessment? *(262)*_____

   _____

   _____

3. What is the best position in which to place the patient for lung auscultation? *(263)*_____

   _____

PRIORITY SETTING

Directions: Indicate the order of priority in which you would begin actions for the following scenario. (262-264)

Scenario: You are performing a physical assessment of the respiratory system.

_____   a.   Instruct the patient to breathe deeply and slowly through the mouth.

_____   b.   Observe the head and look for facial puffiness over the sinus area.

_____   c.   Note the posture and the way abdominal muscles are used.

_____   d.   Note skin color.

_____   e.   Move your stethoscope to compare one side of the chest to the other.

_____   f.   Place the diaphragm of the stethoscope against the skin with moderate pressure.

REVIEW QUESTIONS FOR THE NCLEX® EXAMINATION

Directions: Choose the best answer(s) for the following questions.

1. Evaluation of the effectiveness of deep-breathing and coughing is best done by: *(270-272)*
   1. auscultating the lungs bilaterally both before and after.
   2. assessing the color and amount of secretions produced.
   3. observing the respiratory rate and quality afterward.
   4. asking the patient whether he is breathing more easily.

2. When performing a respiratory assessment, which action(s) should be performed? *(Select all that apply.)* *(262-264)*
   1. Inquire about exposure to respiratory inhalants.
   2. Obtain a throat culture and a sputum specimen.
   3. Auscultate the lungs bilaterally.
   4. Assess the patient's knowledge of respiratory disease.
   5. Assess color of mucous membranes.
   6. Assess the rate and quality of respirations.
   7. Check for use of accessory muscles.
   8. Look for signs of anxiety or restlessness.

Copyright © 2013, 2009 by Saunders, an imprint of Elsevier Inc. All rights reserved.

3. The patient has chest congestion and the nurse instructs him to increase fluid intake. What is the best rationale for this intervention? *(270, 274, Table 13-4)*
    1. Fluids help to decrease the cough reflex.
    2. Coughing may cause dehydration.
    3. Fluid helps to thin secretions.
    4. Congestion increases the chance for sepsis.

4. The nurse notes in the medical record that the patient has orthopnea. Which intervention would the nurse use to address this condition? *(272)*
    1. Offer the patient extra pillows.
    2. Assist the patient to turn every 2 hours.
    3. Obtain an order for continuous oxygen.
    4. Monitor the patient after mild exertion.

5. What is an objective sign of long-term decreased oxygenation? *(263)*
    1. Chest pain with deep inspiration
    2. Paroxysmal nocturnal dyspnea
    3. Rapid respiratory rate
    4. Clubbed fingers

6. Which position is best for the patient undergoing a thoracentesis? *(267, Table 13-3)*
    1. Sitting up, leaning forward on an overbed table
    2. Side-lying, affected side up, head slightly raised
    3. Side-lying, affected side down, head flat
    4. High Fowler's position

7. An elderly patient with a severe respiratory infection is seen in the emergency department. The physician orders an IV of $D_5\frac{1}{2}NS$ 1000 mL over 12 hours. The IV tubing delivers 10 drops per mL. At what drip rate should this IV be administered? _____

8. Indicate on the diagram where you would place the stethoscope to begin the respiratory assessment. *(264)*

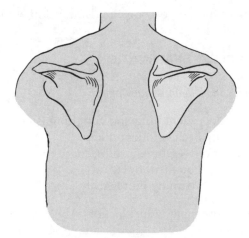

9. When a patient is scheduled for a lung ventilation and perfusion scan, which nursing action is pertinent? *(266, Table 13-3)*
    1. Keep the patient NPO for 6 hours after the test.
    2. Assist the patient to remove metal jewelry from neck/head area.
    3. Be certain the patient is well hydrated pretest.
    4. Explain need for isolation related to radioactive substance.

Copyright © 2013, 2009 by Saunders, an imprint of Elsevier Inc. All rights reserved.

10. The patient has just returned from having a bronchoscopy. The nurse would intervene if the nursing student performs which action? *(261, 266, Table 13-3)*
    1. Takes the patient's vital signs.
    2. Obtains food and fluids for the patient.
    3. Raises the head of the bed to 30 degrees.
    4. Auscultates the lung fields.

11. The nurse is caring for a patient with emphysema. What is the most essential point in administering oxygen to this patient? *(262-272)*
    1. Instructing the patient to call for assistance as needed.
    2. Initiating continuous pulse oximetry monitoring.
    3. Frequently checking the skin underneath the cannula.
    4. Ensuring that oxygen flow is set at the correct rate.

12. Which instruction set should the nurse give to the patient in order to obtain a good sputum specimen? *(265, Table 13-3)*
    1. Perform mouth care just before giving the specimen.
    2. No fasting or other special preparation is required.
    3. The specimen should be obtained in the morning before eating.
    4. Cough deeply and spit the specimen into a clean container.

13. A patient with a long history of smoking and emphysema has a nursing diagnosis of Ineffective health maintenance related to the inability to stop smoking. Which outcome statement is the best? *(266, 271-272, Table 13-3, Table 13-4)*
    1. Patient will list three health reasons to stop smoking.
    2. Patient will receive smoking cessation information.
    3. Patient will explain how smoking became a habit.
    4. Patient will verbalize two strategies to stop smoking.

14. Which sputum characteristic is the greatest immediate concern? *(263, Table 13-1)*
    1. Thick, tenacious, "ropey" and difficult to cough up
    2. Frothy, pinkish or blood-tinged
    3. Scant, sticky, and rust-colored
    4. Yellow or grayish-yellow with a foul odor

15. The nurse is preparing to give a patient an influenza vaccination. Which patient statement is the biggest concern? *(261)*
    1. "I am afraid of needles; could I have the inhaled form?"
    2. "I recently stopped smoking and I seem to be coughing a lot."
    3. "I have a lot of allergic reactions to many common foods."
    4. "I have a history of chronic congestive heart failure."

CRITICAL THINKING ACTIVITIES

1. Describe particular ways you would adjust your teaching for an elderly patient who needs to be taught to use an incentive spirometer and cough effectively.

2. Within your extended family, determine the risk factors for respiratory disorders.

Copyright © 2013, 2009 by Saunders, an imprint of Elsevier Inc. All rights reserved.

STEPS TOWARD BETTER COMMUNICATION

VOCABULARY BUILDING GLOSSARY

Term	Definition
malaise'	(noun) general feeling of bodily discomfort
refrain'	(verb) to avoid doing something
dysphag'ia (dis fa' jee ah)	(noun) difficulty swallowing
hypocapnea	deficiency of carbon dioxide in the blood
hypercapnea	excess of carbon dioxide in the blood
surfactant	an agent that reduces fluid surface tension
naris, *plural* nares	nostril
adventitious (ad ven ti' shus)	accidental, occasional; abnormal, outside of the usual place
apneusis (ap nu' sis)	long inspiration unrelieved by expiration

COMPLETION

Directions: Complete the following sentences using the glossary words above.

1. Bronchitis is usually evident upon auscultation of the lungs because _____ sounds are present.

2. The elderly patient seemed to have a general feeling of _____.

3. A(n) _____ is used to make soaps more effective, as well as being found natu-rally in the body.

4. Please _____ from smoking near the entryway.

MATCHING

Directions: Match the combining form or abbreviation on the left with its meaning on the right.

1. _____   -itis
2. _____   -oscopy
3. _____   MRI
4. _____   CT

a. Magnetic resonance imaging
b. Computed tomography
c. Inflammation
d. Process of visually examining

TERMINOLOGY

Directions: Identify the correct term for each definition.

1. Examination of the larynx: _____

2. Sinuses next to the nose: _____

Copyright © 2013, 2009 by Saunders, an imprint of Elsevier Inc. All rights reserved.

3. Abnormal lung sounds: _____

4. Oxygen-deficient: _____

5. Difficulty breathing: _____

PRONUNCIATION

Directions: Practice saying these words with a partner.

1. **"l"** as the initial sound: (Curl the tip of your tongue and place it against the back of your front teeth. Air will flow around the sides of your tongue.)

laryngi'tis	le'sions	lung
larynx	lined	

2. **"l"** as the final sound:

cell	na'sal	tonsil
fron'tal	or'al	vo'cal
muco'sal	skull	

COMMUNICATION EXERCISE

A. With a partner, practice an explanation to an elderly person of the steps she should take to avoid contracting a URI (immunization, staying out of crowds, prompt treatment of any symptoms, avoid youngsters with coughs and colds, maintain adequate rest and nutrition, good handwashing).

B. Switch roles and explain to a youngster how to avoid catching and spreading respiratory diseases (covering coughs—cough into elbow, disposing of tissues, handwashing—sing the ABC song 2–3 times to expand alveoli, don't go to school or parties when you are sick or contagious, stay away from crowded places).

Copyright © 2013, 2009 by Saunders, an imprint of Elsevier Inc. All rights reserved.

Care of Patients with Disorders of the Upper Respiratory System

Answer Key: Textbook page references are provided as a guide for answering these questions. A complete answer key was provided to your instructor.

SHORT ANSWER

Directions: Provide a short answer for the following questions.

1. List three common symptoms of sinusitis. *(279-280)*

    a. _____

    b. _____

    c. _____

2. List five self-care measures that patients can use when they have a cold. *(279)*

    a. _____

    b. _____

    c. _____

    d. _____

    e. _____

APPLICATION OF THE NURSING PROCESS

Upper Respiratory Disorders

Directions: Provide a short answer for the following questions.

1. Write one expected outcome for each of the following nursing diagnoses.

    a. Impaired verbal communication related to inability to speak due to tracheostomy

    _____

    b. Risk for aspiration related to impaired swallowing

    _____

    c. Ineffective airway clearance related to physical alteration in airway (tracheostomy)

    _____

Copyright © 2013, 2009 by Saunders, an imprint of Elsevier Inc. All rights reserved.

2. List two nursing interventions for each of the following nursing diagnoses for a patient who has undergone a laryngectomy. *(283-284)*

   a. Ineffective airway clearance related to throat surgery: _____

   _____

   b. Impaired verbal communication related to loss of voice: _____

   _____

   c. Risk for injury related to aspiration: _____

   _____

COMPLETION

Directions: Fill in the blanks to complete the statements.

1. A nursing intervention to help promote drainage in the patient with acute sinusitis is _____

   _____. *(279)*

2. Warning signs of cancer of the larynx include _____

   _____. *(283)*

3. When cleaning the tracheostomy site and tube, the nurse must be careful not to allow _____

   _____. *(286)*

4. The nurse's chief concern for the postoperative tonsillectomy patient is _____

   _____. *(281)*

5. One way to detect postoperative bleeding in the tonsillectomy patient is to observe for frequent

   _____. *(281)*

6. When suctioning a tracheostomy, the nurse must use totally _____ technique. *(286)*

7. If a radical neck dissection must be performed, a(n) _____ is performed at the

   same time. *(284)*

PRIORITY SETTING

1. You are assigned the following patients:
   - M.S., a preoperative patient scheduled for surgery at 10:00 AM
   - O.T., an early tonsillectomy (adult) who was admitted due to excessive bleeding
   - M.R., a postlaryngectomy patient with a tracheostomy who is first-day postoperative

Directions: Indicate the order of priority in which you would do the following: (Use 1, 2, 3.)

_____ Assess O.T.'s status.

_____ Assess M.R.'s status.

_____ Provide preoperative care for M.S. including the preoperative checklist.

Copyright © 2013, 2009 by Saunders, an imprint of Elsevier Inc. All rights reserved.

2. Which patient should be your first priority? _____
   a. The patient with the tracheostomy who is having considerable difficulty breathing.
   b. The postoperative patient just arriving on the unit from surgery.
   c. The radical neck dissection patient who is complaining of considerable pain.

REVIEW QUESTIONS FOR THE NCLEX® EXAMINATION

Directions: Select the best answer(s) or fill in the blank with the correct word(s) for the following questions.

1. The priority assessment for any patient with any problems of the upper airway is: *(277, 279)*
   1. anxiety and pain.
   2. adequacy of oxygenation.
   3. presence and thickness of nasal and oral secretions.
   4. signs of dyspnea.

2. A patient comes to the emergency department with a nosebleed. Which is the appropriate action? *(280)*
   1. Applying ice to the back of the neck.
   2. Having the patient tip the head way back, hyperextending the neck.
   3. Packing the nose with gauze.
   4. Applying pressure to the nose with the thumb and forefinger.

3. When drugs are prescribed for treatment of rhinitis and sinusitis, which type(s) of drugs would be included? *(Select all that apply.) (277-280, Table 14-1)*
   1. Decongestants
   2. Bronchodilators
   3. Antihistamines
   4. Antitussives
   5. Antipyretics
   6. Mucolytics

4. Which statement regarding rhinitis and the elderly patient is true? *(279)*
   1. Complementary and alternative therapies are ineffective in the older adult.
   2. Antihistamines and decongestants should be used with caution.
   3. Antipyretics and antibiotics are not used because of risk of allergic reactions.
   4. Viral rhinitis is self-limiting and comfort measures are not necessary.

5. The patient with acute pharyngitis has a nursing diagnosis of Discomfort and pain related to inflammation. Which intervention would the nurse use for this diagnosis? *(280-281)*
   1. Advise to use warm saline gargles.
   2. Obtain a throat culture.
   3. Monitor the patient's temperature.
   4. Assess the potential for aspiration.

6. The patient reports a long history of smoking and now complains of hoarseness and a lump-like feeling in the throat. Which question is the most relevant to collect data about possible signs of throat cancer? *(283)*
   1. Are you coughing up green or gray sputum?
   2. Do you experience any wheezing after exercise?
   3. Does the lump in your throat disappear when you swallow?
   4. Have you had hoarseness for more than 3 weeks?

Copyright © 2013, 2009 by Saunders, an imprint of Elsevier Inc. All rights reserved.

7. The patient is being discharged after undergoing a rhinoplasty for a nasal fracture. Which discharge instruction would the nurse question? *(282)*
   1. Use a humidifier at home to decrease mucosal dryness.
   2. Take ibuprofen every 6 hours for pain.
   3. Apply a cool compress over the nose and face.
   4. Use a stool softener as needed to avoid straining.

8. In the immediate postoperative period after a tonsillectomy, what is the highest priority? *(281)*
   1. Pain control
   2. Adequate hydration
   3. Prevention of aspiration
   4. Treatment of nausea

9. A patient undergoing sinus surgery has a preoperative piggyback of cefazolin (Ancef) ordered. 500 mg of the drug is dissolved in 50 mL of IV solution. The powdered drug was mixed with 10 mL of sterile water before it was added to the IV solution. The drug is ordered to be administered over 20 minutes. The IV tubing delivers 10 drops per mL. The IV should run at _____ per minute.

10. When suctioning a tracheostomy, infection control guidelines indicate that you should use: *(Select all that apply.) (286-288)*
    1. sterile glove(s).
    2. sterile drape.
    3. mask.
    4. face shield.
    5. sterile water.
    6. sterile suction catheter.

11. The nurse is caring for patients who have been diagnosed with laryngeal cancer. Which patient is likely to have the best outcome after medical treatment? *(283)*
    1. An elderly man with a long history of smoking and difficulty swallowing
    2. A middle-aged man who reported having persistent hoarseness
    3. A young man who complains of a pain in the region of the Adam's apple
    4. An elderly woman who reports weakness and difficulty breathing

12. A man eating in a restaurant suddenly stands up and grasps his throat with his hands. What is the priority action? *(281-282)*
    1. Call 911 and stay with the man.
    2. Direct the man to cough forcefully.
    3. Start cardiopulmonary resuscitation.
    4. Initiate abdominal thrusts (Heimlich maneuver).

13. The nurse observes that a patient is having severe respiratory distress. Which action should be delegated to the nursing assistant? *(281-282)*
    1. Calling the physician
    2. Staying with the patient
    3. Obtaining an Ambu bag
    4. Setting up suction equipment

14. A patient with a new tracheostomy has a nursing diagnosis of Ineffective airway clearance. What is the most likely etiology for this problem? *(286)*
    1. Improper suctioning technique
    2. Failure of the tracheostomy tube
    3. Inadequate oral hygiene
    4. Inability to cough up secretions and mucus

Copyright © 2013, 2009 by Saunders, an imprint of Elsevier Inc. All rights reserved.

15. A patient's wife reports that her husband frequently snores. Which question would the nurse ask to identify another symptom of obstructive sleep apnea? *(282)*
    1. "Does he wake suddenly at night?"
    2. "Does he have shortness of breath on waking?"
    3. "Does he complain of a sore throat in the evening?"
    4. "Does he go to bed early or late in the evening?"

CRITICAL THINKING ACTIVITIES

Scenario: A 76-year-old male patient possibly has laryngeal cancer. He is to undergo diagnostic testing and then, if cancer is diagnosed, he will have a laryngectomy.

1. What diagnostic tests would most likely be done for this patient? *(283)*

2. If the patient has a laryngectomy and a tracheostomy, how would you provide a means of communication? *(289)*

3. What criteria would you use to determine when the patient's tracheostomy needs suctioning? *(286)*

4. What are the two most important principles to be observed when suctioning? *(286)*

STEPS TOWARD BETTER COMMUNICATION

VOCABULARY BUILDING GLOSSARY

Term	Pronunciation	Definition
diligent	dil' ah jent	(adj.) hardworking, dedicated at all times
vigilant	vij' ah lent	(adj.) watchful, alert to danger
prevalent	prev'a lent	(adj.) commonly occurring, widespread
susceptible	sus cep'ti ble	(adj.) easily affected by something—physical or emotional
patent	pa' tent	(adj.) open

Copyright © 2013, 2009 by Saunders, an imprint of Elsevier Inc. All rights reserved.

COMPLETION

Directions: Fill in each blank with the appropriate word from the Vocabulary Building Glossary to complete the statement.

1. Immediate postoperative care of a tonsillectomy patient focuses on maintaining a _____ airway and observing for hemorrhage.

2. To prevent a respiratory infection in a tracheostomy patient, the nurse must be _____ with hand hygiene before suctioning.

3. The elderly are very _____ to upper respiratory infections.

4. When a patient suffers from dysphagia, the nurse must be _____ for signs of aspiration when the patient is eating or drinking.

5. The idea of the value of immunization is very _____ in Western culture.

SHORT ANSWER

Directions: Write the word to match the definition.

1. nosebleed: *(280)*_____

2. removal of the adenoids: *(281)* _____

3. inflammation of the sinuses: *(279)* _____

IDIOMATIC USAGES

Idioms are phrases used in everyday speech that do not translate literally from one language or culture to another. Below are some common English language idioms.

"Catching" a cold means getting a viral infection.

"Stuffier" means becoming more congested.

"Dull" can mean mentally slow, as well as referring to a soft, toneless sound. The opposite would be "sharp, clear" for all of these meanings.

A "magic slate" is a board covered with wax and a plastic sheet on top that can be written on with a stylus. The words show, but are erased when the sheet is lifted so that it can be reused.

PRONUNCIATION

In English, the consonant sound **"l"** is found at the beginning, middle, or end of words. It is made by putting the tip of the tongue against the back of the top front teeth with the lips open a little. The tongue lies in the bottom of the mouth and the air comes out on both sides. The voice is used.

Copyright © 2013, 2009 by Saunders, an imprint of Elsevier Inc. All rights reserved.

Directions: Practice saying these words with a partner.

1. **"l"** as the middle sound:

air-filled	irregular'ity	physiol'ogy
al'lergy	malig'nant	plaque
car'tilage	max'illary	pol'yps
cil'ia	mobil'ity	re'flex
cold	mus'cle	swal'lowed
eld'erly	olfact'ory	swell'ing
epiglot'tis	pa'late	til'ted
flu	pal'lor	ulcera'tion
glot'tis	pal'pate	
inflamma'tion	par'ticles	

2. **"l"** is silent:

calm	half	talk
could	should	would

SPELLING AND PRONUNCIATION SKILLS

ph = f

When the letters **"ph"** occur in the same syllable in English, they are pronounced like **"f."** They may occur at the beginning, middle, or end of words. The sound is made by touching the top teeth with the bottom lip. Air is blown out between the lip and the teeth.

Directions: Practice saying the following words.

dysphagia	esophageal	facial	frontal
esophagus	pharynx	lymph	

Copyright © 2013, 2009 by Saunders, an imprint of Elsevier Inc. All rights reserved.

Care of Patients with Disorders of the Lower Respiratory System

chapter **15**

Answer Key: Textbook page references are provided as a guide for answering these questions. A complete answer key was provided to your instructor.

REVIEW OF ANATOMY AND PHYSIOLOGY

Terminology

Directions: Match the term on the left with its best description on the right. (see Chapter 13)

1. _____	Diffusion	a.	Movement of air from outside body to alveoli
2. _____	Tidal volume	b.	Amount of gas in air one can exhale after maximal inhalation
3. _____	Vital capacity	c.	Amount of gas either inhaled or exhaled with each breath
4. _____	Resistance	d.	Chiefly determined by radius or caliber of airway
5. _____	Perfusion	e.	Prevents collapse of lung by stabilizing alveoli and decreasing capillary pressure
6. _____	Surfactant	f.	Passage of fluid through vessels of an organ
7. _____	Ventilation	g.	Takes place between gas in alveolar space and blood in capillaries of lung

APPLICATION OF THE NURSING PROCESS

Directions: List specific nursing actions that could be planned for a patient.

1. List four points to include in the assessment of a patient with a cough. *(see Chapter 13)*

   a. _____

   b. _____

   c. _____

   d. _____

2. Name four interventions that can help prevent pneumonia. *(296)*

   a. _____

   b. _____

   c. _____

   d. _____

Directions: Provide a nursing action to alleviate the problem.

3. Data: "My husband coughs as hard as he can, but he just can't get the phlegm up from his lungs." *(see Chapter 13)*

    Nursing action: _____

4. Data: "It seems that I have to come to the hospital at least twice a year for an infection in my lungs. I suppose there is nothing I can do about it now that I have chronic bronchitis and emphysema." *(303)*

    Nursing action: _____

5. Data: "I get short of breath just trying to take a bath and put on my clothes. Here at the hospital, there is someone wanting to do something to me every time I turn around. I wish I could get some rest." *(296)*

    Nursing action: _____

SHORT ANSWER

Directions: Describe the nursing action to be implemented for each of the following patient situations.

1. Anxiety about a scheduled bronchoscopy. *(see Chapter 13)*

    Nursing action: _____

2. A patient tells you his sputum is streaked with blood following his bronchoscopy. *(see Chapter 13)*

    Nursing action: _____

3. You are asked to assist with a thoracentesis and pleural biopsy and to watch the patient after the procedure. *(see Chapter 13)*

    a. How would you prepare the patient?_____

    _____

    b. How would you monitor the patient after the procedure? _____

    _____

4. List four signs or symptoms to note during data collection when caring for a patient with a lower respiratory disorder. *Example: Sits leaning forward with shoulders elevated. (293-297)*

    a. _____

    b. _____

    c. _____

    d. _____

5. Name three reasons why problems of nutrition and hydration are common in patients with respiratory disease. *(see Chapter 13)*

    a. _____

    b. _____

    c. _____

Copyright © 2013, 2009 by Saunders, an imprint of Elsevier Inc. All rights reserved.

6.   List five signs of respiratory alkalosis. *(see Chapter 13)*

   a.   _____

   b.   _____

   c.   _____

   d.   _____

   e.   _____

COMPLETION

Directions: Fill in the blanks to complete the statements.

1.   _____ is an extensive inflammation of the lung with either consolidation of the lung tissue as it fills with exudate or interstitial inflammation and edema. *(296)*

2.   _____ occurs when the fluid within the pleural cavity becomes infected and the exudate becomes thick and purulent. *(298)*

3.   The most common fungal lung infections are _____ and _____. *(298)*

4.   The fatigue that is often present in patients with respiratory disease is usually caused by a deficit in the _____ supply to the tissues. *(see Chapter 13)*

5.   Excessively high concentrations of inhaled oxygen can bring about collapse of the alveoli because of an interruption in production of _____, which stabilizes the alveoli. *(323)*

PRIORITY SETTING

Directions: It is 7:15 AM. Your patients have the following needs. In what order would you try to meet them? Number in order of priority. Discuss your answers with a classmate and state your rationale.

_____   a.   A patient post-thoracotomy is complaining of pain in spite of using his PCA pump.

_____   b.   A patient needs clean gown and towels to shower. She is scheduled for surgery at 8:00 AM.

_____   c.   A patient with pneumonia did not get his breakfast tray and is asking for it.

_____   d.   A nursing assistant has just told you that a patient is febrile.

_____   e.   A patient with a tracheostomy needs suctioning.

REVIEW QUESTIONS FOR THE NCLEX® EXAMINATION

Directions: Select the best answer(s) or fill in the blank with the answer for the following questions.

1.   Safety factors for administering oxygen to the patient with chronic obstructive pulmonary disease (COPD) include: *(304)*
   1.   auscultating the lungs when the patient coughs.
   2.   keeping oxygen flow below 2 L per minute.
   3.   placing the patient in a recumbent position.
   4.   filling the humidifier with warm tap water.

Copyright © 2013, 2009 by Saunders, an imprint of Elsevier Inc. All rights reserved.

2. A nursing intervention that can *best* help prevent respiratory failure in the patient with compromised lung function is to: *(315)*
   1. encourage at least 3000 mL of fluid intake per day.
   2. assist with all activities of daily living (ADLs) to prevent excess fatigue.
   3. have the patient turn, cough, and deep-breathe at least every 2 hours.
   4. administer an expectorant to help clear airways.

3. Evaluation of the effectiveness of deep-breathing and coughing is done by: *(Select all that apply.)* *(see Chapter 13)*
   1. auscultating the lungs bilaterally both before and after.
   2. assessing the color and amount of secretions produced.
   3. observing the respiratory rate and quality afterward.
   4. asking the patient whether he is breathing more easily.
   5. assessing the pulse oximetry reading.
   6. listening to the character of the patient's voice.

4. The nurse is assessing the patient for early stage emphysema. What sign would the nurse look for? *(303)*
   1. Dyspnea
   2. Pale skin color
   3. Yellow, tenacious sputum
   4. Rapid, pounding pulse

5. The nurse is assessing the patient with a chest tube. Which finding indicates that there may be a problem with the apparatus? *(316-317)*
   1. There is bloody drainage in the collection chamber.
   2. There is continuous bubbling in the water seal chamber.
   3. There is rigorous bubbling in the suction chamber.
   4. The water level fluctuates in the water seal chamber with breathing.

6. The nursing diagnosis for a patient with tuberculosis is Noncompliance with medication therapy. However, the etiology of the problem is unclear. What is the priority nursing action? *(298-301)*
   1. Suggest that the patient wear a mask until the problem is resolved.
   2. Notify the public health department to follow up on exposed family and friends.
   3. Assess the patient's understanding of the therapy and treatment plan.
   4. Engage the family to remind the patient to take the scheduled doses.

7. Your pneumonia patient is encouraged to increase his fluid intake. He had 340 mL at breakfast, 60 mL with pills, 280 mL midmorning, 410 mL with lunch, and 240 mL midafternoon. How much more fluid does he need to reach the goal of 3000 mL for the day? _____

8. When administering respiratory medications to a patient, which medication should be administered *last*? *(see Chapter 13)*
   1. Albuterol (Proventil)
   2. Montelukast (Singulair)
   3. Robitussin cough syrup
   4. Advair discus

9. The laboratory results for an arterial blood gas results shows that patient has respiratory alkalosis. Before calling the physician, what additional assessment information is the most relevant? *(see Chapter 13)*
   1. Current setting of the supplemental oxygen
   2. Pulse oximetry reading on room air
   3. Respiratory rate and breathing pattern
   4. Patient's subjective feeling of dyspnea

Copyright © 2013, 2009 by Saunders, an imprint of Elsevier Inc. All rights reserved.

10. What is a major intervention to prevent further lung damage in the patient with chronic respiratory disease? *(303-304)*
    1. Institute a plan to balance rest and activity.
    2. Convince the patient to quit smoking.
    3. Teach proper breathing techniques.
    4. Teach ways to maintain optimal health.

11. There is an order for a pneumonectomy patient to "avoid turning patient onto unoperated side." What is the best rationale for this order? *(316)*
    1. Tension pneumothorax and mediastinal shift could occur.
    2. Position would cause kinking of the chest tubes.
    3. Patient could have increased chest excursion.
    4. The stomach and intestines will cause distention.

12. The nurse is checking the oxygen delivery system at the beginning of the shift. What is included in the assessment of the system and equipment? *(Select all that apply.)* *(323-325)*
    1. Check to make sure that the oxygen flow rate is less than 3L/min.
    2. Observe the tubing for kinks or blockage.
    3. Make sure that the tubing and connections are not touching the floor.
    4. Verify that the flow rate is set according to the physician's order.
    5. Make sure that the oxygen source or tank is not combustible.

13. Which nutritional suggestion would the nurse give to a COPD patient? *(304)*
    1. Restrict fluids to prevent fluid overload and possible pulmonary edema.
    2. Perform mild exercise just before eating to stimulate appetite.
    3. Eat three regular meals a day, but limit protein intake.
    4. Cook when feeling most energetic and freeze extra portions.

14. A postoperative patient suddenly and unexpectedly becomes very anxious and complains of dyspnea. What is the priority nursing action? *(see Chapter 13)*
    1. Encourage expression of feelings.
    2. Assess for other symptoms.
    3. Notify the RN or MD.
    4. Tell the patient to calm down.

15. The nurse is caring for a trauma patient and notes that with inhalation a portion of the chest is drawn inward and with exhalation, the portion expands outward. What is the significance of this observation? *(see Chapter 13)*
    1. This is a normal and expected pattern of chest movement.
    2. The patient is having excessive pain that is interfering with respiration.
    3. Several ribs are fractured and patient should be turned onto the affected side.
    4. This pattern is associated with a pneumothorax or hemothorax.

CRITICAL THINKING ACTIVITIES

A patient who had been living in Southeast Asia for the past 2 years has just been diagnosed with tuberculosis. He is complaining of night sweats, fatigue, and weight loss. He has a cough. *(298-301)*

1. Therapy for tuberculosis consists of several medications. What medications would you expect to be prescribed? What teaching points are especially important for this patient?

Copyright © 2013, 2009 by Saunders, an imprint of Elsevier Inc. All rights reserved.

2. At what point will this patient no longer be considered contagious?

3. What are the reasons that tuberculosis is increasing in the United States?

STEPS TOWARD BETTER COMMUNICATION

VOCABULARY BUILDING GLOSSARY

Term	Definition
re′coil	to move back quickly; to return with force to an original position
flar′ing	getting wider; extending outward at the edges or tips
pursed (purst)	rounded, gathered together (as when lips are ready to blow out a candle or to whistle)
com′bustion (kŏm bust -shŭn)	burning or fire
suscep′tible (su sep′ ti bel)	likely or probably will be affected; at risk of; prone to catch sickness
aggres′sive care	vigorous, strong; frequent care that follows all guidelines
cor′relate	link together two or more things; fit together into a pattern (e.g., *correlate* the symptoms with the disease)
ag′gravate	to cause to increase; to make worse
paradox′ical (par ah dok′ si kel)	something that looks contradictory but is true; two things that are working opposite of usual; contrary to what is normal or expected
hall′mark	sign, criteria; standard signal or feature of some condition
fluc′tuate	to change, vary up and down
cal′ibrate	to measure exactly, usually with markings
occlud′ed	blocked
emerging	rising or coming up

PRONUNCIATION OF DIFFICULT TERMS

Directions: Practice pronouncing the following words:

Term	Pronunciation	Definition
kyphosis	ki fo′ sis	abnormal outward curvature of the spine; hunchback
scoliosis	sko lee o′sis	S-type curvature of the spine
empyema	em pie ee′ ma	accumulation of pus in a body cavity
hemoptysis	he mop′ti sis	coughing and spitting of red, frothy blood
hematemesis	hem ah tem′e sis	vomiting of blood

Copyright © 2013, 2009 by Saunders, an imprint of Elsevier Inc. All rights reserved.

COMPLETION

Directions: Fill in the blanks with the appropriate words from the Vocabulary Building Glossary to complete the statements.

1. Learning to breathe with _____ lips helps decrease dyspnea for the patient with emphysema.

2. People with chronic respiratory disease are more _____ to respiratory infections than the general public.

3. When a chest tube is functioning properly, the fluid in the water seal chamber will _____ with each breath.

4. Oxygen is *not* explosive; however, oxygen does support _____.

5. When several ribs are fractured, _____ chest motion will be observed.

6. When respiratory distress is occurring, the nurse may observe _____ of the patient's nostrils.

7. A(n) _____ of acute respiratory distress syndrome (ARDS) is respiratory failure.

8. The Center for Disease Control monitors _____ infectious diseases, such as SARS.

9. When turning a patient who is attached to a ventilator, the nurse must be careful to check to see that the ventilator tubing is not _____.

10. Patients with severe _____ or _____ of the spine often have restrictive lung disease.

WORD ATTACK SKILLS

Directions: Look at the word elements defined below and then break the listed words into their word parts using vertical lines. Write the meaning of each word as in the example below:

anti/venom   *an agent that counteracts the effect of a poison from snake or insect bite.*

-oid: resembling

-megal/o: enlargement

-osis: condition

anti-   against

1. Cytomegalovirus: _____

2. Immunocompromised:_____

3. Immunosuppressive: _____

4. Antiinfective: _____

5. Coccidioidomycosis:_____

Copyright © 2013, 2009 by Saunders, an imprint of Elsevier Inc. All rights reserved.

COMMUNICATION EXERCISE

Directions: Here is an example of what you would say to teach a patient ways to prevent the spread of a respiratory infection.

"You can help prevent the spread of your respiratory infection by washing your hands frequently with soap and warm water. Cover your mouth when you cough or sneeze. Throw away used tissues immediately and wash your hands again. Be careful not to touch objects after coughing or sneezing before you wash your hands. Try to sit and stand several feet away from other people while your nose is running and you are coughing and sneezing. Stay out of crowded places."

Directions: With a peer, practice performing a respiratory assessment.

Take and record the respiratory history. Document your physical assessment findings. Ask your instructor to review your documentation of the assessment.

_____

_____

_____

_____

_____

_____

Copyright © 2013, 2009 by Saunders, an imprint of Elsevier Inc. All rights reserved.

The Hematologic System

chapter

16

Answer Key: Textbook page references are provided as a guide for answering these questions. A complete answer key was provided to your instructor.

REVIEW OF ANATOMY AND PHYSIOLOGY

Completion

Directions: Fill in the blanks to complete the statements.

1. The type of blood cell responsible for the transport of oxygen is the _____
   _____. *(332)*

2. Erythropoiesis must continue throughout life because the average life span of a red blood cell is
   _____. *(332)*

3. An infection in the body stimulates the production of _____, resulting in
   _____. *(332)*

4. A(n) _____ infection prompts the production of lymphocytes. *(333)*

5. The major functions of thrombocytes is to promote _____. *(333)*

6. Bone marrow activity decreases by about _____ percent as years advance. *(334)*

7. The storage and release of blood and the removal of old blood cells are major functions of the
   _____ and _____. *(332, 334)*

8. Basophils in response to allergens release _____. *(333)*

COMPLETION

Age-Related Changes Affecting the Hematologic System

Directions: Complete each of the following statements.

1. A problem that might be encountered by the decrease in plasma volume after age 60 is:

   _____

   _____ . *(334)*

Copyright © 2013, 2009 by Saunders, an imprint of Elsevier Inc. All rights reserved.

2. The elderly are at greater risk for infection because _____

    _____ . *(334)*

3. Anemia, when it occurs, takes longer to resolve in the elderly because _____

    _____ . *(334)*

4. Changes in blood coagulation make the elderly person more at risk for _____

    _____ . *(334)*

SHORT ANSWER

Causes and Prevention of Hematologic Disorders

Directions: Provide a short answer for each of the following questions.

1. Inherited disorders that interfere with normal blood function are: *(334-335)*

    a. _____

    b. _____

    c. _____

2. Genetic tendencies for hematologic problems in these groups are: *(334)*

    a. African-Americans: _____

    b. Scandinavian descent: _____

    c. Middle-Easterners: _____

3. Drugs that can cause particular blood dyscrasias (abnormalities) are: *(334-335)*

    a. Procainamide may cause: _____

    b. Furosemide may cause: _____

    c. Quinidine may cause: _____

    d. Oral contraceptives may cause: _____

4. Nutritional deficiencies that may interfere with erythropoiesis are: *(335)* _____

    _____

5. Lifestyle factors that can help prevent anemia are: *(335-340)* _____

    _____

    _____

6. You can help prevent excessive blood loss by: *(343)* _____

    _____

Copyright © 2013, 2009 by Saunders, an imprint of Elsevier Inc. All rights reserved.

7. Two ways you can help prevent blood dyscrasias are: *(335-336)*

   a. _____

   _____

   b. _____

   _____

SHORT ANSWER

Assessment and Diagnostics

Directions: Briefly answer the following.

1. List the five kinds of data that should be obtained during history-taking for assessment of a patient with a blood disorder. *(339)*

   a. _____

   b. _____

   c. _____

   d. _____

   e. _____

2. State the possible cause or condition usually associated with each of the following. *(Example: Tarry stools: intestinal bleeding)*

   a. Jaundice: *(339)* _____

   b. Bruises and petechiae: *(339)*_____

   c. Polycythemia: *(339)*_____

   d. Sore and bleeding gums: *(339)*_____

   e. Smoky, brownish urine: *(339-340)*_____

   f. Swollen and painful joints: *(340)*_____

   g. Weakness and intolerance to physical activity: *(340)*_____

   h. Irritability, dizziness, and difficulty concentrating: *(340)* ____

3. Inquiring about occupation and hobbies is important to a hematologic history because: *(339)*

   _____

   _____

4. If during assessment, a patient's urine is noted to be a brown tea color, it could indicate that

   _____ is occurring. *(339-340)*

Copyright © 2013, 2009 by Saunders, an imprint of Elsevier Inc. All rights reserved.

5. Two nursing responsibilities for obtaining a urine specimen for Bence-Jones protein are: *(338, Table 16-1)*

    a. _____

    b. _____

6. When blood collection is performed, nursing responsibilities are to: *(336)*

    a. _____

    b. _____

    c. _____

7. On the blood count differential, allergy may be indicated by the presence of _____
    _____. *(337-338, Table 16-1)*

8. A d-Dimer blood test is useful for diagnosing _____. *(338, Table 16-1)*

PRIORITY SETTING

Directions: You have been asked to obtain a blood sample for a CBC from a patient in the ambulatory clinic. Number the following tasks in the order in which you would perform them. Consider that a task may be performed more than once. (see Skill 16-1 on Evolve)

_____   a. Obtain the needed supplies.

_____   b. Place the label the specimen tube.

_____   c. Don latex gloves.

_____   d. Write the information on the specimen label.

_____   e. Send the specimen to the laboratory.

_____   f. Perform the venipuncture.

_____   g. Cover the wound.

_____   h. Identify the patient using two identifiers.

_____   i. Remove the gloves.

_____   j. Fill out the laboratory requisition slip.

_____   k. Stop bleeding at the site.

_____   l. Perform hand hygiene.

_____   m. Explain what you are going to do to the patient.

REVIEW QUESTIONS FOR THE NCLEX® EXAMINATION

Directions: Choose the best answer(s) for the following questions.

1. A diagnostic test commonly used to detect inflammation is: *(336-337, Table 16-1)*
    1. platelet count.
    2. monophage count.
    3. activated partial thromboplastin time.
    4. erythrocyte sedimentation rate.

Copyright © 2013, 2009 by Saunders, an imprint of Elsevier Inc. All rights reserved.

2. Erythropoiesis cannot occur normally if: *(Select all that apply.)* *(332)*
   1. bone marrow activity is suppressed.
   2. there is a lack of vitamin K.
   3. there are insufficient amino acids available.
   4. the diet does not include sufficient green and yellow vegetables.
   5. vitamin E is insufficient.
   6. linoleic acid is not present.

3. The normal range for platelets in adults is _____ mm^3. *(334)*

4. The elderly who live alone are at high risk of poor nutrition due to problems with: *(Select all that apply.)* *(336)*
   1. cooking ability.
   2. vision or arthritis.
   3. financial means.
   4. mobility.
   5. chronic diseases that cause fatigue.
   6. cooking equipment.

5. When gathering assessment data you would: *(Place the choices in proper sequence.)* *(339-340)*
   _____ 1. inspect the skin for abnormal color.
   _____ 2. inquire about family hereditary diseases.
   _____ 3. check scleral and conjunctival color.
   _____ 4. inquire about headaches or palpitations.
   _____ 5. inquire about ease of bleeding.
   _____ 6. measure vital signs.
   _____ 7. check for swollen or painful joints.
   _____ 8. check condition of fingernails and hair.

6. Yellowed skin or sclera and conjunctiva may occur from: *(Select all that apply.)* *(339)*
   1. anemic state.
   2. excess bilirubin in the blood.
   3. inadequate platelet function.
   4. hemolysis.
   5. excess consumption of carrots.

7. A sign of spleen enlargement is: *(340)*
   1. feeling of fullness in upper left abdomen.
   2. complaints of stomach pain from pressure.
   3. decreased erythrocyte count.
   4. an upper left quadrant lump felt upon palpation.

8. When a patient is anorexic, things that may interfere with eating are: *(343)*
   1. providing socialization during meals.
   2. odors in the room.
   3. serving small frequent meals and snacks.
   4. providing mouth care before each meal.

9. People who have a blood abnormality may be prone to bleeding problems and _____. *(340)*

10. When a patient has a prolonged clotting time, after drawing blood, you should: *(342)*
    1. apply pressure for 2 full minutes.
    2. have the patient apply pressure to the site until the bleeding stops.
    3. apply pressure for 5–10 minutes.
    4. use a styptic pencil to stop the bleeding.

Copyright © 2013, 2009 by Saunders, an imprint of Elsevier Inc. All rights reserved.

11. Activity intolerance and fatigue occur with some hematologic disorders because: *(340, 343)*
    1. too many blood cells make blood thicker and circulation sluggish.
    2. a deficiency of hemoglobin decreases the oxygen-carrying capacity of the blood.
    3. oxygen molecules will not attach to faulty erythrocytes and can't reach the cells.
    4. oxygen cannot diffuse through alveolar membrane thickened by abnormal cells.

12. The patient with a blood abnormality is at higher risk for infection. Therefore, the nurse should make which intervention a priority? *(340)*
    1. Treat pain immediately.
    2. Correct nutritional deficiencies.
    3. Use aseptic technique.
    4. Prevent undue fatigue.

CRITICAL THINKING ACTIVITIES

1. If you came upon an auto accident, stopped to help, and found someone on the ground spurting blood from the upper thigh, what would you do first? After that, what would you do? *(343)*

2. You have been assigned to a recent postoperative patient who has just had a thoracotomy. You know that postoperative hemorrhage is always a potential complication. What would you specifically assess to assure yourself as best you can that a postoperative hemorrhage is not occurring? *(339-343)*

STEPS TOWARD BETTER COMMUNICATION

VOCABULARY BUILDING GLOSSARY

Term	Definition
ag'gregate	(verb) bring separate parts together in a group, to combine together
brought on	caused to occur , induced by, emerged from
clot	a thickened mass of liquid, especially of blood
perni'cious (per nish' us)	having a very harmful effect
pleth'ora	red complexion caused by excessive blood

COMPLETION

Directions: Fill in the blanks with the appropriate words from the Vocabulary Building Glossary above to complete the statements.

1. When a cut occurs and a blood vessel is damaged, platelets _____ as part of the clotting process.

Copyright © 2013, 2009 by Saunders, an imprint of Elsevier Inc. All rights reserved.

2. _____ anemia is caused by an inability of the body to absorb vitamin B_{12} from the intestinal tract.

3. Fibrinogen is another factor in addition to platelets that works to form a blood _____.

4. Patients suffering from polycythemia vera often display _____.

5. Lymphedema may be _____ by the lymph node extraction that accompanies a radical or modified mastectomy.

PRONUNCIATION

Directions: With a peer, practice pronouncing the following words. Use each word in an appropriate sentence.

Term	Pronunciation	Definition
dyscra'sia	dis kray' zee ah	imbalance in the elements of something
erythropoi'etin	a rith' ro poy' e tin	hormone that stimulates red blood cell production
erythropoie'sis	a rith' ro poi ee' sis	red blood cell production
fatigue'd	fa teeg' d	very tired, completely weary, exhausted
parenterally	pah ren' ter ah lee	by a route other than the digestive tract
pete'chia	pa tee' ki a	round red spot
splenomeg'aly	splen' o meg' a lee	enlargement of the spleen
throm'bocytope'nia	throm' bo si to pee' ne ah	decrease in the number of platelets

MATCHING

Directions: Match the prefix or suffix on the left with its correct meaning on the right.

1. _____ -cyte a. have affinity for
2. _____ -chrom b. normal, usual
3. _____ -phils c. negative prefix (not or without)
4. _____ a- d. white
5. _____ normo- e. cell
6. _____ gran- f. large, long
7. _____ neo- g. color
8. _____ mono- h. sole, one
9. _____ macro- i. grain, particle
10. _____ leuko- j. new, young
11. _____ erythro- k. red

Copyright © 2013, 2009 by Saunders, an imprint of Elsevier Inc. All rights reserved.

SHORT ANSWER

Directions: Write the meaning of each word, referring to the word elements in the exercise above. Use your dictionary as needed.

1. Macrophage: _____

2. Monochrome:_____

3. Leukocytosis: _____

4. Erythropoietin: _____

5. Granulocyte: _____

6. Neutrophil:_____

7. Agranulocyte: _____

8. Normochromic: _____

Copyright © 2013, 2009 by Saunders, an imprint of Elsevier Inc. All rights reserved.

Care of Patients with Hematologic Disorders

chapter

17

Answer Key: Textbook page references are provided as a guide for answering these questions. A complete answer key was provided to your instructor.

COMPLETION

Hematologic Disorders

Directions: Fill in the blanks to complete the statements.

1. An individual with pernicious anemia does not produce _____, which is essential to the production of erythrocytes. *(347)*

2. Treatment of pernicious anemia consists of _____. *(349)*

3. The primary difficulty caused by anemia is failure to meet the _____ _____. *(346)*

4. Sickle cell trait occurs when the individual has _____. *(353)*

5. When both parents have sickle cell trait, the chances of their children having sickle cell disease rise to _____%. *(353)*

6. The symptoms suffered during a sickling crisis are the result of _____ _____. *(353)*

7. Leukemias are characterized by _____ _____. *(355)*

8. Leukemia patients receiving chemotherapy should avoid eating _____. *(357, Nursing Care Plan 17-1)*

9. There is a hereditary link for _____ leukemia. *(355)*

10. Patients who are anemic and receiving iron therapy should increase their intake of vitamin C because it helps _____. *(366-367)*

11. Management of classic hemophilia is by transfusion of _____. *(361)*

12. When a patient has an iron-deficiency anemia, treatment consists of _____ _____ _____. *(364-367)*

Copyright © 2013, 2009 by Saunders, an imprint of Elsevier Inc. All rights reserved.

13. When a patient is anemic, oxygen levels tend to drop because of the deficiency of _____ present in the blood. *(366)*

14. Side effects of oral iron therapy include _____
_____. *(366)*

15. Aplastic anemia may be caused by _____, a(n) _____ or
a(n) _____. *(352)*

16. A blood loss of as little as _____ mL can cause hypovolemic shock. *(346)*

17. The classic signs and symptoms of hypovolemic shock are _____
_____
_____. *(348, see also Chapter 45)*

18. The patient experiencing hypovolemic shock is positioned _____
_____. *(see Chapter 45)*

19. Nutritional anemia is caused by inadequate _____, _____, or _____
_____. *(347)*

APPLICATION OF THE NURSING PROCESS

Directions: Write an expected outcome and list three nursing measures for each of the following nursing diagnoses commonly found in patients with blood disorders.

1. Altered tissue perfusion related to decreased red blood cells and hemoglobin

   Expected outcome: _____
   _____

   a. _____

   b. _____

   c. _____

2. Risk for infection related to decreased or abnormal white blood cells

   Expected outcome: _____
   _____

   a. _____

   b. _____

   c. _____

Copyright © 2013, 2009 by Saunders, an imprint of Elsevier Inc. All rights reserved.

3. Activity intolerance related to fatigue and weakness

    Expected outcome: _____

    _____

    a. _____

    b. _____

    c. _____

4. Risk for injury related to possible hemorrhage

    Expected outcome: _____

    _____

    a. _____

    b. _____

    c. _____

5. List interventions you would place on the teaching plan for the 35-year-old female patient who has iron-deficiency anemia. *(351)*

    _____

    _____

    _____

    _____

    _____

    _____

Copyright © 2013, 2009 by Saunders, an imprint of Elsevier Inc. All rights reserved.

PRIORITY SETTING

Your patient is to receive a transfusion of packed red cells. Place the following actions in the order in which you would do them. *(363-364)*

_____ a. Prime the filter and IV tubing with normal saline.

_____ b. Hook up the unit of packed cells to the IV tubing.

_____ c. Check the orders.

_____ d. Stay with the patient.

_____ e. Obtain the blood bag from the blood bank.

_____ f. Check the size of the IV cannula that is in place already.

_____ g. Check the patient's identification with the blood bag and the relevant papers.

_____ h. Establish that the IV site is patent.

_____ i. Verify the blood unit numbers and the patient's blood bracelet with another nurse.

_____ j. Set the correct drop rate for the blood to flow for the first 15 minutes.

_____ k. Take the baseline vital signs.

_____ l. Inquire if the patient has ever had a transfusion reaction.

_____ m. Perform hand hygiene.

_____ n. Don impermeable gloves.

_____ o. Attach the blood IV tubing to the IV cannula.

_____ p. Take the vital signs again.

_____ q. Reset the drop rate to the calculated flow rate.

REVIEW QUESTIONS FOR THE NCLEX® EXAMINATION

Directions: Choose the best answer(s) for the following questions.

1. An important part of assessment of the patient with an iron-deficiency anemia is: (*Select all that apply.*) *(351)*
   1. determining if there is a family history of this type of problem.
   2. determining if there is abnormally high blood loss with menstruation.
   3. asking if the patient takes any vitamins.
   4. determining if the patient is a strict vegetarian.
   5. checking to see if any drugs that cause hemolysis are being taken.
   6. obtaining a thorough dietary history of what the patient normally eats.

2. Independent care for the patient admitted with severe anemia should include: *(348-349)*
   1. interventions to conserve the patient's energy.
   2. obtaining blood specimens for diagnostic testing.
   3. administering ordered blood products.
   4. assessing the patient for signs of depression.

3. When the nurse administers a form of iron to the anemic patient, she keeps in mind that iron: *(366-367)*
   1. comes in many different forms and strengths.
   2. should be given through a straw if in liquid oral form.
   3. usually leaves a bad aftertaste in the mouth.
   4. is more quickly effective in the intravenous form.

Copyright © 2013, 2009 by Saunders, an imprint of Elsevier Inc. All rights reserved.

4. When a blood transfusion is given to an elderly patient, to prevent fluid overload, blood units should be: *(363)*
   1. administered 2 hours apart.
   2. warmed before infusion.
   3. administered over 4 hours.
   4. restricted to 2 units per 24 hours.

5. A patient with chronic iron-deficiency anemia may have _____ nails. *(348)*

6. A treatment often used for polycythemia vera is: *(354-355)*
   1. iron therapy.
   2. vitamin C.
   3. phlebotomy.
   4. aspirin.

7. Nursing interventions for the patient with idiopathic thrombocytopenic purpura must include measures to: *(359-360)*
   1. prevent spontaneous bleeding.
   2. increase the number of red blood cells.
   3. prevent health care–associated infection.
   4. encourage better nutrition.

8. Teaching to prevent aplastic anemia includes: *(352)*
   1. encouraging the patient to get regular blood counts performed.
   2. teaching patients proper nutrition to build blood cells.
   3. teaching people to avoid skin exposure to household and garden chemicals.
   4. encouraging avoidance of any drug that might cause the disorder.

9. A high-priority goal for the planning of care for the patient with aplastic anemia is: *(352)*
   1. prevention of fatigue.
   2. assistance with activities of daily living (ADLs).
   3. prevention of infection.
   4. alleviation of pain.

10. When gathering data to support a diagnosis of leukemia, the nurse knows that the most common symptoms are: *(355-356)*
    1. excessive bleeding, headaches, and chills.
    2. exposure to known toxic agents that cause the disorder.
    3. fatigue, malaise, and frequent infections.
    4. viral infection, nausea, and decreased hemoglobin.

11. One of the first signs of disseminated intravascular coagulation is: *(362)*
    1. blood clotting that interferes with circulation in the extremities.
    2. chest pain from tiny blood clots throughout the lungs.
    3. continued bleeding from an injection site, ecchymoses, and petechiae.
    4. bleeding from the mouth, nose, and other body orifices.

12. When administering more than one unit of blood by transfusion, the nurse must: *(363)*
    1. change the filter for each new unit to be transfused.
    2. wait at least 1 hour between administration of units.
    3. allow the second unit to warm to room temperature before hanging it.
    4. administer at least 250 mL of normal saline between units given.

Copyright © 2013, 2009 by Saunders, an imprint of Elsevier Inc. All rights reserved.

13. Subtle signs of a transfusion reaction may be: *(364)*
    1. somnolence and confusion.
    2. bradycardia and increased blood pressure.
    3. backache and a feeling of anxiety.
    4. irritability and headache.

14. Leukapheresis is performed to: *(364)*
    1. wash antigens from the bloodstream.
    2. separate neutrophils from the blood.
    3. treat all types of leukemia.
    4. treat certain types of immune disorders.

15. Which statement is true about bone marrow transplant? *(364, 366)*
    1. There is a 50% chance of HLA match between siblings.
    2. 200 mL of bone marrow is needed for the transplant.
    3. A potential complication for the donor is excessive blood clotting.
    4. Engraftment of the transplanted bone marrow takes 2–5 weeks.

16. A chemotherapy drug used for chronic myelogenous leukemia but not other leukemias is
    _____. *(356)*

17. The basis for having elderly adults take a low-dose aspirin daily is: *(355)*
    1. the blood of the elderly tends to coagulate more easily.
    2. aspirin stimulates the bone marrow to produce new cells.
    3. aspirin assists the uptake of iron from the intestinal tract.
    4. aspirin helps prevent the ecchymoses common in the elderly.

18. The order is to infuse 2 units of packed red cells. One unit contains 195 mL and the other contains 210 mL. The blood is to infuse over 4 hours. The blood IV tubing setup delivers 10 gtts/mL. At what rate should the infusion run? _____

CRITICAL THINKING ACTIVITIES

Scenario A: S.T. is a 37-year-old black man who has sickle cell disease. He has frequent episodes of pain. His anemia has been managed with transfusions on several occasions. He has signs of chronic renal failure. He has been prescribed pentoxifylline (Trental), oxycodone/acetaminophen (Roxicet), and folic acid (Folvite). At the hematology clinic this morning, his Hgb was 6.9 g/dL. He was transfused with 2 units of packed red cells over 3 hours and then sent home. About an hour and a half later, he developed dyspnea. His wife called 911 and he arrived at the emergency department with oxygen by mask.

1. How would you describe sickle cell disease? How is it related to race? *(353)*

2. What is the mechanism by which patients with sickle cell disease develop anemia? *(353)*

3. Why should the admitting nurse inquire about his pain and the need for medication? *(353-354)*

Copyright © 2013, 2009 by Saunders, an imprint of Elsevier Inc. All rights reserved.

Scenario B: P.W., age 12, has hemophilia B (Christmas disease). His mother brought him to the emergency department because of considerable pain and swelling in his left knee. He states that he bumped the knee on a desk at school. A CBC shows Hgb of 10.4 g/dL and a deficiency of clotting factor IX.

1. Describe how this X-linked recessive trait for hemophilia is transmitted. *(361)*

2. Explain why this patient has a bleeding problem when injured. *(361)*

3. What is the expected treatment for P.W.? *(361-362)*

STEPS TOWARD BETTER COMMUNICATION

VOCABULARY BUILDING GLOSSARY

Term	Definition
clump	(noun) a cluster, group of pieces; a small pile of things (verb) pieces gather or stick together in a group
dire (dīr)	very serious; having dangerous or threatening consequences
enhance'	increase, improve; give better opportunity
har'vest	to collect something for use
meti'culous	extremely careful
mit'igate	(verb) reduce, lessen, alleviate
modal'ity, -ies	a particular system or arrangement, a method
sic'kle	a crescent shape, like a new moon; a farm tool with a curved blade

COMPLETION

Directions: Fill in the blanks with the appropriate words from the Vocabulary Building Glossary above to complete the statements.

1. When extensive bleeding occurs during surgery, extra fluids are given to _____ the effect of the blood loss.

2. When a patient develops leukopenia, the nurse must use _____ aseptic technique to prevent infection.

3. When an injury occurs to tissue, platelets _____ to help stop bleeding.

Copyright © 2013, 2009 by Saunders, an imprint of Elsevier Inc. All rights reserved.

4. An oxygen deficit will cause red blood cells to _____ in patients with sickle cell disease.

5. When leukemia is diagnosed, the patient and physician must choose an appropriate

    _____ of treatment.

6. When a leukemia patient suffers an episode of bleeding, the consequences may be _____.

7. Using strict asepsis when caring for a patient with a blood dyscrasia will _____ the chances of preventing infection.

8. Before a bone marrow transplant, the physician must _____ marrow from a matching donor.

GRAMMAR POINTS

The word **"by"** + the **-ing** form of a verb is often used when talking about how something happens, or the method of doing something. An object or phrase is usually required to complete the sentence.

Example: Nurses help patients by teaching about drug side effects.

Directions: Complete each sentence using "by" plus the -ing forms of the following verbs:

cautioning	undergoing
reporting	following
asking	suppressing
using	destroying
wearing	administering

1. After giving a narcotic, nurses help prevent patient falls _____ patients not to get up without assistance.

2. Patient information is relayed to the oncoming shift _____ on the condition, treatments, and complaints of patients by the nurses leaving.

3. A thorough history is obtained _____ the patient several specific questions.

4. A nurse complies with Standard Precautions _____ gloves whenever contact with body fluids is likely.

5. The nurse is protected from contamination _____ a waterproof gown, gloves, and goggles when irrigating a wound.

6. A patient fights leukemia _____ chemotherapy treatment.

7. The immunosuppressed patient prevents infection _____ strict guidelines to avoid contact with pathogens.

8. Many types of chemotherapy work _____ replication of the malignant cells.

Copyright © 2013, 2009 by Saunders, an imprint of Elsevier Inc. All rights reserved.

9. Radiation therapy works _____ malignant cells.

10. Hypovolemic shock is treated _____ fluids and blood.

COMMUNICATION EXERCISE

Directions: With a partner, make a list of the most important points to use in teaching the patient and the family about 1) prevention of infection, 2) prevention and treatment of bleeding episodes, and 3) appropriate nutrition. Then orally "teach" your partner about these issues.

_____

_____

_____

_____

CULTURAL POINT

Be aware that some religions prohibit blood transfusions, and other people are very suspicious of the procedure. Approach a patient carefully to determine his or her feelings about transfusions.

Copyright © 2013, 2009 by Saunders, an imprint of Elsevier Inc. All rights reserved.

Student Name_____ Date_____

Answer Key: Textbook page references are provided as a guide for answering these questions. A complete answer key was provided to your instructor.

REVIEW OF ANATOMY AND PHYSIOLOGY

Labeling

Structures of the Circulatory System

Directions: On the figure below, label the structures of the circulatory system. Then, using arrows, indicate the pathway that blood follows through the system. Explain the diagram and pathway to a partner. **(372)**

superior vena cava	inferior vena cava	pulmonary artery
pulmonary vein	mitral valve	tricuspid valve
pulmonic valve	aortic valve	right atrium
right ventricle	left atrium	left ventricle
aorta		

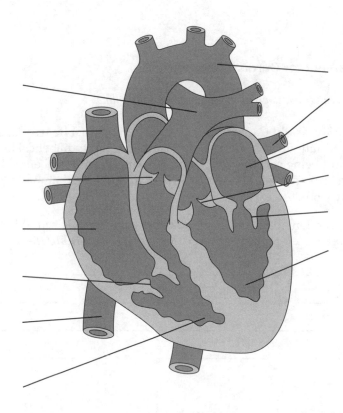

Copyright © 2013, 2009 by Saunders, an imprint of Elsevier Inc. All rights reserved.

COMPLETION

Directions: Fill in the blanks to complete the statements.

1. Cardiac output depends on the heart _____, the amount of blood returning to the _____, the strength of _____, and the _____ to the ejection of the blood. *(373)*

2. The right coronary artery supplies the _____, _____, _____, and the _____. *(373)*

3. _____ equals the amount of blood pumped out of the heart each minute. *(373)*

4. The aging heart becomes _____, resulting in decreased _____ in the elderly. *(375)*

5. A(n) _____ is the difference between the apical and radial pulse rates when they are counted at the same time. *(386)*

6. A weight gain of 3 lbs. or more in a(n) _____ period indicates fluid retention. *(394)*

7. The doctor orders furosemide (Lasix) oral liquid 20 mg PO every morning. The pharmacy delivers a 100-mL bottle of furosemide with a concentration of 40 mg/5 mL. How many mL should you give the patient? _____ mL

SHORT ANSWER

Risk Factors and Assessment for Cardiac Disorders

Directions: Read the clinical scenario and answer the questions that follow.

Scenario: Mr. Nielsen is a 58-year-old Caucasian banker. He reports that he was having difficulty doing his usual 2-mile walk because of fatigue and shortness of breath. He is pre-diabetic. He tells you, "At first, I thought it was just stress and being sort of overweight, drinking too much beer, and eating too much rich food. I decided to make an appointment because my wife reminded me that my father and grandfather died of heart disease in their early 60s."

1. You are collecting information about cardiac risk factors from Mr. Nielsen. What are four nonmodifiable risk factors related to the development of heart disease? *(376, 377, Table 18-1)*

   a. _____

   b. _____

   c. _____

   d. _____

Copyright © 2013, 2009 by Saunders, an imprint of Elsevier Inc. All rights reserved.

2. List five modifiable risk factors that Mr. Nielsen has just indicated in the scenario. What information can you give him about modifying the factors that he has just mentioned? *(376-377, Table 18-1)*

    a. _____

    b. _____

    c. _____

    d. _____

    e. _____

3. What diagnostic tests would you expect Mr. Nielsen to undergo? *(377-384, Table 18-2)*

    a. Laboratory: _____

    b. Diagnostic: _____

    _____

    _____

4. List at least six things that should be included in the physical assessment of a patient like Mr. Nielsen, who may have a cardiac disorder. *(385-388)*

    a. _____

    b. _____

    c. _____

    d. _____

    e. _____

    f. _____

COMPLETION

Diagnostic Testing for Cardiac Disorders

Directions: Fill in the blanks to complete the statements.

1. Ultrasound Doppler flow studies are conducted to detect a(n) _____ in the vessel or to determine the _____ of the vessel. *(384)*

2. Coronary angiography requires injection of a(n) _____. *(380, Table 18-2)*

3. The purpose of a stress echocardiogram is to detect _____
   _____. *(379, Table 18-2)*

4. Explain to the patient that during impedance plethysmography, he may feel some discomfort related to _____. *(382, Table 18-2)*

5. Myoglobin level is performed to detect damage to the _____ from a(n) _____ _____ infarction. *(383, Table 18-2)*

Copyright © 2013, 2009 by Saunders, an imprint of Elsevier Inc. All rights reserved.

APPLICATION OF THE NURSING PROCESS

Changes with Aging

Directions: Read the scenario and provide the answers to the following questions.

Scenario: You are working in an extended-care facility and Mrs. Wiabo is one of your elderly patients. Mrs. Wiabo is in stable condition, but she has several chronic health problems, including hypertension and occasional problems with fluid retention.

1. List at least six changes in the cardiovascular system associated with aging. *(377, 386)*

    a. _____

    b. _____

    c. _____

    d. _____

    e. _____

    f. _____

2. List at least five interventions (including assessments) to use with patients like Mrs. Wiabo who have fluid retention. *(394)*

    a. _____

    b. _____

    c. _____

    d. _____

    e. _____

    f. _____

3. Which nursing diagnosis is top priority for Mrs. Wiabo? *(388-393)*
    a. Chronic low self-esteem related to activity intolerance
    b. Knowledge deficit related to disease process, medications, and self-care
    c. Imbalanced fluid volume, risk for, related to heart failure
    d. Impaired social interaction related to being away from family

4. What is the best expected outcome for the nursing diagnosis chosen in question 3? *(389-392)*
    a. Patient will verbalize signs and symptoms of medication side effects within 7 days.
    b. Patient will be able to perform ADLs within 2 months.
    c. Patient's urine output will be within normal range day to day.
    d. Patient will not gain more than 1 lb. in any 24-hour period.

Copyright © 2013, 2009 by Saunders, an imprint of Elsevier Inc. All rights reserved.

PRIORITY SETTING

Directions: Read the scenario and prioritize the steps to perform the procedure. (387)

Scenario: You are preparing to take a routine blood pressure on an ambulatory patient at a clinic. You have never taken a blood pressure on this patient before and the patient does not remember his last blood pressure reading. You must use an ordinary manual blood pressure cuff (i.e., not a blood pressure machine). Put the following steps in the correct order to perform the procedure.

_____   a.   Palpate the brachial artery.

_____   b.   Select the correct cuff size.

_____   c.   Center the bladder cuff over the brachial artery.

_____   d.   Listen until the sounds stop.

_____   e.   Report abnormal findings to the RN or MD.

_____   f.   Release cuff and wait 30–60 seconds.

_____   g.   Deflate cuff slowly and smoothly to obtain a correct diastolic reading.

_____   h.   Record your findings as soon as you obtain the reading.

_____   i.   Support the patient's arm, on which the cuff is placed, at heart level.

_____   j.   Ensure the patient has not smoked or had caffeine for the past 30 minutes.

_____   k.   Place the bell of your stethoscope over the brachial artery.

_____   l.   Tighten the screw clamp; inflate cuff 30 mm above the palpated pressure.

_____   m.   Obtain a palpated systolic blood pressure.

REVIEW QUESTIONS FOR THE NCLEX® EXAMINATION

Directions: Choose the best answer(s) for the following questions.

1. The patient with elevated cholesterol and two or more cardiac risk factors should be advised to work at keeping the LDL at or below: *(377)*
    1.   150 mg/dL.
    2.   73 mg/dL.
    3.   120 mg/dL.
    4.   210 mg/dL.

2. The nurse knows that in order to correctly perform the procedure for taking an apical pulse, the pulse must be counted for: *(386)*
    1.   15 seconds.
    2.   30 seconds.
    3.   1 minute.
    4.   2 minutes.

3. The nurse has observed that the patient's jugular veins are prominent when the patient is in an upright position. This finding is associated with which of following cardiovascular disorders? *(393)*
    1.   Congestive heart failure
    2.   Cardiac dysrhythmia
    3.   Angina pectoris
    4.   Aortic aneurysm

Copyright © 2013, 2009 by Saunders, an imprint of Elsevier Inc. All rights reserved.

4. When obtaining a patient's blood pressure, the nurse knows that if the blood pressure cuff is too narrow, the blood pressure will be: *(387)*
   1. unaffected by the equipment.
   2. falsely elevated.
   3. lower than expected.
   4. the same in both arms.

5. When planning care for a patient with a cardiovascular problem, it is important to plan activities to: *(388, 392-393)*
   1. promote cardiac output.
   2. prevent venous occlusion.
   3. prevent edema and fluid retention.
   4. promote rest and relieve fatigue.

6. The nurse is evaluating the patient's peripheral pulses. Which intervention(s) should be included in a routine assessment? *(386-387)*
   1. Note rate and rhythm and mark the location.
   2. Take radial pulse on the patient's dominant side.
   3. Compare pulses bilaterally; note volume and strength.
   4. Elevate the extremity and check the pulse.

7. What is considered the best indicator of fluid buildup? *(393)*
   1. Pitting edema
   2. Decreased urinary output
   3. 3 lbs. weight gain in 24 hours
   4. Low serum sodium

8. A patient has a nursing diagnosis of Impaired tissue integrity related to an ulcer from decreased circulation. An appropriate nursing intervention would be: *(394-395)*
   1. increase fluid intake to 3000 mL per day.
   2. promote adequate protein in the diet.
   3. administer the prescribed diuretic to decrease edema.
   4. allow to ventilate feelings about the disease process.

9. When planning nursing care, the nurse knows that many heart medications need to be given as close to the prescribed time as possible. The best rationale for this practice is to: *(385)*
   1. complete shift duties in a timely fashion.
   2. prevent adverse response to medications.
   3. avoid confusing your elderly patients.
   4. maintain a steady blood level of the drug.

10. Which statement by the patient's wife indicates a need for further discussion about modifiable risk factors for cardiac disorders? *(377, Table 18-1)*
    1. "He can't lose weight because his parents were obese."
    2. "He could have up to two alcoholic drinks per day."
    3. "He could take a relaxation or meditation class for stress."
    4. "His blood pressure should be lower than 120/80."

11. The nurse is caring for a patient with Activity intolerance related to chronic heart failure. Which activity(ies) would be best to assign to the nursing assistant? *(393)*
    1. Observe the patient for fatigue and shortness of breath when ambulating.
    2. Assist the patient with limited morning hygiene such as washing face and brushing teeth.
    3. Explain to the family why taking long walks on the hospital grounds is not feasible at this time.
    4. Obtaining assistive devices that would help the patient to conserve energy and strength.

12. When working with patients with lower limb arterial disorders, you know that _____ _____ are contraindicated. *(395)*

Copyright © 2013, 2009 by Saunders, an imprint of Elsevier Inc. All rights reserved.

CRITICAL THINKING ACTIVITIES

Scenario: Mrs. Eoyang is an elderly female who comes to the clinic after experiencing some mild chest pain. She is accompanied by her husband. You are attempting to perform the PQRST for pain assessment. Mr. Eoyang keeps answering for his wife, even though she is alert and oriented and seems capable of answering for herself. She sits quietly and smiles at you, but allows her husband to do the talking despite your best efforts.

1. What is the PQRST pain assessment? *(386, Table 18-3)* _____

   _____

   _____

   _____

2. What other assessment questions would you ask? *(384-388)* _____

   _____

   _____

   _____

3. What are your personal feelings about this type of situation? _____

   _____

   _____

4. What factors (i.e., cultural, social, age, psychological) might help to explain Mr. and Mrs. Eoyang's behavior? *(377, Table 18-1)*

   _____

   _____

   _____

   _____

   _____

   _____

Copyright © 2013, 2009 by Saunders, an imprint of Elsevier Inc. All rights reserved.

STEPS TOWARD BETTER COMMUNICATION

VOCABULARY BUILDING GLOSSARY

Term/Phrase	Pronunciation	Meaning
a whooshing or purring sound	whoosh' ing	a sound like quickly moving air
equipment used should be calibrated	cal' i bray ted	marked with correct units of measure
appear pale and mottled	mot' tled	marked with irregular patches of color
condition indicative of gangrene	in dic' a tive	showing signs of, suggesting
excoriations	ex co ri ay' shuns	scratches or abrasions on skin
it is a good gross assessment	gross ah ses' ment	general and broad, not specific
circulation is occluded by constriction	oc clud' ed	blocked
assessment and staging of edema	stay' jing	determining the extent or phase of a disease or condition
dependent edema	de pen' dent	hanging down, which can cause swelling
impede, impedance	im pede'	to block, to get in the way of
precipitate; precipitating event	pre cip' i tate	to cause to start
assess mentation	men tay' shun	mental activity
collaborate with patients/colleagues	col lab' o rate	to work together with in both planning and action

COMPLETION

Directions: Using the vocabulary above, prepare five sentences. Leave the vocabulary word space blank, and ask a classmate to complete the sentence with the correct word.

1. _____

2. _____

3. _____

4. _____

5. _____

Copyright © 2013, 2009 by Saunders, an imprint of Elsevier Inc. All rights reserved.

VOCABULARY EXERCISE

Descriptors, Descriptive Terms, Special Uses

Directions: The words listed below are used to describe the quality and character of a patient's pulse. If you are not sure of the meaning of some of the words, ask your instructor to explain, or to let you hear an example.

Descriptors of pulse qualities:

full	fast	absent
strong	irregular	hammer-like
weak	regular	normal
thready	erratic	fleeting
bounding	diminished	moderate
rapid	distant	1+, 2+, 3+, 4+ (designates strength)
slow	barely palpable	

Directions: Evaluate the expected pulse of the following three people and write out your assessment findings using the descriptive terms.

Person 1: Radial pulse of someone who has just run a race: _____

_____

Person 2: Pedal pulse of someone with arterial vascular disease: _____

_____

Person 3: Apical pulse of a patient with heart disease who has a dysrhythmia: _____

_____

COMMUNICATION EXERCISE

History-Taking and Documenting Assessment

1. What are the things you would need to ask about in history-taking that would provide information about a cardiovascular patient? What objective observations could you make that would also provide information?

    _____

    _____

    _____

2. With a peer, practice cardiac assessment by asking questions about the risk factors in Table 18-1 of the textbook. Write out the questions you will use. Take turns asking and then answering the questions. Take notes and document your assessment findings. Ask your partner or the instructor to critique your documentation.

    _____

    _____

    _____

    _____

    _____

Copyright © 2013, 2009 by Saunders, an imprint of Elsevier Inc. All rights reserved.

COMMUNICATION EXERCISE

Directions: With a partner, discuss some things you would say to a patient in each of these cases.

1. The patient is in pain and you want to interact therapeutically with active listening.

   _____

   _____

   _____

   _____

   _____

2. Mr. Johnson wants a hot water bottle on his feet because they are cold.

   _____

   _____

   _____

3. Miss Bennett does not want anything to eat or drink, but her medications are to be taken with food.

   _____

   _____

   _____

4. Explain to a family the risks to cardiac health that cannot be controlled or modified and those risks that can be modified.

   _____

   _____

   _____

CULTURAL POINT

African-Americans and females have different experiences with heart conditions and symptoms than those usually described for Caucasian males. Be sure that you learn what these differences are and pay attention to the symptoms of these people.

Copyright © 2013, 2009 by Saunders, an imprint of Elsevier Inc. All rights reserved.

Care of Patients with Hypertension and Peripheral Vascular Disease

chapter

19

Answer Key: Textbook page references are provided as a guide for answering these questions. A complete answer key was provided to your instructor.

COMPLETION

Hypertension

Directions: Fill in the blanks to complete the statements.

1. Long-term hypertension may lead to death from damage to the _____, _____, and _____. *(398)*

2. Prehypertension is a systolic pressure of _____ or a diastolic pressure of _____. *(399, Table 19-1)*

3. Hypertension can be secondary to and symptomatic of other diseases, such as those affecting the blood supply to the_____ and _____. *(399)*

4. Nicotine has a major impact on blood vessels and blood pressure by producing _____. *(406, 411)*

5. Hypertension is diagnosed when an elevated blood pressure is taken at least _____ and averaged on two different occasions, _____ weeks apart. *(401)*

6. The physician examines blood vessels in the _____ to detect signs of persistent hypertension. *(401)*

Copyright © 2013, 2009 by Saunders, an imprint of Elsevier Inc. All rights reserved.

SHORT ANSWER

Hypertension

Directions: Read the following scenario and answer the questions that follow.

Scenario: You are participating in a health fair that includes blood pressure screening for hypertension and dispensing information about healthy lifestyle habits. In addition, interested people are inquiring about how to recognize potential symptoms and various types of treatment, including medication for hypertension.

1. List four specific ways in which a person with mild hypertension might help reduce his blood pressure without taking any antihypertensive drugs. *(401)*

    a. _____

    b. _____

    c. _____

    d. _____

2. List subjective symptoms and objective data that would be significant in the assessment of a patient with hypertension. *(400-401)*

    a. Subjective symptoms: _____

    _____

    b. Objective data: _____

3. The target is to maintain a blood pressure at or below _____. *(401)*

4. List specific patient information in each of the following areas for the patient with mild hypertension: self-care and keeping blood pressure under control.

    a. General lifestyle changes: *(400-401, 404-406)* _____

    _____

    _____

    _____

    _____

    _____

    b. Dietary advice: *(400-401, 404-406)* _____

    _____

    _____

5. List three drug classifications that may be used in the treatment of hypertension and give an example of each classification. *(401-402, Table 19-3)*

    _____

    _____

    _____

Copyright © 2013, 2009 by Saunders, an imprint of Elsevier Inc. All rights reserved.

APPLICATION OF THE NURSING PROCESS

Caring for a Patient with Arterial Insufficiency

Directions: Read the scenario and provide the answers to the following questions.

Scenario: Mrs. Thompson is a secretary and has worked for an engineering firm for 25 years. She has gained several pounds over the holidays and has started walking to try and lose some weight. She reports that she has noticed leg cramps after walking just a couple of blocks. The pain stops when she stops walking for several minutes. The physician tells her that she may have a mild arterial insufficiency that can be treated with exercise and possible medication if her symptoms worsen.

1. What questions would you ask her to determine risk factors for arterial insufficiency? *(409-411)*

   a. _____

   b. _____

   c. _____

2. List five signs and symptoms that would indicate diminished *arterial* blood flow in the peripheral vessels. *(409-410)*

   a. _____

   b. _____

   c. _____

   d. _____

   e. _____

3. You are assessing Mrs. Thompson and checking the "6 Ps." What are the "6 Ps"? *(408)*

   a. _____

   b. _____

   c. _____

   d. _____

   e. _____

   f. _____

4. The doctor tells Mrs. Thompson that she has intermittent claudication. You explain to her that intermittent claudication is characterized by: *(407)*
   a. edema of the lower legs.
   b. cramping pain occurring with walking that eases with rest.
   c. warm, reddened areas on the lower legs.
   d. pale, cold feet.

5. What are three major nursing goals for patients like Mrs. Thompson? *(410-411)*

   a. _____

   b. _____

   c. _____

Copyright © 2013, 2009 by Saunders, an imprint of Elsevier Inc. All rights reserved.

6. List five self-care measures that could be taught to Mrs. Thompson to help her cope with impaired peripheral circulation. *(409-411)*

   a. _____

   b. _____

   c. _____

   d. _____

   e. _____

7. Write evaluation criteria that would indicate that the interventions are successful and the expected outcome is being met for Mrs. Thompson for the following expected outcome: *(411)*

   Patient will verbalize three self-care measures to protect tissues from injury due to decreased arterial flow after a patient teaching session.

   a. _____

   b. _____

   c. _____

PRIORITY SETTING

Directions: Read the scenario and prioritize as appropriate.

Scenario: You are caring for Mr. Elisandro, who has been admitted for a diagnosis of deep vein thrombosis, and he is currently on bedrest and receiving IV heparin. He has anti-embolism (TED) hose in place, with sequential compression devices (SCDs).

1. In the morning, you enter Mr. Elisandro's room and you find that the IV heparin has been turned off. Mr. Elisandro tells you that "somebody came in during the evening and took the IV pump away." What is your priority action? *(416)*
   a. Quickly obtain a new pump and restart the heparin.
   b. Report the incident to the charge nurse.
   c. Obtain a physician's order for partial thromboplastin time (PTT) and activated partial thromboplastin time (aPTT).
   d. Check the physician's orders to see if heparin was discontinued.

2. Mr. Elisandro is lying in bed. His TED hose are in place, but the SCDs are at the bottom of the bed. He tells you that the new nursing assistant removed them during morning hygiene. What is your priority action? *(416)*
   a. Replace the SCDs; talk to the nursing assistant about the purpose of SCDs.
   b. Instruct the nursing assistant on how to replace the SCDs.
   c. Teach the patient how to replace them and to call for assistance as needed.
   d. Report the incident to the nursing educator and the charge nurse.

3. While you are assessing Mr. Elisandro after lunch, you note several abnormal findings. Which assessment finding is the priority? *(414-416)*
   a. Bleeding of the gums and petechiae
   b. Dyspnea and tachypnea
   c. Increasing pain in the calf
   d. Pitting edema of the affected limb

Copyright © 2013, 2009 by Saunders, an imprint of Elsevier Inc. All rights reserved.

4. Based on your determination of the priority assessment finding (#3 above), which action will you take first? *(415-416)*
   a. Check the PTT and aPTT results.
   b. Obtain equipment to give oxygen.
   c. Assess the quality/onset of calf pain.
   d. Measure the circumference of the limb.

REVIEW QUESTIONS FOR THE NCLEX® EXAMINATION

Directions: Choose the best answer(s) for the following questions.

1. When assessing a patient for possible peripheral vascular disease (PVD), which is a prime contributing factor? *(406)*
   1. History of structural defects in the arteries.
   2. History of excessive alcohol intake.
   3. History of inflammation of the veins.
   4. History of cigarette smoking.

2. A nursing assessment that is most important in the care of a patient with a deep vein thrombosis is to assess for: *(415-416)*
   1. pale, cool extremity.
   2. decreasing level of consciousness.
   3. sudden shortness of breath.
   4. sudden acute pain.

3. A secondary cause of peripheral arterial disorders is: *(407)*
   1. diabetes mellitus.
   2. a sedentary lifestyle.
   3. rheumatic fever.
   4. hypertension.

4. It is most important to teach the patient with chronic venous stasis to sit with the legs: *(421)*
   1. crossed.
   2. straight.
   3. elevated.
   4. dependent.

5. The nurse is teaching the patient about dietary sources of potassium. Which food group is the best dietary source for potassium? *(403, Box 19-1)*
   1. Milk, cheese, and eggs
   2. Beef, turkey, and tomatoes
   3. Whole-grain bread and cereals
   4. Lettuce, cabbage, and onions

6. An acute sign of inadequate blood supply to the feet is: *(400-402, 413-414)*
   1. excessive hair growth.
   2. reddened, warm skin.
   3. brittle, thick toenails.
   4. pale, cool, mottled skin.

Copyright © 2013, 2009 by Saunders, an imprint of Elsevier Inc. All rights reserved.

7. The patient is taking digoxin and a thiazide diuretic. This combination of medications increases the risk for cardiac dysrhythmias related to: *(402, Table 19-3)*
   1. hypokalemia.
   2. hypotension.
   3. hyperkalemia.
   4. hypertension.

8. When evaluating continuous intravenous heparin therapy for a patient with a deep vein thrombosis, the nurse assesses for: *(416)*
   1. the degree of discomfort the patient is experiencing.
   2. the results of the prothrombin time laboratory test.
   3. signs of internal and external bleeding.
   4. nausea and anorexia due to the medication.

9. The medication cilostazol (Pletal) is used for patients experiencing intermittent claudication to: *(409)*
   1. relax vessel walls and increase blood flow to the legs.
   2. decrease the possibility of platelet aggregation.
   3. decrease foot and leg edema.
   4. dissolve any clots in the vessels of the legs.

10. Upon assessment, signs of abdominal aortic aneurysm include: *(411)*
    1. higher blood pressure in the legs than in the arms.
    2. bounding popliteal pulses and warm, pink skin.
    3. an enlarged abdomen with decreased bowel sounds.
    4. back pain and possibly a visible pulsation of the abdomen.

11. Factors that contribute to the formation of varicose veins include: *(Select all that apply.)* *(419)*
    1. gaining too much weight.
    2. family history of diabetes.
    3. family history of atherosclerosis or hypertension.
    4. standing regularly for long periods of time.
    5. congenital heart problems.
    6. pregnancy.

12. When providing postoperative care for a patient following a carotid endarterectomy, which of following assessment findings is the priority concern? *(413)*
    1. Increasing hoarseness
    2. Loss of appetite
    3. Presence of a bruit
    4. Nausea

13. Teaching for a patient discharged on warfarin (Coumadin) includes keeping appointments for frequent laboratory tests to check the: *(416)*
    1. serum heparin level.
    2. activated partial thromboplastin time or partial thromboplastin time.
    3. platelet aggregation test.
    4. International Normalized Ratio value and/or prothrombin time.

CRITICAL THINKING ACTIVITIES

Scenario: You are working with several patients who are to receive heparin. Perform the following math calculations to determine the correct dose or to verify the setting of the IV infusion.

Copyright © 2013, 2009 by Saunders, an imprint of Elsevier Inc. All rights reserved.

1. The patient is on an IV heparin drip for treatment of a deep vein thrombosis. The IV heparin bag (25,000 units/250 mL) is in place with a pump. It is set to infuse at 8 mL/hour. The physician has ordered 800 units/hour. Is the pump setting correct or incorrect? _____

2. The doctor orders 5000 units SQ heparin for postoperative prophylaxis. The pharmacy delivers a 10-mL vial of heparin sodium (5000 units/mL). How many mL should you give? _____

3. The pharmacy delivers a premixed bag of heparin 20,000 units/500 mL. How many units are in 1 mL? _____

4. The patient is on an IV heparin drip. The IV heparin bag (10,000 units/100 mL) is in place with a pump. It is set to infuse at 10 mL/hour. The physician has ordered 1000 units/hour. Is the pump setting correct or incorrect? _____

STEPS TOWARD BETTER COMMUNICATION

VOCABULARY BUILDING GLOSSARY

Term	Pronunciation	Definition
bar'orecep'tor	bar o re sep' tor	sensory receptor stimulated by changes in pressure
claudica'tion	klaw di kay' shun	pain in leg muscles, limping or lameness
depen'dent	de pen'dent	hanging down
incom'petent	in com'pe tent	not able to perform the function or job
ischemia	is kee' me a	insufficient blood in a part
periph'eral	pa rif' ah ral	on the outer edges
poten'tiated	po ten' shee ay ted	made more powerful (two drugs may react together to be more powerful)
synco'pe	sing ko' pee	temporary loss of consciousness, fainting
tor'tuous	tor' chew us	twisted, winding
viscos'ity	vis cos' i tee	thickness of a liquid
noncompli'ant	non com ply'ant	does not follow instructions
"silent" symptoms		symptoms that the patient is unable to observe or feel
side effect		result of a treatment or medication that is an addition to the intended effect

COMPLETION

Directions: Fill in the blanks with the appropriate words from the Vocabulary Building Glossary to complete the statements.

1. When taking a blood pressure, the arm should be at the level of the heart rather than _____

   _____.

Copyright © 2013, 2009 by Saunders, an imprint of Elsevier Inc. All rights reserved.

2. When the nurse assessed the patient's arm before trying to start an intravenous infusion, the veins were found to be _____.

3. The patient who is polycythemic has increased blood _____.

4. The patient with swollen, dusky feet probably has _____ vascular disease.

5. Many hypertensive patients are _____ with therapy because they do not notice any symptoms of high blood pressure.

6. The patient who has peripheral arterial vascular disease often experiences _____ _____ when walking.

7. A(n) _____ signals the brain about changes in blood pressure.

8. When a vein develops varicosities, it becomes _____.

9. The effect on blood pressure is _____ when an antihypertensive is combined with a diuretic medication.

10. Hypertension often causes only _____.

11. When a thrombosis occurs in a vessel, _____ develops distal to it.

12. Carotid occlusion may cause _____ in the patient.

13. Hypokalemia is a(n) _____ of many diuretics.

WORD ATTACK SKILLS

Combining Forms

These combining forms are used in words found in Chapter 18 of the textbook:

angi/o	vessel, channel
vaso	vessel, duct
sclero	hard, hardening
ven/o	vein
thromb/o	blood clot
sta/	make stand, stop
sten/	narrow, compressed

Directions: Write the meanings of the following words constructed from the combining forms above. Use your dictionary as necessary.

1. Vasospasm:_____

2. Vasodilator: _____

3. Vasoconstriction: _____

4. Vasopressor:_____

Copyright © 2013, 2009 by Saunders, an imprint of Elsevier Inc. All rights reserved.

5. Vasomotor: _____

6. Sclerosis: _____

7. Venogram: _____

8. Venous: _____

9. Thrombectomy: _____

10. Thrombosis: _____

11. Thrombus: _____

12. Stasis: _____

13. Stent: _____

Copyright © 2013, 2009 by Saunders, an imprint of Elsevier Inc. All rights reserved.

Care of Patients with Cardiac Disorders

Answer Key: Textbook page references are provided as a guide for answering these questions. A complete answer key was provided to your instructor.

COMPLETION

Cardiac Disorders

Directions: Fill in the blanks to complete the statements.

1. A(n) _____ is used for patients who have repeated episodes of life-threatening ventricular fibrillation or cardiac asystole (arrest). *(442)*

2. The signs and symptoms of mitral valve disorders are _____, _____, _____, and _____. *(445)*

3. A myocardial infarction may lead to heart failure because damage to the muscle causes _____ _____. *(427-428, see also Chapter 21)*

4. Valve surgery is performed on the dysfunctional valve when the person's _____ _____. *(446)*

5. A sign of pericarditis that can be heard during auscultation of the heart is _____ _____. *(443)*

6. _____ imbalances may cause serious cardiac dysrhythmias. *(434)*

7. Untreated strep throat may lead to _____ and _____ disease. *(445)*

8. An elderly patient with a history of heart failure can experience a relapse from a(n) _____. *(432)*

Copyright © 2013, 2009 by Saunders, an imprint of Elsevier Inc. All rights reserved.

APPLICATION OF THE NURSING PROCESS

Care of the Patient with Congestive Heart Failure

Directions: Read the scenario and provide the answers to the following questions. (427-435)

Scenario: Mrs. Jackson, age 68, has congestive heart failure. She has been admitted to the hospital for complaints of severe dyspnea, generalized edema, weakness, and fatigue. Her physician has ordered bedrest, up to bathroom PRN, in chair for 30 minutes three times a day, and oxygen at 5 L/min for dyspnea. Mrs. Jackson is also receiving digoxin (Lanoxin) 0.25 mg daily, hydrochlorothiazide (a diuretic), and Isordil (a venous dilator). Her daily sodium intake is limited to 1000 mg.

1. List objective and subjective data that would help assess Mrs. Jackson's status with regard to dyspnea, edema, and peripheral circulation.

    a. Dyspnea: Subjective data:_____

    _____

    Objective data: _____

    _____

    b. Edema: Subjective data: _____

    _____

    Objective data: _____

    _____

    c. Peripheral circulation: Subjective data: _____

    _____

    Objective data: _____

    _____

2. Upon admission, which of the following nursing diagnoses is a priority for Mrs. Jackson? *(432-433)*
    a. Activity intolerance related to decreased perfusion
    b. Risk for injury related to complications of CHF
    c. Decreased cardiac output related to ineffective cardiac pumping
    d. Dyspnea, gas exchange, impaired, related to fluid in lung tissue

3. List three nursing actions you would expect to find on Mrs. Jackson's nursing care plan for "Decreased cardiac output related to ineffective cardiac pumping" during her hospitalization. *(431-434)*

    a. _____

    b. _____

    c. _____

4. An appropriate task to assign to the nursing assistant would be to: *(431-434)*
    a. ask the patient if she needs extra pillows to prevent orthopnea.
    b. assist the patient to turn every 1–2 hours.
    c. determine if Mrs. Jackson needs partial or full assistance with ADLs.
    d. check the sacral area for edema and skin breakdown.

Copyright © 2013, 2009 by Saunders, an imprint of Elsevier Inc. All rights reserved.

5. Mrs. Jackson lives with her husband, daughter, and four grandchildren. Before she is discharged, she will need instruction in self-care and her family will need instruction so they can give her support and encouragement. She has been told by her physician to work up to walking at least 1 mile per day, to continue taking her digoxin and diuretic, to stay on her sodium-limited diet, and to lose 25 pounds. Identify at least five points that should be included in the teaching plan for Mrs. Jackson and her family so that she can remain relatively symptom-free once she returns home. *(432-434)*

   a. _____

   b. _____

   c. _____

   d. _____

   e. _____

6. Which of the following statements by Mrs. Jackson indicates that she understands the implications of digoxin toxicity? *(430, 447, Table 20-4)*
   a. "I will report nausea, vomiting, and anorexia."
   b. "I can eat bananas and citrus to counteract side effects."
   c. "I can skip a dose if I experience side effects."
   d. "I should carry digoxin immune (Digifab) as an antidote."

7. Mrs. Jackson is prescribed digoxin 0.50 mg daily. The pharmacy delivers a bottle with 50 Lanoxin tablets of 0.25 mg/tablet. Has the pharmacy delivered the correct medication? _____ If so, how many tablets should Mrs. Jackson take? _____

PRIORITY SETTING

Directions: Read the scenario and prioritize as appropriate.

Scenario: You are caring for Mr. Hijazi, an elderly gentleman who was admitted for heart failure related to mitral valve disease. During the morning assessment you find that his condition seems to have deteriorated compared to yesterday. You find several abnormalities. *(444-445)*

1. Which assessment finding is the most important?
   a. Absent peripheral pulses
   b. Frothy sputum and orthopnea
   c. Confusion and irritability
   d. Fever and tachycardia

2. Based on your assessment findings, Mr. Hijazi appears to be having complications due to heart failure and he is exhibiting the signs and symptoms of acute pulmonary edema. Rank according to priority of action: _____ *(431)*
   a. Report your findings to the RN/physician.
   b. Administer oxygen and morphine per standing orders.
   c. Place the patient in a high Fowler's position.
   d. Provide reassurance and support.

Copyright © 2013, 2009 by Saunders, an imprint of Elsevier Inc. All rights reserved.

REVIEW QUESTIONS FOR THE NCLEX® EXAMINATION

Directions: Choose the best answer(s) for the following questions.

1. Which would the patient most likely report when experiencing atrial fibrillation? *(437-438)*
   1. Low blood pressure
   2. Headaches and fatigue
   3. Feelings of palpitations
   4. An irregular pulse rate

2. Medications that the nurse might administer to a patient with atrial fibrillation include: *(438-439, Table 20-4)*
   1. digoxin and Coumadin.
   2. potassium and Tenormin.
   3. lidocaine and calcium.
   4. aspirin and Isordil.

3. A patient is receiving digoxin. To evaluate the effectiveness of the medication, the nurse would check: *(439, Table 20-4)*
   1. pulse rate and breath sounds.
   2. digoxin and potassium laboratory values.
   3. blood pressure and respirations.
   4. weight loss and appetite.

4. Early signs of heart failure include: *(428-429)*
   1. weight gain and dyspnea on exertion.
   2. a wet cough and severely swollen ankles.
   3. cyanosis, fatigue, and dyspnea.
   4. an irregular pulse rate and elevated blood pressure.

5. When the nurse is administering digoxin, she should always first: *(430, 447, Table 20-4)*
   1. assess the amount of weight gain or loss.
   2. question the patient about fatigue and dizziness.
   3. check for signs of hypokalemia.
   4. be certain that the patient has a full stomach.

6. A patient with third-degree heart block will demonstrate: *(436)*
   1. a very slow pulse.
   2. a spike in blood pressure.
   3. edema in the lower extremities.
   4. rapid breathing and diaphoresis.

7. Upon assessment of the patient with aortic stenosis, the nurse might find which sign that differs from other valve disorders? *(445)*
   1. Cardiac murmur
   2. Pulsus paradoxus
   3. Dyspnea upon exertion
   4. Widened pulse pressure

8. The postoperative care of a patient who has received a permanent pacemaker includes: *(Select all that apply.)* *(441)*
   1. Monitor heart rate and rhythm and check vital signs.
   2. Perform dressing changes and care for the insertion site.
   3. Check peripheral pulses proximal to the insertion sites.
   4. Check level of consciousness frequently in the immediate postoperative period.
   5. Teach the patient to count his pulse for a full minute.
   6. Teach patient that full recovery takes about 12 weeks.

Copyright © 2013, 2009 by Saunders, an imprint of Elsevier Inc. All rights reserved.

9. When planning care for a patient who needs dietary modifications to improve heart health, the nurse would include teaching to: *(447-448)*
   1. include 12 grams of fiber in diet each day.
   2. include only foods that contain no trans-fats.
   3. avoid drinking any coffee or iced beverages.
   4. decrease the sodium and fat intake.

10. You are helping a patient with atrial fibrillation ambulate and she wobbles and tells you, "I'm suddenly quite dizzy." Which action should you take first? *(437)*
    1. Tell her to take a few slow deep breaths.
    2. Take her blood pressure.
    3. Assess her pulse rate and rhythm.
    4. Help her to sit down.

CRITICAL THINKING ACTIVITIES

Scenario: You are assigned to work on a telemetry unit. There is a telemetry technician who is monitoring the patients from a remote location; however, there is a monitor at the nurse's station that is displaying the ECG rhythm for each patient. Although the technician will call if he notes a problem, the nurses are responsible to also be able to recognize arrhythmias and respond accordingly.

Directions: Identify the EKG rhythms and answer the related questions. (435-440)

1. Rhythm strip #1

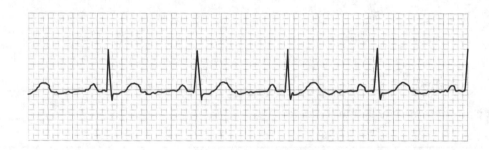

   a. Identify this rhythm. _____

   b. What is the appropriate action to take? _____

   _____

Copyright © 2013, 2009 by Saunders, an imprint of Elsevier Inc. All rights reserved.

2. Rhythm strip #2

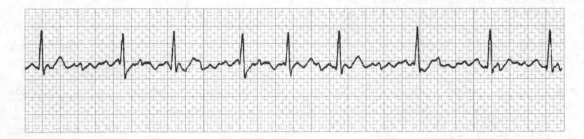

a. Identify this rhythm. _____

b. Explain why patients who have this arrhythmia may be on Coumadin.

_____

_____

3. Rhythm strip #3

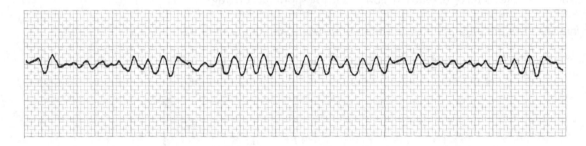

a. Identify this rhythm. _____

b. What is the appropriate action to take? _____

_____

4. Rhythm strip #4

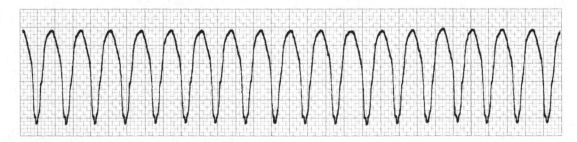

a. Identify this rhythm. _____

b. What are two medical treatments that could be ordered to treat this arrhythmia?

_____

_____

Copyright © 2013, 2009 by Saunders, an imprint of Elsevier Inc. All rights reserved.

5. Rhythm strip #5

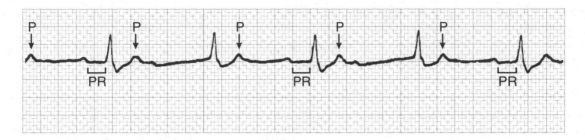

a. Identify this rhythm. _____

b. Explain in your own words why this rhythm may cause your patient to have a change in mental status.

_____

_____

STEPS TOWARD BETTER COMMUNICATION

VOCABULARY BUILDING GLOSSARY

Term	Pronunciation	Definition
inva'sive	in vay'sive	involving the puncture or cutting of the skin, or putting an instrument into the body
telem'etry	te lem' e tree	measuring data with radio waves and electronic equipment
engorg'ed	en gorj' d	filled to the limit; swollen
bloated	blow' tid	to be swollen, larger than normal
quiver	kwiv' er	to vibrate with a small, rapid motion
hyper'trophy	hi per' tro fee	extra growth, thickened
cardiomyop'athy	kar dee o mi op' ah thee	disorder of heart muscle that prevents it from pumping effectively
a'trioventric'ular	a' tree o ven trik' you lar	relating to an atrium and ventricle of the heart
fib'rilla'tion	fib' ri la' shun	small, rapid, irregular muscle contractions; quivering
intersti'tial	in ter stish' al	spaces in the tissue between the cells

Copyright © 2013, 2009 by Saunders, an imprint of Elsevier Inc. All rights reserved.

COMPLETION

Directions: Fill in the blanks with the appropriate words from the Vocabulary Building Glossary to complete the statements.

1. During ventricular fibrillation, the heart _____.

2. The patient whose heart rate is being monitored is hooked up to a(n) _____ unit that transmits the EKG pattern to the monitor in the nurse's station.

3. _____ or increased growth of left ventricle muscle may be hereditary.

4. When congestive heart failure occurs, the lung vessels become _____ with blood and fluid leaks into the interstitial spaces.

5. A cardiac catheterization is a(n) _____ type of test.

6. The major problems exhibited by patients with _____ are heart failure and dysrhythmias.

7. If the SA node fails to pace the heart, the _____ node may take over.

8. Patients can be treated for chronic atrial _____, but ventricular _____ is life-threatening.

9. The patient who experiences right-sided congestive heart failure develops a swollen liver and may feel _____.

10. Edema results if body fluids in the intravascular fluid compartment begin to leak into the _____ compartment.

WORD ATTACK SKILLS

Combining Forms

Here are some important combining forms found in this chapter:

cardi/o	heart
my/o	muscle
sin/o	a space or channel
vas/o	vessel
end/o	inside

Copyright © 2013, 2009 by Saunders, an imprint of Elsevier Inc. All rights reserved.

COMMUNICATION EXERCISE

You are advising Mrs. Perryman who has complained of pain in her legs due to varicose veins. She also has high blood pressure. (Practice the dialogue with a partner.)

Mrs. Perryman:	My legs hurt—and look at these ugly varicose veins! My feet and legs hurt at the end of the day. They are swollen. And I get so tired!
Nurse:	Would you like me to work out a plan with you that might help?
Mrs. Perryman:	Oh, yes! That would be wonderful.
Nurse:	I would like you to wear these support hose—but no tight underwear or pants or garters that would cut off the circulation. If you can put the hose on in the morning while you are still in bed it would help.
Mrs. Perryman:	Why is that?
Nurse:	If you put them on before your legs swell, it helps keep the circulation flowing. When your legs hang off the edge of the bed they swell with the blood flowing to them.
Mrs. Perryman:	That makes sense.
Nurse:	When you are sitting, I would like you to keep your feet elevated if you can. Do you get much exercise?
Mrs. Perryman:	No, not very much.
Nurse:	Let's see if you can do more walking. You can begin with just 15 minutes at a time. If you could do swimming or water aerobics it would be a big help.
Mrs. Perryman:	Where could I do that?
Nurse:	The YMCA and the parks department sometimes have programs. I can check into it and let you know. Are you a smoker?
Mrs. Perryman:	No, not for years.
Nurse:	That's good, because smoking constricts the blood vessels even more. About your diet—if we can get you on a low-salt, low-fat, heart-healthy diet that will help a lot. I will show you how to read the food labels. That's it—diet, exercise, wearing support hose, and keeping your legs elevated.
Mrs. Perryman:	That sounds like a lot to do.
Nurse:	Yes, it is, but you will feel so much better—and it could even save your life! Next week when I visit, we will see if we can tell the difference in your blood pressure, too.

Copyright © 2013, 2009 by Saunders, an imprint of Elsevier Inc. All rights reserved.

Care of Patients with Coronary Artery Disease and Cardiac Surgery

Answer Key: Textbook page references are provided as a guide for answering these questions. A complete answer key was provided to your instructor.

TERMINOLOGY

Directions: Define the following terms relative to the heart.

1. Angina pectoris: *(453-454)*_____

2. Coronary insufficiency: *(452)* _____

3. Drug-eluting stent: *(464)* _____

4. Myocardial infarction: *(451-458)*_____

5. Infarction: *(458)* _____

6. Ischemia: *(453)*_____

COMPLETION

Directions: Fill in the blanks to complete the statements.

1. As the coronary vessels narrow, the patient may experience symptoms of ischemia such as

   _____ and _____. *(451)*

2. Women are more likely to experience heart attacks after reaching _____; however, poor

   _____ habits, _____ lifestyle, and _____ levels of stress contribute to

   development of cardiovascular disease earlier in life. *(456)*

3. For women, the main symptoms of a heart attack may be diffuse chest pain, extreme fatigue, and tender-

   ness to touch or a burning or tingling sensation, which may be mistaken for _____

   _____. *(455)*

4. Any activity that increases the heart's workload increases its need for _____. *(453)*

5. The prognosis of the patient who suffers an acute myocardial infarction (MI) depends on the

   _____ of the artery obstructed, the location, and the _____ of

   heart tissue that is damaged. *(458)*

Copyright © 2013, 2009 by Saunders, an imprint of Elsevier Inc. All rights reserved.

6. Another treatment method for occlusion of a coronary artery other than coronary artery bypass graft is the procedure called _____. *(464)*

7. To lower cholesterol and maintain a healthy diet, it is recommended to eat fish at least _____ a week. *(453)*

8. A thrombolytic agent must be administered within _____ hours of experiencing the symptoms of MI, in order to prevent or decrease damage to the heart muscle. *(460)*

9. After receiving a heart transplant, the patient must take _____ for life. *(466)*

10. Two constant potential complications that the heart transplant patient must deal with are _____ and _____. *(466, 469)*

11. The doctor orders IV fluid for a postoperative patient to infuse at 125 mL/hour. The drop factor is 10 gtts/mL. What is the drip rate? _____

12. Omega-3 fatty acids have been found to _____ in patients with hyperlipidemia. *(453)*

13. If a person is suspected of having a heart attack at home, besides immediately calling 911 and having the person lie down, it is wise to give the person _____. *(459-460)*

TABLE ACTIVITY

Cardiac Surgeries

Directions: Fill in the blocks below with the type of surgery that matches the description. The first block has been done for you.

Type of Surgery	Description
Coronary artery bypass graft (CABG)	Surgery bypasses the blocked artery, replacing it with sections of a vein or artery taken from another part of the patient's body *(465)*
	Does not require stopping the heart's activity, and therefore does not require using the heart-lung machine *(466)*
	Invasive and similar to the procedure used for cardiac catheterization where a catheter is introduced through the femoral vessel *(464)*
	Accomplished with a mechanical or biological device *(see Chapter 20)*
	Performed for selected patients who have end-stage left ventricular failure resulting from cardiomyopathy *(466)*

Copyright © 2013, 2009 by Saunders, an imprint of Elsevier Inc. All rights reserved.

APPLICATION OF THE NURSING PROCESS

Care of a Patient with Angina Pectoris

Directions: Provide the answer to the following questions.

Scenario: Mr. Souza, age 62, is admitted to the hospital with chest pains. Over the past year, he has gradually become more fatigued and uncomfortable whenever he exerts himself. His admitting diagnosis is possible angina pectoris.

1. What specific questions would you ask when taking Mr. Souza's history that could be helpful in assessing his cardiovascular status? *(451, 455)*

    a. _____

    b. _____

    c. _____

    d. _____

2. Two nursing diagnoses on Mr. Souza's nursing care plan are Pain and Knowledge deficit. List three specific nursing interventions appropriate for each nursing diagnosis.

    Pain related to decreased coronary artery circulation: *(455)*

    a. _____

    b. _____

    c. _____

    Knowledge deficit related to self-care: *(455)*

    a. _____

    b. _____

    c. _____

3. Which objective data indicate(s) that Mr. Souza's level of physical activity is appropriate to his recovery? *(455)*
    a. Patient asks for assistance when he becomes fatigued.
    b. Patient's heart rate and respiratory rate are stable after ambulation.
    c. Patient's activity is observed by the physical therapist.
    d. Family tells you that he is walking like he used to prior to hospitalization.

Copyright © 2013, 2009 by Saunders, an imprint of Elsevier Inc. All rights reserved.

PRIORITY SETTING

Directions: Read the scenario and prioritize as appropriate.

You are working in an extended-care facility. Mr. Ido is walking down the hall and reports to you that he is having angina. He has a PRN order for sublingual nitroglycerine and he asks you to assist him with the medication that is on his bedside table. Prioritize the steps in administering the nitroglycerine. *(454-455)*

_____   a. If the pain has not eased or if BP increases, administer a second tablet.

_____   b. Give one tablet, placed under the tongue, wait 5 minutes.

_____   c. Notify the physician regarding pain.

_____   d. Assist the patient to lie in bed.

_____   e. Wait 5 minutes, reassess pain.

_____   f. Obtain a baseline BP.

_____   g. Reassess pain and recheck BP.

_____   h. Administer a third tablet if pain persists.

_____   i. Recheck BP; it should have decreased.

REVIEW QUESTIONS FOR THE NCLEX® EXAMINATION

Directions: Choose the best answer(s) for the following questions.

1. The risk factors that lead to a higher incidence of atherosclerosis include: *(Select all that apply.)* *(451)*
    1. High levels of high-density lipoproteins
    2. Cigarette smoking
    3. A history of hypertension and diabetes mellitus
    4. Age (> age 40), gender, and race
    5. Women on oral contraceptives or estrogen replacement therapy

2. What is the most significant in diagnosing damage to the myocardium? *(459)*
    1. Elevated level of troponin
    2. Elevated level of creatine phosphokinase (CPK)
    3. Elevated level of creatine phosphokinase-MB (CK-MB)
    4. Elevated level of lactate dehydrogenase (LDH)

3. The patient taking lovastatin (Mevacor) for treatment of hypercholesterolemia should have follow-up because of the potential for: *(454, Table 21-1)*
    1. nephrotoxcity.
    2. cardiotoxicity.
    3. hepatotoxicity.
    4. ototoxicity.

4. The patient presents in the emergency department with severe chest pain. Which drugs are likely to be prescribed during the initial emergency care? *(454, 455, 459-460, Table 21-1)*
    1. Morphine, oxygen, nitrates, aspirin
    2. Beta-blockers, clopidogrel (Plavix)
    3. Simvastatin (Lipitor), lorazepam (Ativan)
    4. Oxygen, dobutamine (Dobutrex)

Copyright © 2013, 2009 by Saunders, an imprint of Elsevier Inc. All rights reserved.

5. Which statement by the patient indicates a need for additional teaching about taking his nitroglycerine? *(455)*
   1. "I should try to sit or lie down before I take a tablet."
   2. "If I get a headache, I should not take any more."
   3. "I can take up to three tablets before I call my doctor."
   4. "The tablets should be stored in a dark bottle."

6. When an elderly person sustains an MI, symptoms expressed are often: *(459)*
   1. severe chest pain, nausea, and dizziness.
   2. dyspnea, nausea, confusion, or indigestion.
   3. pain in the arms and clammy skin.
   4. palpitations, chest pain, and fatigue.

7. The physician is considering using fibrinolytic therapy such as t-PA (Activase) for a patient who has come into the ED experiencing an MI. Which information is most important to relay to the physician? *(460)*
   1. History of hypertension
   2. History of hemorrhagic stroke
   3. Symptom onset 3 hours ago
   4. Intraspinal surgery during childhood

8. Which criteria would indicate that the interventions after an MI are helping meet the expected outcome of "patient will suffer no further cardiac damage"? *(460-461)*
   1. Lessened chest pain
   2. Conscious and interacting appropriately
   3. Maintained in sinus rhythm without PVCs
   4. No complaints of heartburn

9. For a patient who is taking a statin drug, an important teaching point to include would be to: *(453-454, Table 21-1)*
   1. report muscle tenderness or pain that persists for more than a few days.
   2. increase consumption of grapefruit juice to supply K^+.
   3. have follow-up appointments to monitor platelet count.
   4. discontinue medication when the target weight goal is met.

10. You are ready to begin your patient assessments after receiving report. Which patient will you assess first? *(464-469)*
    1. A 36-year-old with mitral stenosis scheduled for a balloon valvuloplasty later in the morning
    2. An 82-year-old one day postoperative after coronary bypass surgery who has a temperature of 100.5° F
    3. A 52-year-old with cardiomyopathy who developed chest pain and shortness of breath during shift change
    4. A 63-year-old who had coronary angioplasty yesterday afternoon who has had occasional chest pain since the procedure

11. There are several patients on a busy cardiac rehabilitation unit who need assistance. Which task would be appropriate to assign to the nursing assistant?
    1. Find out why a depressed patient is not doing his physical therapy.
    2. Answer a family member's question about how to contact a local support group.
    3. Escort a patient who has been discharged home to his wife's car.
    4. Listen to a patient who is complaining about the bad hospital food.

12. After a myocardial infarction, the patient is monitored for cardiogenic shock. A sign that cardiogenic shock is impending might be: *(461-462)*
    1. crackles in the lungs upon auscultation.
    2. slowing of the pulse rate.
    3. a cardiac arrhythmia.
    4. decreasing urine flow to 20 mL per hour.

Copyright © 2013, 2009 by Saunders, an imprint of Elsevier Inc. All rights reserved.

CRITICAL THINKING ACTIVITIES

Scenario A: You are at the local park for a neighborhood picnic. You notice that Mrs. Grandville, a middle-aged obese woman, is holding her hand over her chest. She tells you that she is "having a little indigestion from the potato salad;" however, you notice that she is breathing faster than normal and she appears anxious. On further questioning, she admits to chest pressure, but she says that she will just drive herself home and rest. She declines your offer to help or your advice about going to the hospital.

1. What coping mechanism is Mrs. Grandville using to respond to the symptoms? (458-459)

   _____

2. Explain in your own words how the use of this coping mechanism affects her decision-making.

   _____

   _____

   _____

3. Write a brief dialogue that you could use with Mrs. Grandville so that she can make an informed decision.

   _____

   _____

   _____

   _____

   _____

   _____

Scenario B: You are making home visits to Mr. Ketauna, an elderly patient who has chronic cardiomyopathy. The family reports that Mr. Ketauna is mentally active, although he is somewhat depressed, because over the past several years his quality of life has steadily been decreasing. They are considering asking the doctor if he would be a candidate for a heart transplant. You suggest that the family talk to the doctor and you decide to do some research to help clarify their concerns.

1. List at least five of the criteria for heart transplant. *(466)*

   a. _____

   b. _____

   c. _____

   d. _____

   e. _____

Copyright © 2013, 2009 by Saunders, an imprint of Elsevier Inc. All rights reserved.

2. What are some of the ethical implications for the above criteria when trying to determine who will or will not receive an organ transplant?

_____

_____

_____

_____

_____

_____

_____

3. In your own words, discuss some adjustments that the family and the prospective recipient would have to make while waiting on the transplant list.

_____

_____

_____

_____

_____

_____

_____

_____

STEPS TOWARD BETTER COMMUNICATION

VOCABULARY BUILDING GLOSSARY

Term	Definition
col lat′er al	(adj.) parallel, secondary
com pen′ sa tor y	(adj.) making up for, counterbalancing
com′pro mise	(noun) a settlement between two sides that both agree on; (verb) 1. to make such an agreement; 2. to expose to danger by unwise action
e′ti ol′o gy	(noun) the cause, origin
ex′tra cor por′e al	(adj.) outside the body
fi′brous	(adj.) made of fibers, long thin strands of tissue
prog no′sis	(noun) an advance indication, a forecast or prospect of the probable outcome
wean, weaning (ween)	(verb) a gradual withdrawal

Copyright © 2013, 2009 by Saunders, an imprint of Elsevier Inc. All rights reserved.

COMPLETION

Directions: Fill in the blanks with the appropriate word from the glossary above to complete the statements.

1. The pathology report will help determine the _____ of the disease.

2. _____ plaques build up in the arteries, occluding the blood flow.

3. The _____ for the patient depends on the size and location of the obstruction in the artery.

4. The oxydemands from exertion may _____ the coronary circulation of an elderly person.

5. Patients whose bodies have a strong _____ mechanism may have a well-developed _____ circulation.

6. When the heart-lung machine is used to pump and oxygenate the blood, the procedure is called _____ circulation.

7. After surgery, _____ from the ventilator is begun if oxygenation is adequate.

MATCHING

Directions: Match the abbreviation on the left with the correct meaning on the right.

1. _____ CAD   a. Coronary care unit
2. _____ CHF   b. Percutaneous transluminal coronary angioplasty
3. _____ CK   c. Myocardial infarction
4. _____ CCU   d. Coronary artery bypass graft
5. _____ ECG   e. Congestive heart failure
6. _____ MI   f. Acute coronary syndrome
7. _____ CVP   g. Central venous pressure
8. _____ PAP   h. Metabolic equivalents
9. _____ PCWP   i. Creatine kinase
10. _____ PTCA   j. Coronary artery disease
11. _____ CABG   k. Pulmonary artery pressure
12. _____ IABP   l. Pulmonary capillary wedge pressure
13. _____ ACS   m. Intra-aortic balloon pump
14. _____ MET   n. Electrocardiogram

Copyright © 2013, 2009 by Saunders, an imprint of Elsevier Inc. All rights reserved.

COMMUNICATION EXERCISE

The following words are often used to describe the pain associated with these conditions:

angina pectoris: dull, tightness, ache

acute myocardial infarction: sudden, severe, crushing, burning, pressure, squeezing, knife-like (left arm more frequently indicated)

1. Can you give two reasons why people often have heart attacks while shoveling snow?

    a. _____

    b. _____

2. Unscramble this sentence:

    consumed Grapefruit when be not a juice should drug taking statin.

    _____

Copyright © 2013, 2009 by Saunders, an imprint of Elsevier Inc. All rights reserved.

The Neurologic System

Answer Key: Textbook page references are provided as a guide for answering these questions. A complete answer key was provided to your instructor.

REVIEW OF ANATOMY AND PHYSIOLOGY

Terminology

Directions: Match the term on the left with the correct statement, function, or definition on the right.

1. _____ Pyramidal tracts *(474)*
2. _____ Accommodation *(488)*
3. _____ Subarachnoid space *(475)*
4. _____ Nerve stimulus *(474)*
5. _____ Neurotransmitter *(476)*
6. _____ Dysphagia *(493)*
7. _____ Myelin sheath *(477)*
8. _____ Synapse *(476)*
9. _____ Meninges *(475)*
10. _____ Reflex arc *(474)*

a. Space between two neurons
b. Covering of nerves that insulates them
c. Physical, chemical, or electrical event that changes cell membrane and conducts as an electrical impulse along nerve pathway
d. Path traveled by a stimulus from point of stimulus through the spinal cord and back to effector site
e. Protective membranes that cover the brain and help protect the spinal cord
f. Conduction pathways, beginning in the cerebral cortex and ending in the spinal cord, that control skeletal muscle movement
g. Space through which cerebrospinal fluid travels and where villi help regulate amount of circulating fluid
h. Secreted at the synapse
i. Eye lens adjustment for seeing at different distances
j. Difficulty swallowing

Matching

Directions: Match the part of the brain on the left with its function(s) on the right. (There may be more than one answer for each.) (473, Table 22-1)

1. _____ Cerebrum
2. _____ Cerebellum
3. _____ Thalamus
4. _____ Hypothalamus
5. _____ Midbrain (brain stem)
6. _____ Pons (brain stem)
7. _____ Medulla oblongata

a. Mediates visual and auditory reflexes
b. Responsible for balance
c. Controls body temperature
d. Center of thinking and consciousness
e. Relay between spinal cord and cerebrum
f. Controls appetite and water balance
g. Helps regulate respiration
h. Regulates heartbeat, respiration, and blood pressure
i. Responsible for coordination of movement
j. Links nervous system and endocrine system
k. Control center for swallowing
l. Responsible for judgment and learning

Copyright © 2013, 2009 by Saunders, an imprint of Elsevier Inc. All rights reserved.

SHORT ANSWER

Changes that Occur with Aging

1. Reaction time is slowed with aging because there is a(n) _____ _____. *(478)*

2. Although the ability to learn is not affected by aging, the process of learning is _____. *(478)*

3. Continued intellectual function in the healthy elderly is promoted by _____ _____. *(478)*

4. With aging there is often a decrease in _____ memory, but often _____ _____ is unaffected. *(478)*

SHORT ANSWER

Directions: Answer the following questions in the spaces provided.

1. List specific observations that should be made while conducting a routine "neuro check." *(488)*

    a. Level of consciousness: _____

    _____

    _____

    b. Motor function: _____

    _____

    _____

    c. Pupillary reactions: _____

    _____

    _____

COMPLETION

Nursing Management

Directions: Fill in the blanks to complete the statements.

1. Pyramidal tracts control _____. *(474)*

2. Reflexes cause _____ movements. *(479-480)*

3. A normal response to scraping an object across the sole of the foot will result in _____ _____ of the toes. *(480)*

Copyright © 2013, 2009 by Saunders, an imprint of Elsevier Inc. All rights reserved.

4. A diagnostic test for a possible herniated lumbar disc is called a(n) _____
   _____. *(483, Table 22-6)*

5. A potential side effect of the radiopaque contrast medium used for many diagnostic x-rays is
   _____. *(482, Table 22-6)*

6. A quick way to assess the facial nerve is to ask the patient to _____. *(480, Table 22-5)*

7. When the pupil of one eye is increasing in size, it indicates _____
   _____. *(487-488)*

SHORT ANSWER

Directions: Answer the following questions in the spaces provided.

1. List three specific things you might notice a patient doing that could indicate poor coordination and balance, and write them as if you were documenting them on the patient's chart. *(479)*

   a. _____

   b. _____

   c. _____

2. List four reasons why a lumbar puncture is performed. *(481, Table 22-6)*

   a. _____

   b. _____

   c. _____

   d. _____

3. Describe what an electroencephalogram (EEG) is and what it is *not*. *(481, Table 22-6)*

   _____

   _____

   _____

   _____

   _____

4. List at least four pieces of information you think would be significant during an admission assessment of a patient's neurologic status. This information would be obtained while taking the patient's health history. One example would be recent infections affecting the sinuses or face. *(486-489)*

   a. _____

   b. _____

   c. _____

   d. _____

Copyright © 2013, 2009 by Saunders, an imprint of Elsevier Inc. All rights reserved.

REVIEW QUESTIONS FOR THE NCLEX® EXAMINATION

Directions: Choose the best answer(s) for the following questions.

1. Parasympathetic stimulation may cause a change in vital signs demonstrated by: *(476, Table 22-3)*
   1. increased pulse rate.
   2. slowed pulse rate.
   3. decreased blood pressure.
   4. decreased respiratory rate.

2. Promotion of blood pressure control can help prevent brain damage from: *(479)*
   1. medications.
   2. stroke.
   3. myocardial infarction.
   4. atherosclerosis.

3. Tests for coordination and balance check areas controlled by: *(479)*
   1. tendons and muscles.
   2. the pons and medulla.
   3. the left cerebral hemisphere.
   4. the cerebrum and cerebellum.

4. A test that measures electrical activity of skeletal muscle is _____. *(481, Table 22-6)*

5. You are caring for a patient who sustained a head injury in an accident. Assessment reveals the following signs. Which sign would be the most important to report immediately? *(487-489)*
   1. Weak hand grips
   2. BP rising from 128/78 to 142/88
   3. Restless movements of the extremities
   4. One pupil larger than the other

6. When assessing the accident patient for possible increased intracranial pressure, the nurse should assess the blood pressure for: *(485)*
   1. a steady falling of systolic and diastolic pressure.
   2. signs of a paradoxical pulse.
   3. a drop in diastolic pressure with a rise in systolic pressure.
   4. steady rise in both systolic and diastolic pressure.

7. When a patient with a neurologic problem is confined to a wheelchair and has a nursing diagnosis of Risk for impaired skin integrity, it is important to teach the patient to: *(490, 492, Table 22-9)*
   1. shift weight in the chair every 15 minutes.
   2. flex and extend the arms at least every 2 hours.
   3. deep-breathe and cough periodically.
   4. watch calorie intake so that weight doesn't increase.

8. An appropriate expected outcome for a patient with the nursing diagnosis of Impaired nutrition: less than body requirements related to dysphagia would be: *(491, Table 22-9)*
   1. patient will clearly orally articulate needs within 2 weeks.
   2. patient will eat 90% of each meal within 1 week.
   3. weight loss will not exceed 6 oz. per week of hospitalization.
   4. patient will eat without swallowing difficulty within 1 month.

Copyright © 2013, 2009 by Saunders, an imprint of Elsevier Inc. All rights reserved.

9. Measures that help a patient with dysphagia include: *(Select all that apply.)* **(493)**
   1. check swallowing ability before feeding.
   2. purée foods to ease swallowing.
   3. maintain an upright position for 30 minutes after eating.
   4. keep a nonstressful atmosphere at mealtime.
   5. feed at a steady pace.
   6. refrain from talking while the patient is eating.

10. A high priority of nursing care for the patient who is confused is: **(495)**
    1. enhancing mobility.
    2. providing safety.
    3. adequate nutrition.
    4. promoting sleep and rest.

CRITICAL THINKING ACTIVITIES

1. Why is positioning so important for the patient who is unconscious? **(490, 492, Table 22-9)**

2. What would you teach a patient who is about to have an electromyelogram (EMG)? **(481, Table 22-6)**

STEPS TOWARD BETTER COMMUNICATION

VOCABULARY BUILDING GLOSSARY

Term	Pronunciation	Definition
myriad	mir'i ad	many, a vast number
mechanism	mek'an ism	a method, a process by which something happens
nystagmus	nis tag'mus	rapid involuntary movement of the eyeball
widened pulse pressure		greater difference between systolic and diastolic
mnemonic	ne mon'ik	a device to aid the memory and recall facts

COMPLETION

Directions: Use the correct word from the glossary above to complete the sentence.

1. When checking the eyes, if _____ is found, it indicates an abnormality.

2. A _____ of causes can affect the neurologic system and cause problems.

3. A _____ occurs when the systolic pressure goes up and the diastolic goes down.

Copyright © 2013, 2009 by Saunders, an imprint of Elsevier Inc. All rights reserved.

4. A verse or an abbreviation (e.g., PERRLA) is a good _____ to help recall facts or lists of things.

5. Excess carbon dioxide in the blood is one of the _____ that can cause intracranial pressure to rise after a head injury.

WORD ATTACK SKILLS

Prefixes

Directions: Form a word combining the correct prefix below with the word stem listed. Write the meaning of the word. Use a dictionary as necessary.

Prefix	Meaning
a-, in-, an-, im-	no, not, without, lack of
dys-, dis-, mal-	bad, difficult, wrongly

Word Stem	Combined Word	Meaning
1. -orders	_____	_____
2. -paired	_____	_____
3. -voluntary	_____	_____
4. -noxia	_____	_____
5. -oriented	_____	_____
6. -effective	_____	_____
7. -orientation	_____	_____

Directions: Several words in this chapter have the same prefix. Write the meanings for the following words by attaching the prefix cereb- (brain), dys- (bad, difficult), or hemi- (half, partly) to the suffix listed. Use your dictionary as needed, especially to check correct spelling.

Suffix	Word	Meaning
1. -brum	_____	_____
2. -bellum	_____	_____
3. -bral	_____	_____
4. -paresis	_____	_____
5. -plegia	_____	_____
6. -phasia	_____	_____

Copyright © 2013, 2009 by Saunders, an imprint of Elsevier Inc. All rights reserved.

COMMUNICATION EXERCISES

Dialogue Practice

Directions: Discuss with a partner.

A. With a partner, use the guidelines in the Focused Assessment box on p. 485 in the textbook to perform an assessment. Practice asking each question. Practice charting your assessment.

B. As a second language learner, do you think the steps to help an aphasic person (self talk, parallel talk, expansion, and modeling) would help someone learning a new language? Why or why not? What happens in each of the steps?

Explanations

What would you say to a patient who asked why the doctor does a knee jerk (patellar reflex) test?

_____

_____

Orientation and Function Questions

Directions: Make a short list of questions you could ask an alert patient in order to assess his mental function.

_____

_____

_____

_____

_____

Copyright © 2013, 2009 by Saunders, an imprint of Elsevier Inc. All rights reserved.

Care of Patients with Head and Spinal Cord Injuries

Answer Key: Textbook page references are provided as a guide for answering these questions. A complete answer key was provided to your instructor.

COMPLETION

Head and Spinal Cord Injuries

Directions: Fill in the blanks to complete the statements.

1. When a concussion occurs, there is _____, a disruption in level of consciousness, and _____ regarding the occurrence. *(500)*

2. An acceleration-deceleration injury causes _____ brain injuries. *(501)*

3. Elderly people are more susceptible to subdural hematoma after a bump on the head because the brain tends to _____ within the cranial vault and _____ may be torn. *(501)*

4. A(n) _____ hematoma results after a head injury from rapid leakage of blood from the _____, which quickly elevates _____ _____. *(501)*

5. Ecchymosis behind the ear is termed _____ and indicates _____ _____. *(501)*

6. Initial measures after a head injury include securing a(n) _____ and elevating _____. *(502)*

7. Epidural hematoma occurs _____ and is relieved by _____ _____. *(501)*

8. Traumatic spinal cord injuries occur from compression, _____, _____, or tearing of the cord. *(509)*

9. A complication of spinal cord injury from disruption in the nerve communication pathways between upper and lower motor neurons is _____. *(513)*

10. Following the immediate flaccid paralysis that may occur with spinal cord injury, _____ often occurs. *(513)*

11. To avoid muscle spasms in the spinal cord–injured patient, when positioning the patient, avoid _____. *(513-514)*

12. Autonomic dysreflexia is dangerous because it can cause sudden _____ _____. *(514-515)*

13. A common problem in spinal cord–injured patients is _____ reflux that predisposes to _____. *(515)*

14. Quadriplegia occurs when spinal cord injury occurs at the level of _____. *(509)*

15. If a patient has a cervical spine injury and is in a halo traction device, you should never _____ _____ device. *(516)*

SHORT ANSWER

Intracranial Pressure

Directions: Answer the following questions in the spaces provided.

1. The classic signs of increasing intracranial pressure are _____ _____, _____, _____ and _____ _____. *(507)*

2. The earliest sign of increasing intracranial pressure is usually a change in _____ _____. *(506)*

3. When nursing interventions that may increase intracranial pressure are necessary, it is wise to _____. *(503-504, Nursing Care Plan 23-1)*

4. A priority concern for the nurse caring for a patient after intracranial surgery is _____ _____. *(508, Box 23-2)*

5. Pathophysiologically, a head injury causes swelling and pressure against cerebral veins and arteries that interfere with the flow of blood, causing _____ and _____ of the tissues. *(500-501)*

6. Apneustic breathing has a(n) _____ inspiratory phase or pauses and indicates damage to the _____. *(507)*

7. Pupil changes occur with increasing intracranial pressure because _____ _____. *(507)*

8. Positioning of the patient with increased intracranial pressure is extremely important to help _____ and reduce _____ _____. *(503, 504, 508-509, Nursing Care Plan 23-1)*

Copyright © 2013, 2009 by Saunders, an imprint of Elsevier Inc. All rights reserved.

9. Seven indications that intracranial pressure is rising are: *(508)*

   a. _____

   b. _____

   c. _____

   d. _____

   e. _____

   f. _____

   g. _____

COMPLETION

Back Pain and Ruptured Intervertebral Disk

Directions: Fill in the blanks to complete the statements.

1. Health care workers are prone to back pain just from _____. *(517)*

2. Back pain and disorders can be prevented by proper _____ and the use of _____
   _____ and _____. *(517)*

3. In the elderly, one reason for degeneration of the spinal vertebrae is _____. *(518)*

4. *Chronic back pain* is defined as pain that lasts for more than _____ or occurs on a(n)
   _____. *(518)*

5. Signs of a herniated lumbar disk may include pain radiating down _____ into the
   _____ or _____. *(518)*

6. Signs of a herniated cervical disk may include pain in the _____ and _____,
   radiating down the arm with _____ and _____
   _____. *(518)*

7. Patients who are experiencing back pain should not _____ or _____ for long periods of
   time. *(518-520)*

8. Surgical removal of a damaged disk may be performed by a percutaneous laser _____. *(519)*

9. If a spinal fusion is necessary, a(n) _____ must be performed. *(519)*

10. After spinal surgery, the patient is taught to turn by _____. *(519)*

Copyright © 2013, 2009 by Saunders, an imprint of Elsevier Inc. All rights reserved.

APPLICATION OF THE NURSING PROCESS

Directions: Write a brief answer to each question.

Scenario: Your patient has sustained a closed head injury in an automobile accident and was admitted to the ICU. The priority nursing diagnosis on the care plan is Risk for injury related to potential increased intracranial pressure.

1. Write two appropriate expected outcomes for this diagnosis for this patient. *(505-508)*

    a. _____

    b. _____

2. Nursing interventions that would be carried out to help the patient achieve the expected outcomes would be: *(502-503, 505, 508)*

    _____

    _____

    _____

3. Criteria by which you would evaluate whether the expected outcomes have been met are:

    _____

    _____

PRIORITY SETTING

You are assigned the following patients:

    a. Mr. Hopper, age 23, who has a C-5 injury sustained in a diving accident and is in cervical tongs and on a Roto-Rest type bed.
    b. Mrs. Hernandez, age 48, who has a ruptured disk at L-5. She has just had a diskectomy this morning.
    c. Ms. Chinn, age 72, who suffered a back injury and a pelvic fracture in an automobile accident. She is on bedrest and has paresthesia in her right leg and foot.

Mr. Hopper is complaining of muscle spasms and pain. Mrs. Hernandez calls complaining of nausea. Ms. Chinn calls and asks for help, explaining that she has experienced some incontinence and the bed is wet.

In which order would you attend to these patients' needs? _____

REVIEW QUESTIONS FOR THE NCLEX® EXAMINATION

Directions: Choose the best answer(s) for the following questions.

1. Discharge teaching for the patient who has sustained a concussion should include instructions to: *(500-505)*
    1. take the prescribed analgesic for headache every 4 hours.
    2. lie down flat at home and move around as little as possible.
    3. force fluids to prevent dehydration and infection.
    4. report immediately any severe headache or persistent vomiting.

Copyright © 2013, 2009 by Saunders, an imprint of Elsevier Inc. All rights reserved.

2. Planning for the patient who has sustained a spinal injury would include listing which nursing diagnosis as the highest priority in the care plan? *(512)*
    1. Sensory perception alteration related to spinal contusion
    2. Risk for infection related to trauma to spinal column
    3. Incontinence related to paraplegia
    4. Risk for injury related to inability to move

3. The first priority in assessing the patient with head trauma at an accident scene is determining: *(511)*
    1. whether spinal injury is present.
    2. the level of consciousness using the Glasgow coma scale.
    3. whether the airway is patent.
    4. whether hypotension is present.

4. Baclofen is a drug used to help prevent muscle spasms. The side effects of this drug include: *(Select all that apply.) (514, Table 23-3)*
    1. seizure activity.
    2. diplopia.
    3. rash.
    4. nausea and vomiting.
    5. fatigue.
    6. urinary urgency.

5. Mannitol is an osmotic diuretic that helps decrease intracranial pressure. Nursing interventions for the patient receiving this drug include: *(Select all that apply.) (514, Table 23-3)*
    1. monitor intake and output.
    2. observe for chest pain.
    3. monitor for increasing salivation.
    4. watch for electrolyte imbalances.
    5. check skin turgor.

6. A patient with a daughter who is engaged to be married suffered an accident that left him paraplegic. He says to his minister, "If God will let me just walk my daughter down the aisle for her wedding, I'll never complain about being in this chair again." This indicates which stage of grief or mourning? *(514, Table 23-3)*
    1. Shock and denial
    2. Anger
    3. Bargaining
    4. Depression
    5. Adjustment

7. Mr. Pineda suffered a closed head injury and has increased intracranial pressure. The physician has prescribed mannitol 1 g/kg IV every 6 hours. Mr. Pineda weighs 194 lbs. How many grams of mannitol would be the correct dose to be given every 6 hours? _____ g

8. What is a priority nursing intervention for the patient with a spinal cord injury who is quadriplegic? *(515)*
    1. Preventing over-distention of the bladder
    2. Assessing skin integrity every shift
    3. Using an abdominal binder to raise blood pressure
    4. Providing frequent massage of the legs

9. Autonomic dysreflexia can lead to: *(514-515)*
    1. heat stroke from loss of thermoregulation.
    2. paralytic ileus.
    3. severe muscle cramps.
    4. severe hypertension.

Copyright © 2013, 2009 by Saunders, an imprint of Elsevier Inc. All rights reserved.

CRITICAL THINKING ACTIVITIES

Scenario A: Mr. Schultz sustained a head injury in a bicycle accident. He was admitted to the ICU from the emergency department as his level of consciousness was decreasing. He is arousable, but very drowsy. His vital signs are BP 132/84, P 78, R 16, T. 98.8° F. Vital and neuro signs are ordered every hour. A pulse oximeter is attached and he is placed on a cardiac monitor.

1. What diagnostic tests would most likely be ordered to determine the extent of damage from his head injury? *(502)*

His pulse pressure shows widening after 3 hours, and he is more difficult to arouse.

2. What medications would you expect he might receive? *(502-503, 507-508, 514, Table 23-3)*

His condition worsens and one pupil begins to dilate. He is placed on mechanical ventilation.

3. When suctioning his endotracheal tube, why is it especially important to oxygenate him well beforehand? *(503, 509)*

Scenario B: Mr. Schultz was found to have a subdural hematoma. Burr holes were performed and the hematoma evacuated. You are caring for him postoperatively. *(503)*

1. What would you pay particular attention to when positioning him?

2. Why is it important to maintain a quiet, nonstimulating atmosphere for this patient?

3. Besides increasing intracranial pressure, what is the next complication against which you would direct your nursing care?

Copyright © 2013, 2009 by Saunders, an imprint of Elsevier Inc. All rights reserved.

STEPS TOWARD BETTER COMMUNICATION

VOCABULARY BUILDING GLOSSARY

Term	Pronunciation	Definition
contracoup	con'tra coo'	a counter or opposite blow—the contents of the cranium hit the inside of the skull, then bounce back and hit the other side, causing a second injury or contracoup
noxious	nok'shus	unpleasant and harmful; foul-smelling
precipitating	pre sip'i tay' ting	causing
"goose bumps"		roughness of the skin as the hairs stand erect, caused by cold or fear
"log rolling"		the method of moving or turning a patient by rolling him to one side by using a blanket beneath him to wrap and roll him so that the body moves as one unit; also describes the exchange of assistance to take such action

COMPLETION

Directions: Fill in the blanks with the appropriate words from the Vocabulary Building Glossary above.

1. Bleeding into the brain is a _____ factor for an increase in intracranial pressure.

2. The patient who has a spinal cord injury is repositioned on the side by _____ him as a single unit.

3. Mr. Eagle hit his head hard on the windshield, his head bounced backwards and he ended up with an injury on the front of the brain and a _____ injury on the back of the brain.

4. _____ odors in the room of a patient after brain surgery may cause the intracranial pressure to rise.

5. A reaction seen with autonomic dysreflexia is _____ on the skin.

Copyright © 2013, 2009 by Saunders, an imprint of Elsevier Inc. All rights reserved.

WORD ATTACK SKILLS

Directions: In the combined word form find then write the word stem that joins with the prefix to make the combined word. Write the meaning. Use a dictionary as needed. Two examples are provided.

Prefix	Word Stem	Combined Word	Meaning
dys-	-reflexia	dysreflexia	disordered response to stimuli
under-	-lying	underlying	at the base or bottom of, a cause
oto-	_____	otorrhea	_____
rhino-	_____	rhinorrhea	_____
contra-	_____	contralateral	_____
	_____	contracoup	_____
ipsi-	_____	ipsilateral	_____
hema-	_____	hematoma	_____
hemo-	_____	hemodynamic	_____
hypo-	_____	hypothermia	_____
	_____	hypoxia	_____
hyper-	_____	hyperextension	_____
	_____	hyperreflexia	_____
un-	_____	uninterrupted	_____
poly-	_____	polyuria	_____
vaso-	_____	vasoconstriction	_____
	_____	vasodilation	_____
im-	_____	immobility	_____
in-	_____	innervation	_____
	_____	inability	_____
over-	_____	overdistended	_____
re-	_____	rehabilitation	_____

Copyright © 2013, 2009 by Saunders, an imprint of Elsevier Inc. All rights reserved.

COMMUNICATION EXERCISE

Dialogue Practice

Write out what you might say to the mother of a 16-year-old boy who suffered a head injury to reassure her and involve her in the plan to help her son. Cover why she shouldn't try to keep him awake (sleep is helpful for healing, but he will be aroused periodically to check the level of consciousness). Explain to her how she can help with passive range-of-motion exercises and with keeping his hands in good anatomical position.

_____

_____

_____

_____

_____

_____

_____

Documentation

Document what you told her below:

_____

_____

_____

_____

CULTURAL POINTS

Many cultures have taboos about discussing sexual matters with outsiders or with someone of the opposite sex who is not a spouse. Even in cultures where sex is discussed openly, people may be hesitant to talk about their personal situations and concerns. As a nurse, you will need to be able to interact with patients about sexual problems.

The patient with a spinal cord injury who is paraplegic will surely have sexual concerns. After reading the section in your text about paraplegia, jot notes about the likely concerns your paraplegic male patient/female patient might have. Think about how you would communicate with each patient about sexual concerns.

To overcome your own shyness or inhibitions in discussing sexual matters, ask a classmate to interact with you so that you can practice what you would say to your patient.

Copyright © 2013, 2009 by Saunders, an imprint of Elsevier Inc. All rights reserved.

Care of Patients with Disorders of the Brain

Answer Key: Textbook page references are provided as a guide for answering these questions. A complete answer key was provided to your instructor.

COMPLETION

Seizure Disorders and Epilepsy

Directions: Fill in the blanks to complete each statement.

1. Seizures may occur anytime the _____ is deprived of _____. *(523)*

2. During a grand mal seizure, the person usually loses _____ and _____ tone. *(524)*

3. In partial seizures, _____ is not lost. *(524)*

4. The goal of anticonvulsant therapy is to control the seizures by using the _____ amount of the drug with the _____ side effects. *(525)*

5. Absence or petit mal seizures usually last for _____ and the person re-mains _____. *(524)*

6. IV phenytoin must be mixed with _____ only. *(526)*

SHORT ANSWER

Directions: Complete the following statements.

1. Other than epilepsy, seizures can be caused by: *(523)*_____
   _____
   _____

2. Generalized seizures are characterized by: *(524)* _____ .

3. Automatisms are: *(524)* _____ .

4. The manifestations of epilepsy depend on: *(524)*_____
   _____

5. Status epilepticus is dangerous because: *(524)*_____
   _____

6. When a seizure occurs, note: (List 5 observations) *(526)*_____

_____

_____

_____

_____

MATCHING

Cerebrovascular Accident

Directions: Match the term in the first column with the brief definition in the second column.

1. _____ Aphasia *(532)*   a. Loss or impairment of acquired motor skills

2. _____ Dysphasia *(532)*   b. Unsteadiness or lack of coordination

3. _____ Apraxia *(532)*   c. Inability to recognize an object by sight, touch, or hearing

4. _____ Hemiplegia *(530, 535)*   d. Reduced sensation on one side

5. _____ Atrophy *(560)*   e. Difficulty speaking

6. _____ Ataxia *(532)*   f. Impairment of or difficult speech

7. _____ Hemiparesthesia *(530)*   g. Paralysis of arm and leg on one side

8. _____ Diplopia *(530, 562)*   h. Double vision

9. _____ Dysarthria *(532)*   i. Muscle wasting

10. _____ Agnosia *(532)*   j. Loss of ability to communicate by either spoken or written word

COMPLETION

Directions: Fill in the blanks to complete the sentence.

1. Transient ischemic attacks (TIAs) are warnings that _____ and the patient should be evaluated by medical personnel. *(527)*

2. Individuals most at risk for stroke include those with _____, a history of _____ and _____. *(528)*

3. When a stroke is suspected, ask the person to_____, _____, _____, and answer a simple question. *(535)*

4. The symptoms of a stroke caused by thrombosis occur _____, whereas those caused by embolus occur _____. *(528-530)*

5. An individual who experiences a cerebrovascular accident (CVA) in the right hemisphere of the brain often has paresis or paralysis on the _____ side. *(535)*

Copyright © 2013, 2009 by Saunders, an imprint of Elsevier Inc. All rights reserved.

6. The results of lumbar puncture in a patient who has had a subarachnoid hemorrhage will show _____ in the cerebrospinal fluid. *(532)*

7. The patient with a leaking cerebral aneurysm often presents with _____

    _____ . *(530)*

8. An embolus causing a stroke often arises from the _____ in a patient who has

    _____. *(530)*

9. Structures that can cause an intercerebral hemorrhage are a(n) _____ and a(n)

    _____. *(528, 530)*

10. A subarachnoid hemorrhage often causes _____ of neurologic _____

    and loss of _____. *(528-530)*

COMPLETION

Brain Tumor

Directions: Fill in the blanks with the correct words to complete the statement.

1. Three characteristic signs of a brain tumor are _____,

    _____, and _____. *(540)*

2. An infratentorial brain tumor often causes a loss of _____ and _____

    _____. *(540)*

3. First signs of a brain tumor may include loss of muscular strength and coordination, _____

    loss, _____, _____, or difficulty in speaking clearly.

    (540)

4. Diagnostic tests to verify presence of a brain tumor are _____, _____, and

    _____. *(540)*

5. Two complications of a brain tumor are _____ and _____

    _____. *(541)*

Infections and Inflammatory Disorders of the Nervous System

Directions: Fill in the blank(s) with the correct words to complete the sentence.

1. Meningitis is a(n) _____ of the _____ covering

    the _____ and _____. *(541)*

2. Bacterial meningitis frequently follows a(n) _____ infection. *(540-541)*

Copyright © 2013, 2009 by Saunders, an imprint of Elsevier Inc. All rights reserved.

3. Classic signs of meningitis are _____
_____. *(542)*

4. A(n) _____ rash on the chest and extremities accompanies _____
meningitis. *(542)*

5. Meningitis is confirmed by a(n) _____, where CSF pressure is _____
and glucose is _____. *(542)*

6. For the patient with meningitis, it is important to watch for _____, as well as
neurologic deficits and seizures. *(543)*

7. The signs and symptoms of viral meningitis are _____, _____,
_____, and _____. *(543)*

8. A non-vector transmitted form of encephalitis is _____. *(544)*

9. Encephalitis is spread by vectors such as _____ and _____. *(544)*

10. Post-viral encephalitis is a(n) _____ disorder. *(544)*

APPLICATION OF THE NURSING PROCESS

Directions: List three nursing activities that would be included in the nursing care plan of a patient with each of the following nursing diagnoses.

1. Impaired verbal communication related to cerebrovascular accident: *(535-539)*

   a. _____

   b. _____

   c. _____

2. Self-care deficit related to hemiplegia: (Patient is a 62-year-old male.) *(535-539)*

   a. _____

   b. _____

   c. _____

3. An expected outcome for Self-care deficit related to hemiplegia might be: *(535-539)* _____

_____

4. A long-term expected outcome for the nursing diagnosis of Impaired verbal communication related to cerebrovascular accident would be:

_____

5. Evaluation criteria for the expected outcome in question 4 would be: _____

_____

Copyright © 2013, 2009 by Saunders, an imprint of Elsevier Inc. All rights reserved.

PRIORITY SETTING

Scenario: A patient who has been diagnosed with a thrombotic CVA was admitted yesterday and is assigned to you. The patient has left-sided hemiplegia, particularly of the arm. It is now 7:30 AM. Breakfast is served at 8:00 AM. According to the orders and care plan, you are to carry out the following. Indicate in what order you would perform each task.

_____ a. Neurologic check q 2 h

_____ b. Vital signs q 4 h

_____ c. IV of 0.9% NS at 50 mL/hr

_____ d. Blood glucose via glucometer AC and HS

_____ e. Urine sample to lab for urinalysis

_____ f. Monitor for seizure activity

_____ g. Up in chair three times a day with assistance

_____ h. Assist with bath

REVIEW QUESTIONS FOR THE NCLEX® EXAMINATION

Directions: Choose the best answer(s) to each of the following or supply the missing words to complete the statement.

1. During a seizure, it is important for the nurse to observe: *(526-527)*
   1. the type of aura the patient experiences.
   2. where movement occurs and how it progresses.
   3. the quality and rate of respirations during the seizure.
   4. the position of the patient's arms and legs during the seizure.

2. During a grand mal seizure, you could expect the patient to experience: *(Select all that apply.)* *(524)*
   1. loss of muscle tone.
   2. tonic-clonic movements.
   3. automatisms.
   4. absence for a few seconds.
   5. possible urinary incontinence.
   6. unilateral movements of limbs.

3. The teaching plan for the patient with epilepsy should include: *(Select all that apply.)* *(527)*
   1. refrain from drinking alcohol.
   2. wear a Medic-Alert bracelet or necklace.
   3. do not go anyplace by yourself.
   4. don't become overly tired.
   5. eat bananas to replace potassium loss.
   6. swim only with a partner.

4. Besides small emboli or small blood vessel rupture, a TIA may be caused by _____
   _____. *(527)*

5. Hydrocephalus is a complication after an intercerebral bleed because: *(534)*
   1. blood in the cerebral ventricular system interferes with the resorption of CSF.
   2. excessive amounts of CSF are produced after an intercerebral bleed.
   3. excessive hormone production increases the production of CSF.
   4. the ventricles become blocked by blood clots.

Copyright © 2013, 2009 by Saunders, an imprint of Elsevier Inc. All rights reserved.

6. A CVA occurring on the left side of the brain may cause motor problems: *(535)*
   1. on the left side of the body.
   2. on the right side of the body.
   3. on both sides of the body.
   4. only in the lower extremities.

7. One of the best things for building the self-esteem of the neurologically impaired person is: *(538-539)*
   1. to establish small, accomplishable goals.
   2. time to adapt to body changes.
   3. a way to be a productive member of society.
   4. contact with friends and family.

8. A distinction of migraine headaches is that they often begin with: *(545)*
   1. a headache at the base of the skull radiating upward.
   2. pain in the forehead area that worsens with movement.
   3. sudden, diffuse, excruciating pain in the head.
   4. visual disturbances such as scotoma.

9. An effective treatment to stop a migraine headache for many people is to: *(545)*
   1. place an ice bag on the throbbing area of the head.
   2. lie down in an odor-free, darkened room with the eyes closed.
   3. sit very still in an upright position with the eyes closed.
   4. apply heat packs to the forehead and neck.

10. A patient experiencing status epilepticus is receiving phenytoin IV. He is to receive 18 mg/kg over 24 hours. He weighs 162 lbs. The total amount he should receive is _____. If he is to receive this medication mixed with 500 mL of 0.9% NaCl every 8 hours, each 500 mL IV should contain _____ mg of phenytoin.

CRITICAL THINKING ACTIVITIES

Scenario A: Mrs. Margarita Rosario has been found to have an aneurysm in the brain. She has had headaches for many years, but they have become much worse lately. She also has type II diabetes and hypertension for which she takes several medications. She has been admitted to your unit.

1. How might this aneurysm be treated? *(533)*

2. If the aneurysm begins to leak, what symptoms might Mrs. Rosario have? *(534)*

3. What would you expect the treatment of this patient to be? *(534)*

4. What is your priority nursing responsibility? *(534)*

Copyright © 2013, 2009 by Saunders, an imprint of Elsevier Inc. All rights reserved.

Scenario B: Mr. Tompkins, age 76, suffered a CVA with right hemiplegia. He is in the recovery stage and has been admitted to the rehabilitation institute. He is achieving some feeling in his right arm and leg, but is still unable to walk or use his arm effectively.

1. What particular deficits might this type of CVA have caused that will affect his everyday living? *(534-538)*

2. What therapies would you expect him to undergo at the rehabilitation institute? *(538-539)*

3. What would you do when he has crying spells? *(534-539)*

4. What medications would you expect to be administering related to the CVA? *(533)*

Scenario C: Mr. Hiroshi, age 66, is experiencing sharp, intense paroxysms of facial pain that last for a couple of minutes. The pain occurs on the right side of the face.

1. What questions would you ask Mr. Hiroshi to assess his problem?

2. What do you expect the diagnosis might be?

3. If this is a facial nerve problem, what treatment would you expect the physician might prescribe?

STEPS TOWARD BETTER COMMUNICATION

VOCABULARY BUILDING GLOSSARY

Term	Pronunciation	Definition
seizure	see′ zur	sudden attack or occurrence of a disease; convulsion; caused by abnormal electrical activity in the brain
spasm	spa′ zim	strong involuntary contractions
untoward [effects]	un tord′	inconvenient, awkward, unexpected
groggy	grog′ ee	weak and unsteady, possibly confused (may come from "grog," an alcoholic drink)
intractable [seizures]	in trak′ ta bel	unmanageable, hard to control
susceptible	su sep′ ti bel	likely to be affected by
debilitating	de bil′ ih ta ting	making weak, or feeble; losing energy and ability
ischemia	is ke′ mia	deficiency of blood, or obstruction
aura	or′ a	atmosphere surrounding something; a radiation of light

Copyright © 2013, 2009 by Saunders, an imprint of Elsevier Inc. All rights reserved.

COMPLETION

Directions: Fill in each blank with the appropriate word from the glossary above.

1. When the patient woke up, he seemed a little _____ and wasn't ready to eat his breakfast.

2. The child's legs seemed to be in _____ and she couldn't straighten them.

3. A person who is poorly nourished is more _____ to disease.

4. The man was found on the floor having an apparent _____.

5. The severe seizures are _____ and need to be better controlled.

6. The man was discouraged because his stroke was so _____.

7. The woman usually was warned that a migraine was coming on by the _____ she saw beforehand.

8. The family was surprised by the _____ effects of their father's illness.

COMMUNICATION EXERCISE

Explanations

A. Directions: Can you put these symptoms in lay terms so that the patient's family can understand them?

"Homonymous hemianopsia, hemiplegia or hemiparesis, agnosia, apraxia, aphasia, and dysphagia are some of the problems caused by a CVA."

_____

_____

_____

_____

_____

_____

B. Directions: Explain the difference between a shunt and a stent.

_____

_____

Copyright © 2013, 2009 by Saunders, an imprint of Elsevier Inc. All rights reserved.

PRONUNCIATION SKILLS

Directions: Practice pronouncing these words aloud.

Symptomatology	Sym tow ma tol'o gee
Electroencephalogram	E lec trow' en sef'a low gram
Homonymous hemianopsia	Ho mon'i mus hem'ee ah nop'see a
Cytomegalovirus encephalitis	Cy tow meg'ah low vir'us en sef'a ly'tis

MATCHING

Directions: Choose from the list of definitions at right, and write in the blank space the correct meaning for each word on the left.

1. Idiopathic _____ No known cause

2. Neoplasm _____ Narrowing of the blood vessels

3. Flaccid _____ Tumor

4. Vasoconstriction _____ Both sides

5. Bilateral _____ Limp, hanging loose, weak, soft

COMMUNICATION EXERCISE

Directions: Write a short dialogue or monologue of what you would say to the patient or family in each of these cases. Practice your dialogue with another student.

Provide encouragement for a stroke patient with left-sided hemiparesis who is learning how to walk again. Show patience and encouragement. What would you say if the patient becomes frustrated and angry? Write out some ideas of how you would provide encouragement and how you would handle the anger.

_____

_____

_____

_____

_____

Copyright © 2013, 2009 by Saunders, an imprint of Elsevier Inc. All rights reserved.

Care of Patients with Peripheral Nerve and Degenerative Neurologic Disorders

Answer Key: Textbook page references are provided as a guide for answering these questions. A complete answer key was provided to your instructor.

COMPLETION

Degenerative Neurologic Disorders

Directions: Fill in the blanks to complete the statements.

1. Substances that seem to play a role in the occurrence of Parkinson's disease are _____ _____. *(551)*

2. In patients with Parkinson's disease, there is a deficiency of _____ in the brain causing problems with _____ and _____. *(551)*

3. Four drugs that help control tremor, rigidity, and drooling are _____, _____, _____, and _____. *(553-554, Table 25-1)*

4. Signs and symptoms of multiple sclerosis depend on the extent to which inflammation and scarring of the _____ have occurred. *(557)*

5. Multiple sclerosis is a disease of the central nervous system, and its symptoms are caused by _____ of the nerve fibers. *(557)*

6. When caring for a patient with confusion, it is important for the nurse not to _____ items around in the patient's room. *(559, see also Chapter 48)*

7. Alzheimer's disease progresses at _____ and eventually results in _____. *(559)*

8. Amyotrophic lateral sclerosis is a(n) _____ neuromuscular disease characterized by degeneration of the _____ in the anterior horns of the _____ and the lower cranial nerves. *(559)*

9. Guillain-Barré syndrome usually follows a(n) _____, but can occur after _____ immunization. *(560)*

10. Pathologic changes that occur with Guillain-Barré syndrome are _____, _____, _____, and _____. *(560)*

Copyright © 2013, 2009 by Saunders, an imprint of Elsevier Inc. All rights reserved.

11. When the lower brainstem becomes involved in Guillain-Barré syndrome, the _____ are affected. *(560)*

12. Guillain-Barré syndrome is characterized by the appearance of a(n) _____ _____. *(560)*

13. The patient with Guillain-Barré syndrome suffers paresthesias, muscular aches and cramps, and _____. *(560)*

14. Postpolio syndrome may occur _____ years later and problems may be _____ or _____. *(562)*

15. Huntington's disease is genetically transmitted and is characterized by _____ _____. *(562)*

16. Huntington's disease causes deterioration in _____ capacity and _____ disturbances. *(562)*

17. Myasthenia gravis is a(n) _____ disease manifested by fatigue and muscle exhaustion aggravated by _____ and relieved by _____. *(562)*

18. The purpose of plasma exchange as a treatment for myasthenia gravis is to mechanically remove _____. *(563)*

Copyright © 2013, 2009 by Saunders, an imprint of Elsevier Inc. All rights reserved.

TABLE ACTIVITY

Directions: Complete the following table comparing three neurologic diseases: Parkinson's disease, multiple sclerosis, and myasthenia gravis.

	Parkinson's Disease (551-557)	Multiple Sclerosis (557-559)	Myasthenia Gravis (562-565)
Definition			
Clinical manifestations			
Cause			
Diagnostic measures			
Medical management			
Special nursing concerns and patient problems			

Copyright © 2013, 2009 by Saunders, an imprint of Elsevier Inc. All rights reserved.

PRIORITY SETTING

Scenario: You are assigned to a variety of patients who have several medications to be administered at 8:00 AM. Breakfast is served at 8:00 AM. You plan to start dispensing the medications ordered for 8:00 AM at about 7:45 AM in order to get them all administered on time. Consider the nursing implications of the diagnoses and the drugs to be administered. Decide on the order of priority in which you will give each patient's medications and indicate the numerical order in the blanks provided.

The patients and medications are:

_____ a. Mrs. Hubers, diagnosis of type 2 diabetes and pneumonia. She is to receive Diabinese and Biaxin.

_____ b. Mr. Hunter, diagnosis hypertension and heart failure. He is to receive digoxin, furosemide, and losartan.

_____ c. Ms. Johnson, diagnosis myasthenia gravis. She is to receive Mestinon.

_____ d. Mr. Takura, diagnosis Parkinson's disease. He is to receive Sinemet, Cogentin, and Metamucil.*

*What special nursing implication regarding the administration of Metamucil should be considered?

REVIEW QUESTIONS FOR THE NCLEX® EXAMINATION

Directions: Choose the best answer(s) for the following questions or fill in the blank with the correct answer.

1. Interventions for the patient with moderate Parkinson's disease might include: *(Select all that apply.)* *(554-557)*
   1. allowing extra time to perform tasks.
   2. medicating 15 minutes before meals.
   3. allowing rest periods during meals.
   4. propping up with pillows when resting.
   5. ambulating at least twice a day.
   6. providing an alternative to oral communication.

2. An expected outcome for the patient with Parkinson's disease who has a nursing diagnosis of Risk for injury would be: *(554-557)*
   1. patient will not experience a fall while ambulating before discharge.
   2. patient will not develop a respiratory infection this month.
   3. patient's rigidity will decrease with medication within 2 weeks.
   4. patient will not sustain skin impairment from bedrest before discharge.

3. Patients taking levodopa to control Parkinson's disease should be assessed for the side effect of: *(553-554)*
   1. headache.
   2. gastrointestinal bleeding.
   3. muscle aches.
   4. orthostatic hypotension.

4. Assessment findings of weakness of a leg, blurred vision, spasticity of muscles, and a positive Lhermitte's sign for a patient will most likely lead to a diagnosis of: *(557-558)*
   1. Parkinson's disease.
   2. multiple sclerosis.
   3. myasthenia gravis.
   4. amyotrophic lateral sclerosis.

Copyright © 2013, 2009 by Saunders, an imprint of Elsevier Inc. All rights reserved.

5. When planning nursing care for the patient with multiple sclerosis, remember that the patient: *(557-558)*
    1. fatigues very easily and has the most strength in the afternoon.
    2. may exhibit periods of elated behavior.
    3. will experience more fatigue in a hot environment.
    4. needs increased calories in the diet.

6. Baclofen is used for multiple sclerosis patients to: *(558-559, see also Chapter 24)*
    1. decrease urinary incontinence.
    2. decrease spinal cord inflammation.
    3. decrease muscle spasticity.
    4. control neurologic pain.

7. A nursing intervention for safety of the patient with Guillain-Barré syndrome is to: *(561)*
    1. keep intubation equipment and an Ambu bag at the bedside.
    2. keep the head of the patient's bed elevated 15–30 degrees at all times.
    3. have the patient perform range-of-motion exercises at least three times a day.
    4. keep the room darkened and the environment quiet to prevent agitation of the patient.

8. An appropriate nursing diagnosis for a patient who has postpolio syndrome might be: *(562)*
    1. Incontinence, urinary, related to loss of bladder control.
    2. Self-care deficit, grooming, related to weakness and fatigue.
    3. Pain, severe, related to neurologic disorder.
    4. Risk for aspiration related to difficulty swallowing.

9. When assessing a patient with amyotrophic lateral sclerosis, the nurse would find: *(560)*
    1. difficulty breathing.
    2. bilateral tremors.
    3. ascending paralysis.
    4. weakness of voluntary muscles.

10. Huntington's disease is genetically transmitted and usually causes death within _____ years after signs appear. *(562)*

CRITICAL THINKING ACTIVITIES

Scenario A: Marlene Johnson, age 33, has just been diagnosed with multiple sclerosis. Her doctor thinks she has the relapsing-remitting type. She is a graduate student at the university. She has been having trouble with her vision.

1. What can she expect with this type of multiple sclerosis? *(560)*

2. How would you help her decide what to do about her vision problems, as they are interfering with her studying? *(560)*

3. Her physician has talked with her about using beta-interferon to help control her disease. What could you tell her about this medication? *(558)*

Copyright © 2013, 2009 by Saunders, an imprint of Elsevier Inc. All rights reserved.

Scenario B: Antonio Katsigris, age 46, has recently been diagnosed with myasthenia gravis. He is not familiar with the disease and has many questions.

1. What could you tell him about the disease? *(562-563)*

2. What are the biggest dangers with this disease? *(562-563)*

3. What would you tell him about the usual treatment for the disease? *(563)*

STEPS TOWARD BETTER COMMUNICATION

VOCABULARY BUILDING GLOSSARY

Term	Pronunciation	Definition
collaborate	co lab'o rate	to work together
ascending	a send' ing	going upward
dyspepsia	dis pep'si a	indigestion
plateau	plat oh'	a level time after an increase; a fairly level area of high ground
drooling		water or saliva coming out of the mouth, usually due to lack of muscle control

COMPLETION

Directions: Complete the following sentences with one of the glossary words above.

1. _____ the stairway takes much more energy than descending the stairs.

2. The nursing staff and the physical therapists agreed to _____ on solving the problem.

3. Because of his stroke, Mr. Branson's facial muscles were paralyzed and he had difficulty preventing himself from _____.

4. The patient's rehabilitation efforts seemed to reach a(n) _____ that was difficult to get beyond.

5. Mrs. Johnson's _____ made her irritable after meals.

Copyright © 2013, 2009 by Saunders, an imprint of Elsevier Inc. All rights reserved.

GRAMMAR POINTS

Collaborate is the base verb meaning to work together; **collaborator** is a noun (one of the people who does the working together); **collaboration** is a noun referring to the action of working together; and **collaborative** is an adjective describing the kind of action.

Similarly **drool** is the base verb; **drooler,** a noun, would be a person (not commonly used); **drooling** would be the noun describing the action (from the participle).

COMMUNICATION EXERCISES

a. Dialogue Practice

Think Critically

A patient comes into the clinic complaining about hand tremors and "stiffness" of the joints that started recently, excessive sweating, and some urinary incontinence. You notice that her gait is abnormal. What would be a priority question you would ask her as you start taking her history?

Use the above as the basis for a dialogue. With a partner, practice asking the questions in the Focused Assessment box on p. 554 in the textbook.

b. Explanations

With a partner, practice explaining to a patient with myasthenia gravis why wearing a Medic-Alert emblem/bracelet is a good idea.

CULTURAL POINTS

Directions: For discussion in a group:

People with the disorders described in this chapter have a number of physical manifestations relating to their illness (tremors, lack of muscle control, strange gaits, tics, etc.). How do you think these physical manifestations affect their feelings about going out in public? How are people with such disorders received by the people they meet or who observe them? What nursing problems could this cause?

If there are people in your class from other cultures, ask how people with physical disorders would be treated in their culture. Are there differences among the cultures?

What might you—as medical personnel—be able to do to help the situation?

Copyright © 2013, 2009 by Saunders, an imprint of Elsevier Inc. All rights reserved.

The Sensory System: Eye and Ear

chapter

26

Answer Key: Textbook page references are provided as a guide for answering these questions. A complete answer key was provided to your instructor.

PART 1—THE EYE

REVIEW OF ANATOMY AND PHYSIOLOGY

Terminology

Directions: Match the term on the left with the correct definition, function, or statement on the right. **(568-569, 571)**

1. _____	Pupil	a.	Secretes tears that moisten, lubricate, and cleanse the eye
2. _____	Ciliary body	b.	Sits between lens and retina and contains vitreous humor
3. _____	Iris	c.	Contains processes that produce aqueous humor
4. _____	Anterior chamber	d.	Contain an enzyme that kills bacteria
5. _____	Posterior chamber	e.	Between the lens and the cornea
6. _____	Eyelashes	f.	Eversion of the lower lid that may occur with aging
7. _____	Lacrimal gland	g.	Secrete aqueous humor
8. _____	Tears	h.	Central opening allowing light into interior
9. _____	Suspensory ligaments	i.	Allow for focusing of light on lens and retina
10. _____	Ectropion	j.	Help trap foreign particles, keeping them out of the eye
		k.	Colored portion of the eye

Copyright © 2013, 2009 by Saunders, an imprint of Elsevier Inc. All rights reserved.

LABELING

Directions: Label the following structures on the diagram of the eye. (569)

sclera
pupil
Schlemm's canal
ciliary process
cornea
conjunctiva
anterior chamber
choroid

lens
optic disk
posterior chamber
iris
optic nerve
retina
vitreous body

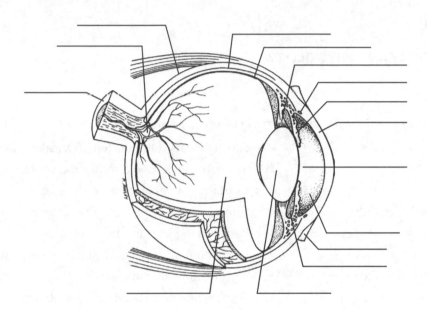

COMPLETION

Prevention of Eye Problems and Diagnostic Tests

Directions: Fill in the blanks with the correct words to complete the statements.

1. Normal eyes do not require _____ or irrigations. *(571)*

2. When using machinery that might cause debris to fly into the eye, _____ should be worn. *(572)*

3. When diagnosed with diabetes mellitus, good control of the disease will help prevent _____. *(572)*

4. _____ is the diagnostic test used to evaluate blood vessel abnormalities in the eye. *(574, Table 26-2)*

5. With aging, the ability of the _____ to dilate decreases, causing difficulty for the older person in going from a(n) _____ into a(n) _____. *(570)*

Copyright © 2013, 2009 by Saunders, an imprint of Elsevier Inc. All rights reserved.

APPLICATION OF THE NURSING PROCESS

Directions: Write a brief answer to each question.

1. List the five danger signals of eye disease that should be looked for upon assessment of each person. *(572)*

   a. _____

   b. _____

   c. _____

   d. _____

   e. _____

2. List five guidelines for assisting a blind person. *(578-579)*

   a. _____

   b. _____

   c. _____

   d. _____

   e. _____

3. What are four important steps in administering eyedrops? *(578)*

   a. _____

   b. _____

   c. _____

   d. _____

REVIEW QUESTIONS FOR THE NCLEX® EXAMINATION

Directions: Choose the best answer(s) for each of the following questions.

1. Fluorescein angiography is used as an assessment tool by the physician. Teaching for the patient about the procedure includes stating: *(575, Table 26-2)*
   1. "the optic nerve will be visualized to determine any problems."
   2. "eye muscle testing will occur during the test."
   3. "the test helps measure visual acuity."
   4. "dye will be injected intravenously and the blood vessels in the fundus examined."

2. When assessing a patient for vision problems, subtle signs of decreasing vision are: *(573, 578)*
   1. becoming less interested in a hobby such as sewing.
   2. developing a bruise on the shin from the open door to the dishwasher.
   3. seeing better when using prescribed glasses.
   4. wanting a light on in the room when watching television.

Copyright © 2013, 2009 by Saunders, an imprint of Elsevier Inc. All rights reserved.

3. An appropriate expected outcome for a patient with a diagnosis of Disturbed visual sensory perception related to injury from a branch would be the patient will: *(577-578)*
   1. instill antibiotic drops three times a day.
   2. wear an eye patch when sleeping.
   3. not develop infection in the affected eye during healing.
   4. wear protective goggles when gardening.

4. An intervention for setting up a dinner tray for a blind person would be to: *(579)*
   1. place the person's hands on each side of the plate.
   2. describe where each type of food is located using the "clock" method.
   3. allow the person to cut up the meat.
   4. make certain there are no shadows in the room.

5. Community teaching for the prevention of eye problems should include: *(Select all that apply.)* *(571-572, 579)*
   1. wearing a hat when outdoors.
   2. wearing sunglasses that block UVA and UVB rays when outdoors.
   3. using eyedrops when returning inside from being in the sun.
   4. eating a diet rich in fruits and vegetables that contain antioxidants.
   5. obtaining regular glaucoma screening after age 40.
   6. cleansing the eyes with eyedrops regularly.

CRITICAL THINKING ACTIVITES

1. Develop a teaching plan on protecting vision for a community or school group. *(571-572, 579)*

2. Explain the Amsler Grid test to your elderly relatives and/or neighbors and perform an assessment for macular degeneration using the grid. *(575, Table 26-2)*

Copyright © 2013, 2009 by Saunders, an imprint of Elsevier Inc. All rights reserved.

PART II—THE EAR

REVIEW OF ANATOMY AND PHYSIOLOGY

Labeling

Directions: Label the diagram of the ear with the following parts. (580)

pinna	malleus	tympanic membrane
semicircular canals	vestibular nerve CN VIII branch	vestibule
auditory meatus	incus	facial nerve
cochlea	cochlear nerve CN VII	
eustachian tube	stapes	

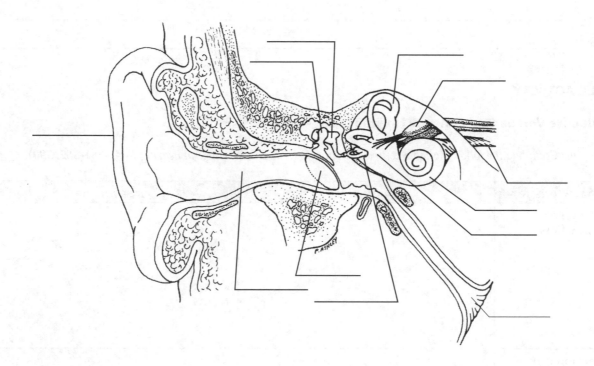

SHORT ANSWER

Prevention of Hearing Loss

Directions: Write a brief answer for each question.

1. How can people protect themselves from hearing damage? *(581-582)*

    a. _____

    b. _____

    c. _____

Copyright © 2013, 2009 by Saunders, an imprint of Elsevier Inc. All rights reserved.

2. What are four signs of hearing loss? *(581-588)*

   a. _____

   b. _____

   c. _____

   d. _____

3. What are five common medications that are potentially ototoxic and may cause hearing loss? *(582-583)*

   a. _____

   b. _____

   c. _____

   d. _____

TABLE ACTIVITY

Conductive Versus Sensorineural Hearing Loss

Directions: Complete the following table comparing conductive and sensorineural hearing loss. *(581-582, 590)*

Characteristic	Conductive	Sensorineural
Location of dysfunction		
Common causes		
Treatment		

Copyright © 2013, 2009 by Saunders, an imprint of Elsevier Inc. All rights reserved.

COMPLETION

The Ear and Hearing Loss

Directions: Fill in the blanks with the correct words to complete the statements.

1. Tuning fork tests measure hearing by _____ conduction or _____

    _____. *(583)*

2. A simple hearing test is the _____ test. *(583)*

3. The Romberg test is performed by having the person stand _____

    _____. *(585)*

4. When eardrops are administered, they should first be _____ or they may cause
    discomfort or dizziness. *(587)*

5. When eardrops are instilled, the patient should remain in the lateral position for _____
    minutes. *(587)*

6. When communicating with a hearing-impaired person, it is best to position yourself
    _____ of the person. *(587-588)*

7. When working with a patient who has a hearing aid, the nurse should make certain that the aid
    _____. *(590)*

8. Many people do not know that hearing aids from a reputable dealer usually have a(n) _____
    _____. *(590)*

9. People who are deaf may _____ themselves because of embarrassment and frustration
    over difficulty in communicating. *(587-588)*

10. Exposure to environmental loud noise causes a(n) _____ hearing loss that is of-
    ten not correctable. *(581)*

REVIEW QUESTIONS FOR THE NCLEX® EXAMINATION

Directions: Choose the best answer(s) for each of the following questions.

1. When assessing a patient who complains of a mild hearing loss, the nurse should *first*: *(585)*
    1. schedule an audiogram.
    2. inspect the ear canal for cerumen.
    3. inquire about past episodes of upper respiratory infection.
    4. lavage the ear canal for clearer vision of the eardrum.

Copyright © 2013, 2009 by Saunders, an imprint of Elsevier Inc. All rights reserved.

2. For the patient undergoing assessment for a hearing loss, the nurse would explain that electronystag-mography is performed in conjunction with: *(584, Table 26-6)*
    1. caloric testing.
    2. the Tine test.
    3. the Rinne test.
    4. an audiogram.

3. Interventions to be used when working with a patient who has a slight to moderate hearing deficit are: *(Select all that apply.) (587-588, 590)*
    1. write everything down for him.
    2. face him and gain his attention before speaking.
    3. speak very loudly and slowly.
    4. be certain that his hearing aid is on if he wears one.
    5. use American sign language to communicate with him.

4. Decreases in hearing often occur with aging because of: *(Select all that apply.) (580)*
    1. vascular changes from diabetes.
    2. loss of elasticity of the tympanic membrane.
    3. nerve cell atrophy in the ear and brain.
    4. arteriosclerosis and decreased blood flow.

5. When irrigating the ear canal to remove cerumen, aim the stream of water above or below the impaction to allow _____ to push out the cerumen. *(585, Figure 26-11)*

CRITICAL THINKING ACTIVITIES

1. Formulate a teaching plan for college students on how to protect hearing.

2. Plan how you would handle the situation if you go to a concert, dance, or other place that has music that is playing too loudly.

STEPS TOWARD BETTER COMMUNICATION

VOCABULARY BUILDING GLOSSARY

Term	Pronunciation	Definition
acuity	ah kyou' i tee	clearness, sharpness
enun'ciate	ee nun' cee at	to speak clearly
opaque	o pak'	light cannot go through it
pitch	pich	degree of highness or lowness of a sound
take it for granted		to not think about something, especially a gift or normal behavior, such as sight, food, or family; to assume a condition will always exist

Copyright © 2013, 2009 by Saunders, an imprint of Elsevier Inc. All rights reserved.

COMPLETION

Directions: Fill in the blanks with the correct words from the Vocabulary Building Glossary to complete the statements.

1. The patient could hear low sounds but had difficulty hearing sounds with a high _____.

2. A cataract makes the lens of the eye _____.

3. After age 70, Joe noticed that the _____ of his hearing had decreased.

4. When a patient has a hearing loss, it is important that the nurse _____ words.

5. After age 40, many people develop decreased visual _____ and need glasses.

6. When hearing loss occurs, it is often the high _____ that are most difficult to hear.

VOCABULARY EXERCISE

Review of Terms and Combining Forms

ophthalm/o	eye
ot/o	ear
aural	relating to the ear
superior	above
inferior	below
lateral	toward the side
medial	central, in the middle

PRONUNCIATION SKILLS

Vestib'ulococh'lear	ves tib' you lo kok' lee ar)
Eusta'chian	you sta' che an

ABBREVIATIONS

OD	right eye
OS	left eye
OU	both eyes

[One way to remember this is to think that right eye (OD) comes first in the alphabet; left eye (OS) comes second in the alphabet, and both eyes (OU) comes last.]

Directions: Practice pronouncing the above words and abbreviations with a peer. Have your partner write down the words or abbreviations as you say them. Check the list for accurate enunciation.

Copyright © 2013, 2009 by Saunders, an imprint of Elsevier Inc. All rights reserved.

COMMUNICATION EXERCISE

With a peer, practice assessment by using the information in the Focused Assessment boxes on p. 585 in the textbook to take a history. Ask your partner questions to help clarify points that require more explanation.

Copyright © 2013, 2009 by Saunders, an imprint of Elsevier Inc. All rights reserved.

Care of Patients with Disorders of the Eyes and Ears

Answer Key: Textbook page references are provided as a guide for answering these questions. A complete answer key was provided to your instructor.

PART 1—THE EYE

COMPLETION

Eye Disorders

Directions: Fill in the blanks with the correct words to complete the statements.

1. The term for inability to see objects close at hand is _____. *(594)*

2. Keratitis may be caused by _____ or _____. *(595)*

3. If a chemical splashes into the eye, the eye should be treated with _____ for

   at least _____ with _____ or _____. *(597)*

4. If a foreign body is stuck into the eye, the best thing to do is to _____ ,

   _____ the eye, and to _____. *(597)*

5. A cataract causes a blurring of vision because the _____ becomes _____

   _____. *(598)*

6. Cataract surgery is performed when the loss of vision _____

   _____ the person's life. *(598)*

7. Glaucoma is often _____ until damage to vision has occurred from _____

   _____ and pressure on the _____. *(602)*

8. The characteristic sign of narrow-angle glaucoma is _____

   _____. *(605)*

9. Drugs used in the treatment of glaucoma act to _____ of

   _____ or decrease _____. *(602)*

10. Uncontrolled glaucoma causes _____. *(604)*

11. The sudden occurrence of flashes of colored light is a sign of _____.

    (606)

Copyright © 2013, 2009 by Saunders, an imprint of Elsevier Inc. All rights reserved.

12. Retinopathy is often a disorder that occurs in patients with diabetes mellitus and is either from

    _____ of blood vessels or _____ of blood vessels with _____. *(608)*

13. Early symptoms of macular degeneration are inability to see _____ of

    _____ and _____. *(609)*

14. The patient who has just had eye surgery should be positioned with the head _____ and

    should not lie on the _____ side. *(611)*

15. When administering preoperative mydriatic eyedrops you should wait _____ minutes between the

    instillation of one drop and the other. *(610)*

APPLICATION OF THE NURSING PROCESS

Directions: Write a brief answer to each question.

1. List five nursing diagnoses frequently encountered for patients with disorders of the eye.

    a. _____

    b. _____

    c. _____

    d. _____

    e. _____

2. Give four assessment findings that may indicate the presence of a cataract. *(598)*

    a. _____

    b. _____

    c. _____

    d. _____

3. Your clinical patient is scheduled for same-day surgery in the ambulatory surgery unit. Eyedrops are ordered to be instilled three times at 15-minute intervals. The patient has just been admitted to the unit. An IV is to be started, a gown put on by the patient, the preoperative checklist is to be completed, and the patient is to be ready for surgery in 60 minutes. In what order of priority should these actions take place?

    _____

    _____

    _____

    _____

    _____

    _____

Copyright © 2013, 2009 by Saunders, an imprint of Elsevier Inc. All rights reserved.

SHORT ANSWER

Retinal Detachment and Eye Surgery

Directions: Read the clinical situation and write brief answers to the questions that follow.

Scenario: Mr. Cox, age 82, is scheduled for a scleral buckle for a retinal detachment. He will be hospitalized at least overnight.

1. Considering the procedure Mr. Cox is undergoing, what should be included in his teaching plan to prepare him for the early postoperative period? *(606)*

    a. _____

    b. _____

    c. _____

    d. _____

    e. _____

2. What safety precautions should be taken during Mr. Cox's hospital stay? *(606-607)*

    a. _____

    _____

    b. _____

    _____

    c. _____

    _____

    d. _____

    _____

3. Name three instructions that should be included in Mr. Cox's discharge teaching specific to the type of surgery he had. *(606-607)*

    a. _____

    _____

    b. _____

    _____

    c. _____

    _____

Copyright © 2013, 2009 by Saunders, an imprint of Elsevier Inc. All rights reserved.

4. List five goals or expected outcomes for nursing interventions in the postoperative care of all patients who have had surgery of the eye.

   a. _____

   b. _____

   c. _____

   d. _____

   e. _____

COMPLETION

Eye Medications

Directions: Fill in the blanks with the correct words to complete the statements. (602-603, Table 27-1)

1. Latanoprost is a(n) _____ medication that works by _____ the pupil.

2. Patients who use pilocarpine should not _____ at _____.

3. Demercarium bromide (Humorsol) works by producing _____, causing an increase in _____.

4. Atropine eye drops are used to _____ the eyes and to _____ the muscles of accommodation.

5. Fluorescein sodium is used to detect _____or _____ on the _____ .

6. When gentamicin (Garamycin) eyedrops are prescribed, the patient should be taught to also use a _____ and _____ each time the face is washed to prevent reinfection.

7. Pred Forte is a(n) _____ eyedrop used to decrease _____ and _____.

8. Fluorescein sodium drops are used to _____ the cornea and if a corneal scratch is present, it will show up as _____.

REVIEW QUESTIONS FOR THE NCLEX® EXAMINATION

Directions: Choose the best answer(s) for each of the following questions.

1. Mrs. Messina is scheduled for a cataract extraction with intraocular lens implant of the right eye. Assessment of Mrs. Messina during preoperative care would include: *(Select all that apply.)* **(598-600)**
   1. food likes and dislikes for dietary selections.
   2. degree of retained vision and history of previous hospitalizations.
   3. ability to instill eyedrops and administer self-care.
   4. ability to understand and follow directions postoperatively.

Copyright © 2013, 2009 by Saunders, an imprint of Elsevier Inc. All rights reserved.

2. Planning for safety needs for a patient with a right cataract extraction and intraocular lens implant in the immediate postoperative period would include: *(Select all that apply.)* **(598-600, 611)**
   1. placing the call light cord and console on her left side.
   2. unplugging the television so that she is not tempted to watch it.
   3. keeping her in bed for 12 hours.
   4. medicating quickly if she becomes nauseous from anesthesia.

3. The priority outcome for the cataract patient with lens implant in the early postoperative period is the patient will have: **(598-600, 611)**
   1. no evidence of nausea or vomiting.
   2. control of pain and discomfort.
   3. prevention of intraocular hemorrhage.
   4. stabilization of vital signs within 4 hours.

4. The *most* important nursing intervention in the recovery period before discharge from the day surgery unit to ensure success of eye surgery is: **(611)**
   1. medicating for pain before it becomes severe.
   2. answering the call light promptly.
   3. assisting the patient to walk to the bathroom.
   4. positioning the patient per orders.

5. The nurse's most important evaluation criterion for interventions to prevent complications of glaucoma surgery is: **(602-605)**
   1. checking the degree of eye pain.
   2. checking security of the eye dressing.
   3. assessing the amount of nausea.
   4. checking the amount of redness of the operative eye.

6. The therapeutic response expected of dorzolamide (Trusopt) is: **(603, Table 27-1)**
   1. dilation of the pupil.
   2. constriction of the pupil.
   3. decreased intraocular pressure.
   4. decreased production of aqueous humor.

7. Mr. Schultz has come to the emergency department with severe eye pain. He is diagnosed with closed-angle glaucoma. The physician orders IV Diamox 150 mg in 200 mL of D_5W to be given over 15 minutes. The vial of the drug contains 500 mg in 2 mL. How many mL would be added to the D_5W for this infusion? _____

PART II—THE EAR

COMPLETION

Ear Disorders

Directions: Fill in the blanks with the correct words to complete the statements.

1. Causes of labyrinthitis include bacterial meningitis, chronic otitis media, or _____. **(613)**

2. Symptoms of labyrinthitis are loss of hearing in the affected ear, severe dizziness with nausea and vomiting, and _____. **(613)**

Copyright © 2013, 2009 by Saunders, an imprint of Elsevier Inc. All rights reserved.

3. A tympanoplasty involves surgical reconstruction of the _____ and _____ to restore middle ear function. *(613)*

4. Besides difficulty hearing, ear problems and deafness are often accompanied by _____, which can cause considerable fatigue in the person. *(613)*

5. Otosclerosis is generally a(n) _____ degeneration of the _____. *(614)*

6. Hereditary deafness is usually due to changes in the _____ of the ear and causes a(n) _____ hearing loss. *(see Chapter 26)*

7. Conductive hearing loss can often be helped by a(n) _____ or corrected with _____. *(614, see also Chapter 26)*

REVIEW QUESTIONS FOR THE NCLEX® EXAMINATION

Directions: Choose the best answer(s) for each of the following questions.

1. When assessing a patient who is complaining of ear pain, the most important question would be: *(612)*
    1. "Have you been listening to loud music?"
    2. "Have you had a recent upper respiratory infection?"
    3. "Are you prone to form a lot of wax in your ears?"
    4. "What have you taken for your pain?"

2. The nurse would expect to implement which order for the patient with Ménière's disease? *(614)*
    1. Keflin 250 mg q 6 hours IV
    2. Lasix 20 mg three times a day
    3. Morphine 4 mg IM q 4 hours PRN pain
    4. Compazine 25 mg IM q 3–4 hours PRN nausea and vomiting

3. The teaching plan for the discharged patient who has Ménière's disease and is prescribed meclizine would probably include which information about the drug? *(614)*
    1. It is a cholinergic medication.
    2. It is a vitamin-drug combination.
    3. There are antihistamine side effects.
    4. It can be taken when you have glaucoma.

4. When evaluating the success of the teaching program on diet for the patient with Ménière's disease, the nurse would assess for avoidance of foods high in: *(614)*
    1. sugar.
    2. fat.
    3. potassium.
    4. sodium.

5. The patient who has had a stapedectomy should be instructed to: *(615)*
    1. keep the head elevated when in bed.
    2. sneeze and cough with the mouth closed.
    3. apply the ear protector for sleep.
    4. sleep with the affected ear up.

Copyright © 2013, 2009 by Saunders, an imprint of Elsevier Inc. All rights reserved.

6. When teaching the elderly patient about care of his hearing aid, you would include which action(s)? *(Select all that apply.)* **(617, see Chapter 26)**
    1. Keep the battery in the hearing aid.
    2. Clean the ear mold regularly with alcohol.
    3. Never put the hearing aid in water.
    4. Open the battery cover when the hearing aid is not in the ear.

7. Meclizine (Antivert) is a drug that is used for patients with Ménière's disease. This drug is used to reduce dizziness and is a(n): **(614)**
    1. anticholinergic.
    2. corticosteroid.
    3. antihypertensive.
    4. beta blocker.

8. Ms. Jaiswal just had a stapedectomy. She has an IV of $D_5\frac{1}{2}$ NS hanging and there are 660 mL left in the bag. It is prescribed to run at 100 mL/hour. The IV tubing delivers 10 drops per mL. You should set the drip rate at _____ gtts/min.

SHORT ANSWER

Tinnitus and Hearing Loss

Directions: Write a brief answer to each question.

1. What are four medical or nursing interventions that might be helpful to the patient with vertigo? **(613-614)**

    a. _____

    b. _____

    c. _____

    d. _____

2. What are four possible causes of tinnitus? **(see Chapter 26)**

    a. _____

    b. _____

    c. _____

    d. _____

3. Can you list four suggestions you might make to help a person deal with chronic tinnitus? **(see Chapter 26)**

    a. _____

    b. _____

    c. _____

    d. _____

Copyright © 2013, 2009 by Saunders, an imprint of Elsevier Inc. All rights reserved.

4. Name two types of therapy that might be useful in the rehabilitation of a person with a hearing loss. *(see Chapter 26)*

    a. _____

    b. _____

CRITICAL THINKING ACTIVITIES

Case Study: Otosclerosis

A 62-year-old female is at the ear, nose, and throat clinic regarding her hearing loss which is getting worse. She has had a progressive loss of hearing since her late 40s. She wears bilateral hearing aids. She can hear better in her left ear than her right ear. Her mother had hearing loss from her 40s on as well. Her evaluation has determined that she has otosclerosis. Treatment options are discussed and she has made a decision to have a stapedectomy of the right ear. *(614-615)*

1. Why is it significant that her mother had early hearing loss?

2. What diagnostic tests would you expect she underwent during the evaluation?

3. Why is the stapedectomy to be done on the right ear rather than the left ear?

4. What preoperative teaching would you do? What would you cover?

Postoperatively, she is nauseous and states that she is quite dizzy when she tries to sit upright. She has meclizine, Percocet, and Compazine ordered. *(614-615)*

5. Which medication would you administer for the nausea? Which for the dizziness?

6. What safety interventions should you implement?

When the external ear dressing is removed, the patient states she can't hear a thing out of the left ear and becomes upset and tearful.

7. What is the probable cause of her inability to hear in that ear now? What could you say to her at this time that might calm her down?

Copyright © 2013, 2009 by Saunders, an imprint of Elsevier Inc. All rights reserved.

STEPS TOWARD BETTER COMMUNICATION

VOCABULARY BUILDING GLOSSARY

Term	Pronunciation	Definition
am'plified	am' plah fĭd	increased, made louder or bigger
ap'titude	ap' tĭ tūd	good ability to do or learn something
bear in mind		remember; think about; consider
catch all	kech' awl	containing a wide variety of different things
phenom'enon	fah nom' ah non	an unusual or interesting fact or occurrence
prompt	prom' t	quickly; on time; exactly when needed

COMPLETION

Directions: Fill in the blanks with the correct words from the Vocabulary Building Glossary to complete the statements.

1. Joan has a special _____ for nursing.

2. Seeing flashing lights after a retinal detachment is an odd _____.

3. The nurse should always _____ that asepsis is always important in caring for patients with an eye or ear surgery.

4. _____ music at concerts may be damaging to the ear and cause a loss of hearing.

5. The term *hearing loss* is a(n) _____ for several different types of physiologic problems.

6. An ear infection should receive _____ medical attention.

GRAMMAR POINTS

Review of Terms and Combining Forms

kerat/o	cornea
phot/o	light
optic, opt/o	vision
os, oste/o	bone
tax/o	order, coordination
toxic, tox/o	poison
opia	vision
humor	any fluid or semifluid in the body

Copyright © 2013, 2009 by Saunders, an imprint of Elsevier Inc. All rights reserved.

PRONUNCIATION SKILLS

Sup' purative	sup' u rah tiv
Trabec' uloplasty	trah bek' you low plas tee
Labyrinthi' tis	lab ĭ rin thy' tis

ABBREVIATIONS

ARMD	age-related macular degeneration
IGF	insulin-like growth factor
LVES	low-vision enhancement system

Practice pronouncing the above words and abbreviations with a peer. Have your partner write down the words or abbreviations as you say them. Check the list for accurate enunciation.

Copyright © 2013, 2009 by Saunders, an imprint of Elsevier Inc. All rights reserved.

The Gastrointestinal System

Answer Key: Textbook page references are provided as a guide for answering these questions. A complete answer key was provided to your instructor.

REVIEW OF ANATOMY

Directions: Label the structures on the diagram of the digestive system. **(621)**

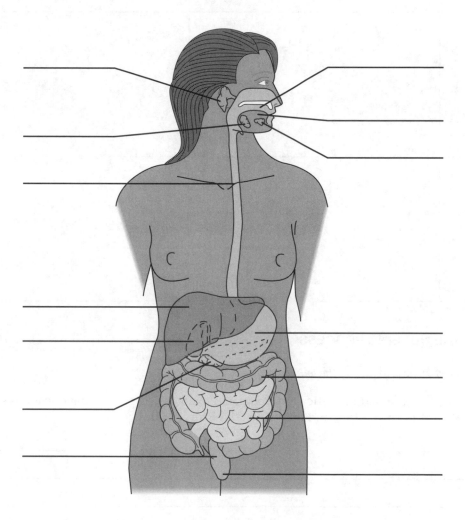

Copyright © 2013, 2009 by Saunders, an imprint of Elsevier Inc. All rights reserved.

TABLE ACTIVITY

Causes and Prevention of Digestive Disorders

Directions: Complete the following table by giving the pathology and preventive measures for various causative factors in the development of digestive disorders. (623-625)

Causative Factors	Pathology (What Occurs)	Preventive Measures
Psychologic and emotional stress and tension		
Mechanical and chemical irritants		
Infectious agents: bacteria, virus, parasites		

APPLICATION OF THE NURSING PROCESS

Directions: Provide a brief answer to each of the following questions.

1. Your patient is scheduled for a diagnostic workup related to epigastric pain. What questions should you ask about the patient's health history and family health history? *(631)*

    a. _____

    b. _____

    c. _____

    d. _____

    e. _____

    f. _____

Copyright © 2013, 2009 by Saunders, an imprint of Elsevier Inc. All rights reserved.

2. Why is checking the color of the urine a part of the gastrointestinal assessment? *(632)* _____

   _____

3. What assessment data might indicate that bile is not reaching the intestine? *(632)* _____

   _____

4. When a patient is experiencing nausea and vomiting, what would be an appropriate nursing diagnosis? *(635-636, Table 28-2)*

   _____

5. When the nursing diagnosis is Constipation related to idiopathic origin, what would be an appropriate expected outcome? *(634, 636, Table 28-2)*

   _____

   _____

6. List three specific nursing interventions for the patient who suffers from constipation. *(634, 636, Table 28-2)*

   a. _____

   b. _____

   c. _____

7. How would you evaluate whether the above interventions were effective? *(634, 636, Table 28-2)*

   _____

   _____

   _____

8. The patient is scheduled for an esophagogastroduodenoscopy (EGD). How would you explain this procedure to her? What special care would she need before and after the procedure? *(627, Table 28-1)*

   a. Procedure: _____

   _____

   _____

   b. Care before EGD: _____

   _____

   _____

   c. Care after EGD: _____

   _____

   _____

Copyright © 2013, 2009 by Saunders, an imprint of Elsevier Inc. All rights reserved.

PRIORITY SETTING

Directions: You are assigned to a newly admitted elderly patient who is suffering from abdominal pain and vomiting.

1. When examining the abdomen, you would perform the steps in a particular order. What order should the examination be performed? *(631-632)*

   _____

   _____

2. As you are performing the abdominal assessment, the patient begins to vomit. What is the priority action?
   1. Assess the emesis for blood, bile, or undigested food particles.
   2. Offer the patient tissues, an emesis basin, and mouth care.
   3. Elevate the head of the bed or assist to a side-lying position.
   4. Administer a prn antiemetic medication.

3. The patient tells you that the pain is "really bad" and seems to be getting worse. What is the first action that you should perform?
   1. Check the time and dose of last administered pain medication.
   2. Reassure the patient that everything that can be done has been done.
   3. Ask the patient to further describe and locate the pain.
   4. Report the worsening of pain to the physician or RN.

REVIEW QUESTIONS FOR THE NCLEX® EXAMINATION

Directions: Choose the best answer(s) for the following questions.

1. The physician schedules a patient for a colonoscopy. In preparing him for this procedure, you explain that: *(628, Table 28-1)*
   1. he will be moderately sedated to minimize discomfort.
   2. the procedure takes only about 6 minutes.
   3. he may have a clear liquid breakfast before the procedure.
   4. he can go back to work as soon as the procedure is over.

2. The nurse is caring for several patients with gastrointestinal problems. Which patient is most likely to need a guaiac (Hemoccult) test? *(625, 629, 631, Table 28-1)*
   1. Patient reports dark amber-colored urine.
   2. Patient reports black discoloration of stool.
   3. Patient vomits small amounts of yellow emesis.
   4. Patient complains of right upper quadrant pain.

3. Which healthy lifestyle choice can decrease the risk of pancreatic cancer? *(625)*
   1. Eat a well-balanced diet.
   2. Obtain 30 minutes of exercise at least 3 times a week.
   3. Refrain from drinking any alcohol.
   4. Refrain from smoking cigarettes.

4. When patients undergo diagnostic tests of the gastrointestinal system, elderly patients in particular must be closely watched for: *(631)*
   1. dehydration and electrolyte imbalance.
   2. nausea and vomiting.
   3. diarrhea.
   4. constipation from contrast media.

Copyright © 2013, 2009 by Saunders, an imprint of Elsevier Inc. All rights reserved.

5. Hyperactive bowel sounds in one quadrant and absent bowel sounds in other quadrants plus nausea and vomiting may indicate: *(632)*
   1. pancreatitis.
   2. cholecystitis.
   3. gastrointestinal bleeding.
   4. intestinal obstruction.

6. Your patient is receiving an IV of $D_5\frac{1}{2}NS$ 1000 mL ordered to run at 150 mL/hr. The IV tubing delivers 15 drops per mL. You would set the IV to run at _____ gtts/min.

7. Your patient is to have a liver biopsy. What teaching point(s) should be included in the instructions? *(Select all that apply.)* *(628, Table 28-1)*
   1. Nothing is allowed by mouth for 4–8 hours prior to the procedure.
   2. Local or general anesthesia will be used.
   3. Patient will be positioned on the right lateral side for the procedure.
   4. The procedure takes about an hour.
   5. It will be necessary to lie on the right side for 1–2 hours postprocedure.
   6. Heavy lifting or strenuous activities are to be avoided for 1–2 weeks.

8. The nurse hears in report that a patient is suspected of having ascites. Which action is the nurse most likely to initiate for this specific condition? *(631)*
   1. Elevate the head of the bed 30-45 degrees.
   2. Assess for pain every 30-60 minutes.
   3. Perform serial measurements of abdominal girth.
   4. Slightly elevate legs and buttocks to help expel flatus.

9. The patient is supposed to be NPO for 12 hours prior to diagnostic testing. The nursing assistant reports that the patient just drank a soda and ate a sandwich. What should the nurse do first? *(631)*
   1. Explain the purpose of NPO to the patient.
   2. Make an incident report that includes all the relevant facts.
   3. Cancel the test and reschedule it for the next day.
   4. Notify the charge nurse and the diagnostic technician.

CRITICAL THINKING ACTIVITIES

Scenario: A 78-year-old is admitted with nausea, vomiting, diarrhea, and dehydration. An IV of D_5RL is started at 125 mL per hour. The patient also has hypertension and osteoarthritis of the knees. The vomiting has stopped, but the patient is still somewhat nauseous.

1. Considering the nausea and vomiting, what measures would you take to help rehydrate the patient? *(635)*

Copyright © 2013, 2009 by Saunders, an imprint of Elsevier Inc. All rights reserved.

2.   Considering the diagnosis of hypertension, what fluids would you need to use with caution in this patient? *(see Chapter 19)*

3.   What nursing measures would you institute because of the diarrhea? *(636)*

STEPS TOWARD BETTER COMMUNICATION

VOCABULARY BUILDING GLOSSARY

Term	Pronunciation	Definition
absorption (noun)	ab sorp' shun	the uptake of a substance into or across tissues
alleviate; alleviating (verb)	a lee'vee ate	to lessen, to make less severe
assimilation (noun)	as sim i lay' shun	the transformation of food into tissue
atrophy (verb)	a' tro fee	to dry up, become withered, waste away

COMPLETION

Directions: Fill in the blanks with the correct words from the Vocabulary Building Glossary to complete the statements.

1.   Taste buds may _____ as a person ages.

2.   Every attempt is made to _____ pain.

3.   Water is _____ from fecal material as it passes through the large intestine.

MATCHING

Directions: Match the abbreviation or word on the left with the correct term on the right.

1.   _____   ERCP
2.   _____   BE
3.   _____   HIDA
4.   _____   UGI
5.   _____   NPO
6.   _____   GI
7.   _____   Mastication
8.   _____   Peristalsis
9.   _____   Metabolism

a.   Upper gastrointestinal
b.   Gastrointestinal
c.   Nothing by mouth
d.   Barium enema
e.   Endoscopic retrograde cholangiopancreatography
f.   Hepatoiminodiacetic acid scan
g.   Converting nutrients to energy
h.   Chewing
i.   Rhythmic squeezing action

Copyright © 2013, 2009 by Saunders, an imprint of Elsevier Inc. All rights reserved.

COMMUNICATION EXERCISE

Scrambled Sentences

Directions: Arrange the words in the correct order to make a sentence.

1. avoided Heavy weeks. are or to be 1–2 activities for lifting for strenuous

   _____

2. be anesthetic or will general used. local A

   _____

3. history have digestive Do a family of problems? you

   _____

CULTURAL POINT

Certain diseases have a genetic predisposition. This means people may tend to inherit that disease from their parents. Because of this, people of certain races or ethnic groups may be more liable to get a particular disease. Genetic predisposition is one reason why taking a family medical history is so important. If you are working in an area with a particular ethnic population (Jewish, Native American, Asian, etc.) be sure to inform yourself and be on the lookout for the related symptoms of diseases that are genetically predisposed to that group. Working with the groups for education and prevention is also recommended.

Copyright © 2013, 2009 by Saunders, an imprint of Elsevier Inc. All rights reserved.

Care of Patients with Disorders of the Upper Gastrointestinal System

Answer Key: Textbook page references are provided as a guide for answering these questions. A complete answer key was provided to your instructor.

REVIEW OF ANATOMY AND PHYSIOLOGY

COMPLETION

Upper Gastrointestinal Disorders

Directions: Fill in the blanks to complete the statements.

1. A surgical procedure for obesity that can be done laparoscopically is _____
    _____. *(641)*

2. In North America, an emphasis on a slim body has been an influence that has contributed to the development of _____ in young women. *(see Chapter 46)*

3. A risk factor for cancer of the esophagus is gastric _____ and the development of
    _____. *(645)*

4. A hiatal hernia is a defect in the wall of the _____. *(645)*

5. About 90% of patients who have GERD have a(n) _____. *(646)*

6. The main cause of gastritis is _____. *(649)*

7. Decreased blood pressure and increased pulse do not occur in the patient with a GI bleed until he has lost more than _____ of his blood. *(651)*

8. When GI bleeding occurs, the hemoglobin and hematocrit readings do not show a drop for _____ hours. *(651)*

9. Dumping syndrome sometimes occurs after the patient has had a(n) _____
    _____. *(657)*

10. Gastritis associated with _____ is common in the patient with kidney failure. *(649)*

11. The surgical procedure of hemiglossectomy is performed for the treatment of
    _____. *(644)*

Copyright © 2013, 2009 by Saunders, an imprint of Elsevier Inc. All rights reserved.

SHORT ANSWER

Ulcer Disease

Directions: Read the clinical situation and answer the questions that follow.

Scenario: Mrs. Galt, age 41, works two jobs to support herself and her children. Recently, she has been skipping meals to save time and money. In the past few months, she has had frequent bouts of heartburn, has lost 15 pounds, and occasionally vomits up blood-streaked, partially digested food. She was seen by a physician at her neighborhood clinic who told her she may be developing a peptic ulcer and that she should eat more regularly and take an antacid when she has heartburn.

1. Although she is suffering from anxiety about her home situation, Mrs. Galt's ulcer is not diagnosed as a stress ulcer. How does a stress ulcer differ from a peptic ulcer? *(650)*

   _____

   _____

Mrs. Galt continues to have epigastric pain and becomes too sick to work. She is admitted to the hospital for a diagnostic workup and treatment.

2. What daily pattern of pain would you expect Mrs. Galt to describe when asked about her pain? *(651)*

   _____

   _____

3. What type of diagnostic test would most likely be performed first? *(651-652)*_____

   _____

4. What are the three major complications of peptic ulcer? *(655)*

   a. _____

   b. _____

   c. _____

5. Her physician prescribes esomeprazole (Nexium) for Mrs. Galt. List the three results that are expected from this drug. *(647, 652, Table 29-1)*

   a. _____

   b. _____

   c. _____

Copyright © 2013, 2009 by Saunders, an imprint of Elsevier Inc. All rights reserved.

6. Mrs. Galt is also told to take an antacid four times a day, to avoid foods that disagree with her, and to return to the outpatient clinic in 3 months for follow-up. What information do you think Mrs. Galt will need to take care of herself properly, recover from her illness, and return to work? *(653, 655, Nursing Care Plan 29-1)*

    a. _____

    b. _____

    c. _____

    d. _____

    e. _____

7. Some patients are not able to respond to medical management and must have surgery. List four surgical procedures that might be performed to treat gastric and duodenal ulcers. *(655-656)*

    a. _____

    b. _____

    c. _____

    d. _____

APPLICATION OF THE NURSING PROCESS

Directions: Provide the answer to the following questions.

Scenario: Mr. Timmons has cancer of the stomach. He has been vomiting and unable to eat and was admitted to the hospital yesterday. He has lost 7 lbs. in the last week. He was started on TPN yesterday afternoon.

1. Which nursing diagnosis would be appropriate for this problem? *(657)*
    a. Altered nutrition, less than body requirements r/t vomiting and inability to keep food in the stomach
    b. Readiness for enhanced fluid balance r/t nausea and vomiting
    c. Deficient fluid volume related to vomiting
    d. Risk for deficient fluid volume related to vomiting

2. Can you write an expected outcome for the correct nursing diagnosis for Mr. Timmons' problem? *(657)*

    _____

3. List three interventions appropriate for Mr. Timmons related to the administration of the TPN. *(660)*

    a. _____

    b. _____

    c. _____

4. What are comfort interventions often used for the patient who is vomiting? *(649, 658)*_____

    _____

    _____

    _____

Copyright © 2013, 2009 by Saunders, an imprint of Elsevier Inc. All rights reserved.

5. What evaluation criteria would be needed to determine whether the interventions are effective and the expected outcome is being met? *(657-660)*

_____

_____

PRIORITY SETTING

Scenario: You are caring for the following patients: Ms. Schultz, a confused elderly lady with gastroenteritis and dehydration; Mr. Hooper, a 45-year-old working man with a bleeding peptic ulcer, Ms. Peterson, a 48-year-old woman who is second-day postoperative after an abdominal surgical procedure for weight control. Which patients have needs that can be delegated to the nursing assistant? Indicate the order you would attend to the following needs of these patients. It is presently 7:45 AM.

_____ a. Ms. Schultz urgently needs to go to the bathroom.

_____ b. Mr. Hooper has just vomited again and has called for his nurse.

_____ c. Ms. Peterson is calling for more pain medication.

_____ d. Ms. Peterson needs assistance with her bath.

_____ e. Mr. Hooper is scheduled for a gastroscopy at 9:30 AM and needs to be prepared.

_____ f. Ms. Schultz has not yet been assessed for this shift.

REVIEW QUESTIONS FOR THE NCLEX® EXAMINATION

Directions: Choose the best answer(s) for the following questions.

1. A nurse hears in report that a patient has stomatitis. Which intervention is the nurse most likely to initiate for this patient? *(643, see also Chapter 8)*
   1. Check for tube gastric residual before feeding.
   2. Assess for a typical 24-hour eating pattern.
   3. Offer frequent mouth care and artificial saliva.
   4. Perform a physical assessment with a skinfold measurement.

2. The nurse is giving care to a patient with a gastrostomy tube. Which nursing intervention is appropriate? *(659, 668, Box 29-1)*
   1. Flush the tube after each feeding.
   2. Instruct the patient to take some practice swallows.
   3. Give only thickened liquids.
   4. Handle the tube using sterile technique.

3. Prior to administering an enteral feeding through a feeding tube, the nurse checks for residual. What is the best rationale for performing this nursing action? *(659-660, Box 29-1)*
   1. Checking for residual is likely to be in the procedural manual.
   2. The appearance of residual should be documented.
   3. Excessive volume can cause regurgitation and aspiration.
   4. Nutritionist bases formula recommendations on residual content.

Copyright © 2013, 2009 by Saunders, an imprint of Elsevier Inc. All rights reserved.

4. Following a stroke, a patient has dysphagia and a nursing diagnosis of Impaired swallowing. What would be the best outcome statement? *(643-644)*
   1. Patient will receive puréed foods and thickened liquids.
   2. Patient will increase swallowing muscle strength.
   3. Patient will control breathing while swallowing.
   4. Patient will keep head tilted back when swallowing.

5. A patient is second-day post-gastrointestinal surgery and has a nasogastric (NG) tube attached to suction. There is little drainage in the suction container after 4 hours. What should the nurse do first? *(658-660)*
   1. Check to see that the NG tube is still in the correct place by checking the mark near the nose.
   2. Try to aspirate some stomach contents.
   3. Irrigate the tube with the ordered amount of solution.
   4. Instill 2 mL of air into the pigtail of the NG tube with a dry syringe.

6. A patient is suspected of having esophageal cancer. Which diagnostic test is the physician most likely to order to make the definitive diagnosis? *(645)*
   1. Esophageal manometry with 24-hour pH monitoring
   2. Gastric analysis and serum tests for *H. pylori*
   3. Upper GI series and check body mass index
   4. Esophagogastroduodenoscopy with biopsy

7. Your patient who has had gastric surgery has an NG tube attached to suction. You have irrigated the tube twice with 30 mL of sterile water. At the end of the shift there is 420 mL of drainage in the container. The NG output for the shift is _____ mL.

8. Proton pump inhibitors such as rabeprazole (Aciphex) work by: *(647, Table 29-1)*
   1. increasing HCl secretion in the stomach.
   2. neutralizing stomach acid.
   3. both neutralizing and suppressing stomach acid.
   4. suppressing the secretion of stomach acid.

9. A nursing implication for esomeprazole (Nexium) is to: *(647, Table 29-1)*
   1. administer the drug only with food.
   2. not to administer the drug with digoxin (Lanoxin).
   3. administer the drug along with an antacid.
   4. do not administer the drug along with orange or grapefruit juice.

10. When caring for a patient with nasogastric suction, you would test the drainage for blood if you found: *(658)*
    1. copious greenish drainage in the container.
    2. coffee ground-like material in the tubing.
    3. complaints of continued nausea by the patient.
    4. a rising blood pressure and pulse rate.

CRITICAL THINKING ACTIVITIES

Scenario A: Mr. Sims comes to the ambulatory clinic because he is having severe heartburn (GERD). He was diagnosed with a hiatal hernia a year ago. You are assigned to take his history and will do the teaching reinforcement that he needs.

1. What questions would you ask him? *(645-646, 649)*

Copyright © 2013, 2009 by Saunders, an imprint of Elsevier Inc. All rights reserved.

2. Describe the specific teaching you would do for this patient. *(645-646, 649)*

Scenario B: The nurse is working in clinic that specializes in treating obesity. The nurse is responsible for assessing patients and teaching about weight management, risk factors, and treatment options.

1. Some factors of obesity are controllable, some are not. What factors contribute to obesity? *(Select all that apply.) (641)*
   1. A high-protein, moderate-fat diet
   2. Vitamin and supplement intake
   3. A diet high in calories and fat
   4. Family genetic make-up
   5. Large dinner plates and growing portion sizes
   6. Prepackaged foods and "fast food"

2. What are the complications of obesity? *(Select all that apply.) (641)*
   1. Hypertension
   2. Diabetes mellitus
   3. Multiple sclerosis
   4. Asthma
   5. Cholelithiasis
   6. Coronary artery disease
   7. Arthritis of the knees

3. A person is considered obese if he or she weighs more than _____ percent above ideal weight for height and body type. *(Fill in the blank.) (641)*
   1. 10%
   2. 30%
   3. 5%
   4. 20%

4. What data would the nurse gather that is specific to the assessment of a patient with obesity? *(642)*

5. Discuss five nonsurgical treatment approaches that may be recommend for weight loss. *(641)*

Copyright © 2013, 2009 by Saunders, an imprint of Elsevier Inc. All rights reserved.

STEPS TOWARD BETTER COMMUNICATION

VOCABULARY BUILDING GLOSSARY

Term	Pronunciation	Definition
regurgitation	ree gurj ah ta' shun	bringing food from the stomach back to the mouth; repeating something without thinking about it
dumping	dump'ing	dropping a mass suddenly
intrinsic factor	intrin'sik fak'tor	glycoprotein necessary for the absorption of vitamin B_{12} from the gastrointestinal system
manifested	man'ifested	showing symptoms of something
adverse	ad'verse	negative, unfavorable
adhere	ad heer'	to follow, to stick to
abound	ah bownd'	exist in great numbers; to be multiple
despite	des pyt'	in spite of; not prevented by

COMPLETION

Directions: Fill in the blanks with the appropriate words from the Vocabulary Building Glossary to complete the statements.

1. Sometimes after a subtotal gastrectomy and vagotomy, _____ syndrome occurs.

2. Recurrent stomach pain, nausea, and _____ may be signs of peptic ulcer.

3. Patients who lack _____ tend to develop pernicious anemia.

4. People trying to lose weight often have problems trying to _____ to their diet.

5. People who regularly take antacids _____ in our society.

MATCHING

Directions: Match the abbreviation on the left with the correct term on the right.

1. _____ GI   a. Milliliter
2. _____ NG   b. Hemoglobin
3. _____ NSAIDs   c. Gastrointestinal
4. _____ mL   d. Nasogastric
5. _____ Hb or Hgb   e. Nonsteroidal antiinflammatory drugs

Copyright © 2013, 2009 by Saunders, an imprint of Elsevier Inc. All rights reserved.

PRONUNCIATION SKILLS

Directions: With a peer, take turns pronouncing these words to increase your ability to speak English clearly.

gas'troesophage'al (gas' tro ee sof ah jee' al)   pertaining to the stomach and esophagus

hy'poglyce'mic (hi' po gli see' mik)   having low serum glucose

mal'occlu'sion (mal' ah cloo' zhun)   top and bottom teeth do not come together properly

meta'bolism (mah tab' ah lizm)   process of the building up and breaking down tissue

The pronunciation of the letters **"ai"** in the two words constraint and contraindicated are different. In the first word, they make the long **"a"** sound because they are in the same syllable and are pronounced together (as in pain and complain). In the second word, they are pronounced separately because they are in different syllables:

con straints (kon strants')

con tra in di ca ted (kon' trah in' di ka' ted)

Copyright © 2013, 2009 by Saunders, an imprint of Elsevier Inc. All rights reserved.

Care of Patients with Disorders of the Lower Gastrointestinal System

Answer Key: Textbook page references are provided as a guide for answering these questions. A complete answer key was provided to your instructor.

SHORT ANSWER

Assessment and Pathophysiology

Directions: Provide brief answers for the following questions.

1. The cause of irritable bowel syndrome is unknown, but several things seems to trigger episodes including: *(664)*

   _____

   _____

2. The pathophysiologic explanation for diverticulitis is: *(668)*_____

   _____

   _____

3. If an elderly person develops appendicitis, the presenting signs and symptoms may differ from those in a younger adult. The older adult may present with only _____

   _____. *(672)*

4. Peritonitis may occur when the appendix ruptures. The pathophysiologic explanation is: *(673)*

   _____

   _____

   _____

5. Hemorrhoids may be internal or external and usually present with: *(685-686)* _____

   _____

COMPLETION

Lower Gastrointestinal Disorders

Directions: Fill in the blank to complete the statement.

1. Severe malabsorption problems of the small intestine often necessitate _____

   _____. *(673-674)*

Copyright © 2013, 2009 by Saunders, an imprint of Elsevier Inc. All rights reserved.

2. An abdominoperineal resection requires a(n) _____ colostomy. *(675, 680)*

3. If a hernia becomes incarcerated, it can cause _____ of the protruding part. *(664)*

4. Instead of surgery, hemorrhoids can sometimes be removed by _____ or _____. *(686)*

5. A diet high in _____ is thought to contribute to the formation of cancer of the colon. *(674)*

LABELING

Ostomies

Directions: Write the correct names of the procedures depicted in the three drawings below. (680)

1. _____

2. _____

3. _____

COMPLETION

Directions: Fill in the blanks to complete the statements.

1. The discharge from an ascending colostomy is normally _____. *(679)*

2. A potential problem for the patient with a sigmoid colostomy is _____. *(680)*

3. An ascending colostomy is usually _____. *(679)*

4. The discharge from an ileostomy is _____. *(680)*

5. An ileostomy is often performed on the patient who has _____. *(680)*

6. A continent ileostomy is drained by _____. *(683)*

7. It is easier to establish a pattern of evacuation to control the flow of fecal material through a(n) _____ colostomy. *(683)*

Copyright © 2013, 2009 by Saunders, an imprint of Elsevier Inc. All rights reserved.

8. In a double-barreled colostomy, the distal stoma leads to the rectum and should discharge only small amounts of _____. *(679)*

9. The colonoscopy shows a small, apparently localized tumor in the upper sigmoid colon. The treatment of choice for this tumor would be _____. *(675)*

SHORT ANSWER

Directions: Write a short answer for each of the following questions.

1. What are two major principles that should be followed to protect the skin around the stoma from irritation and breakdown? *(682)*

   a. _____

   b. _____

2. What is the major reason for irrigating a colostomy? *(683)* _____

   _____

3. What three nursing interventions may help prevent cramping, nausea, and dizziness during a colostomy irrigation? *(682-683)*

   a. _____

   b. _____

   c. _____

4. What three nursing interventions may help a patient prevent or overcome repeated expulsion of gas from the colostomy? *(684-685)*

   a. _____

   b. _____

   c. _____

5. What three nursing interventions may help a patient prevent or overcome obstruction of the ileostomy? *(685)*

   a. _____

   b. _____

   c. _____

6. List four nursing interventions that might be helpful in assisting the patient to adjust psychologically to an ostomy. *(684)*

   a. _____

   b. _____

   c. _____

   d. _____

Copyright © 2013, 2009 by Saunders, an imprint of Elsevier Inc. All rights reserved.

COMPLETION

Medications

Directions: Fill in the answers to the following questions. **(666-667, Table 30-1)**

1. List two important points the nurse should teach the patient who has diphenoxylate hydrochloride (Lomotil) prescribed.

   a. _____

   b. _____

2. What is a contraindication to using a stool softener? _____

   _____

3. Name a major problem with the use of contact laxatives. _____

   _____

4. Give an important nursing implication for administering a histamine receptor antagonist to a patient who is also taking an antacid.

   _____

5. How should a patient who has an antispasmodic prescribed be taught to take it? _____

   _____

6. What should the diabetic patient taking an oral hypoglycemic drug and sulfasalazine be specifically told to prevent a problem?

   _____

   _____

PRIORITY SETTING

Scenario: You are assigned the following patients: Ms. K., a newly admitted female, 68 years old, with probable intestinal obstruction. Mr. P., a 46-year-old male 1 day postoperative for a ruptured appendix and peritonitis. Ms. T., a 72-year-old female with diverticulitis and dehydration. Ms. S., a 56-year-old female patient with Crohn's disease on total parenteral nutrition (TPN). You have just received shift report for the previous shift. Place the following tasks and needs in the order in which you would attend to them.

_____ a. Ms. T. is calling for pain medication.

_____ b. Assessment (data collection) for Ms. T.

_____ c. Wound irrigation and dressing change for Mr. P.

_____ d. Assessment (data collection) for Mr. P.

_____ e. Ms. K. is vomiting, coughing, and calling for help.

_____ f. Assessment (data collection) for Ms. K.

_____ g. Assessment (data collection) of Ms. S. including blood sugar determination.

Copyright © 2013, 2009 by Saunders, an imprint of Elsevier Inc. All rights reserved.

REVIEW QUESTIONS FOR THE NCLEX® EXAMINATION

Directions: Choose or supply the best answer(s) for the following questions.

1. The patient has a diagnosis of irritable bowel syndrome. What symptoms is the patient mostly likely to display? *(665)*
   1. Constipation and/or diarrhea, abdominal pain, bloating
   2. Abnormal pouching out from the abdominal wall or in the groin area
   3. Frequent high-pitched bowel sounds in the area of peristaltic contractions
   4. Rapid dehydration and only slight abdominal distention

2. A female, age 26, has been diagnosed with ulcerative colitis. She is hospitalized prior to intestinal surgery. When gathering data on this patient, the nurse would expect to obtain a history of: *(670-671)*
   1. alternating bowel pattern of diarrhea and constipation.
   2. intolerance to milk and milk products.
   3. episodes of bloody, mucoid diarrhea.
   4. excessive smoking and/or alcohol use.

3. In planning care for a patient with ulcerative colitis, there is a nursing diagnosis of Nutrition, less than body requirements. Which intervention is most appropriate? *(671-672)*
   1. Offer small frequent amounts of high-protein, high-calorie food.
   2. Help the patient to list effective coping mechanisms to deal with weight loss.
   3. Encourage large amounts of favorite and culturally acceptable foods.
   4. Advise the patient to exercise less and adopt a sedentary lifestyle.

4. The nurse is assessing a patient's abdomen and observes an outpouching of tissue on the abdomen. What should the nurse do *first*? *(663-664)*
   1. Immediately report the finding to the RN or the MD.
   2. Ask the patient if this outpouching has recently occurred after lifting.
   3. Push on the outpouching to determine if there is a reducible hernia.
   4. Suggest that the patient make an appointment with a surgeon.

5. What evaluation data indicates that therapy for intestinal inflammation is effective? *(665)*
   1. Decrease in the number of diarrheal stools
   2. Decrease in appetite and food consumption
   3. Decrease in hemoglobin and hematocrit
   4. Decrease in weight and energy

6. Treatment of ulcerative colitis sometimes involves resting the bowel. In this event, the patient is placed on: *(671-672)*
   1. long-term intravenous fluids.
   2. a bland diet for several weeks.
   3. a low-residue diet for 3 weeks.
   4. total parenteral nutrition.

7. When a patient is receiving TPN, the nurse incorporates which safety factor into the plan of care? *(see Chapter 29)*
   1. Never speeding up the TPN solution if it falls behind schedule
   2. Carefully monitoring and assessing intake and output
   3. Changing the peripheral IV site every 48 hours
   4. Monitoring for signs of hypoglycemia during each nursing shift

Copyright © 2013, 2009 by Saunders, an imprint of Elsevier Inc. All rights reserved.

8. The nurse is caring for a postsurgical patient who had abdominal resection with a permanent colostomy. What is the best rationale for immediately initiating deep vein thrombosis (DVT) precautions? *(681-682)*
    1. DVT precautions are always ordered for major surgery patients.
    2. A high lithotomy position is used during surgery.
    3. Anticoagulants were discontinued preoperatively.
    4. The patient will not be able to ambulate for several days.

9. A sign of colon cancer that a patient might experience is: *(675)*
    1. nausea.
    2. excessive gas.
    3. pain after eating.
    4. black stool.

10. Which ostomy patient is most at risk for Impaired skin integrity related to contact with digestive enzymes at the ostomy site? *(679-682)*
    1. Patient with an ileostomy
    2. Patient with sigmoid colostomy
    3. Patient with a double-barreled colostomy
    4. Patient with a continent ileostomy

11. The patient has an order to "force fluids." The intake and output records indicate the following for this shift:

	Intake	Output
0730		650 mL
0800	250 mL	
0900	220 mL	
1000	175 mL	420 mL
1100	225 mL	
1200	110 mL	
1300	455 mL	
1400	180 mL	675 mL
1500	220 mL	

    The intake and output for the shift are: I = _____ O = _____

12. A patient with diverticulitis and dehydration is receiving intravenous fluid. The order reads D_5NS 1000 mL at 150 mL/hr. The available IV tubing delivers 10 gtts/mL. The IV should run at _____ gtts/min.

13. The nurse is caring for a patient who had intestinal surgery. In the immediate postoperative period, what is the priority nursing diagnosis? *(see Chapter 29)*
    1. Risk for deficient fluid volume
    2. Risk for nausea
    3. Risk for infection
    4. Risk for disturbed body image

14. The nurse is observing the new stoma of a patient who recently had a colostomy. Which finding is the nurse most concerned about? *(682)*
    1. There is slight bleeding around the stoma and the stem.
    2. The stoma has a cherry-red color and appears moist.
    3. The stoma has a deepening color of a purplish hue.
    4. There is no fecal output on the second postoperative day.

Copyright © 2013, 2009 by Saunders, an imprint of Elsevier Inc. All rights reserved.

15. The patient with diverticular disease states, "Why can't I eat raspberries? I love them?" What is the best nursing response to the patient's question? *(668)*
    1. The berries can cause a bowel obstruction.
    2. The red color will come out in your stool and look like blood.
    3. The seeds will scratch the mucosa and cause bleeding.
    4. The seeds can get caught in the pouchings and cause inflammation.

16. The nursing student is caring for a patient with a possible appendicitis. The nurse would intervene if the student performed which action? *(672)*
    1. Suggests that the patient rest with the right thigh drawn up
    2. Checks the patient's vital signs, including the temperature
    3. Applies a warm pack to the right lower quadrant for comfort
    4. Explains that food and fluids are not allowed at this time

17. The patient reports that after a bowel movement, the stool is floating in the water. What is the significance of this finding? *(674)*
    1. A stool specimen should be collected for culture and sensitivity.
    2. The patient may not be eating enough fiber in the diet.
    3. There may be a problem with the digestion of fat.
    4. Potentially there is insufficient bile to aid digestion.

CRITICAL THINKING ACTIVITIES

Scenario: Ms. Rubens has had inflammatory bowel disease for the past 5 years. Her specific diagnosis is Crohn's disease. She is tired of feeling ill all the time, the diarrhea episodes, and inability to work full-time. The infliximab (Remicade) infusions don't seem to help much anymore. She is presently anemic, has lost 10 lbs. in the past few months, and is seeking treatment that will help her have an improved lifestyle. She enters the hospital for hyperalimentation with TPN.

1. When you come onto your shift and are assigned this patient, which laboratory values would you check in the medical record? *(671, see also Chapter 29)*

2. How do the signs and symptoms of Crohn's disease differ from those of ulcerative colitis? *(671)*

3. Why is surgery not a first choice for patients with Crohn's disease? *(671-672)*

4. What type of drug is infliximab? What are its major side effects? *(672)*

Copyright © 2013, 2009 by Saunders, an imprint of Elsevier Inc. All rights reserved.

STEPS TOWARD BETTER COMMUNICATION

VOCABULARY BUILDING GLOSSARY

Term	Pronunciation	Definition
adhere	ad heer'	to follow, to stick to
adverse	ad'verse	negative, unfavorable
manifested	man'ifested	showing symptoms of something
mush		a soft, wet mass; consistency of cooked cereal
constraints	kon strayn'ts	limitations
"worry wort"		person who worries about everything
offend'ing	ah fend' ing	causing a problem
gur'gle	ger' gul	sound of water or liquid bubbling (as in boiling or moving over stones)
bout	bowt	a short, difficult period
empathy	em' pa thee	understanding another person's feelings
effluent	ef' floo ent	material discharged or flowing out
blanching	blanch' ing	turning white or light-colored

COMPLETION

Directions: Fill in the blanks with the appropriate words from the Vocabulary Building Glossary to complete the statements.

1. The patient's stool was the consistency of _____.

2. Because the patient worried about every little thing, she was called a(n) _____.

3. The _____ from a new ileostomy must be carefully measured.

4. The patient was having trouble with his ileostomy because he did not _____ to the dietary guidelines.

5. Ostomy patients do worry about _____ those around them with bad odors.

6. The patient's intestinal disease was _____ by frequent bouts of bloody diarrhea.

7. While auscultating bowel sounds, the nurse heard a(n) _____ in the left upper quadrant.

8. The nurse checked the reddened area on the patient's buttocks for _____ when she turned him to determine if a pressure ulcer was developing.

9. The patient who ignores signs of colon cancer may have a(n) _____ outcome.

10. The patient with diverticulitis was experiencing another _____ of severe abdominal pain.

11. The nurse must try to develop _____ for patients who are experiencing a tremendous body image change due to an ostomy.

Copyright © 2013, 2009 by Saunders, an imprint of Elsevier Inc. All rights reserved.

MATCHING

Directions: Match the abbreviation on the left with the correct term on the right.

1. _____ BM
2. _____ IBS
3. _____ IBD
4. _____ TPN

    a. Inflammatory bowel disease
    b. Bowel movement
    c. Total parenteral nutrition
    d. Irritable bowel syndrome

PRONUNCIATION SKILLS

Directions: Practice pronouncing these words with a peer to increase your ability to speak English.

def'ecate (def' ah kayt)   eliminate stool

incon'tinence (in kon' tah nens)   no control over passage of urine or stool

piloni'dal (py lo nydal)   having a core of hair

sa'crococcyg'eal (sa' kro kok sij' ee al)   pertaining to the sacrum and coccyx

CULTURAL POINT

There are a variety of common terms that patients may use for digestive functions. Proper medical terms are listed below in dark print; the other terms are not medical terms and are impolite, but you should understand the meaning when you hear them.

bowel movement (BM), **defecate**, **stool**, **feces**, shit, crap, excreta, poop, dump

gas, **flatus**, **flatulence**, pass gas, pass wind, fart, poop

diarrhea, the runs, the trots

Copyright © 2013, 2009 by Saunders, an imprint of Elsevier Inc. All rights reserved.

Care of Patients with Disorders of the Gallbladder, Liver, and Pancreas

Answer Key: Textbook page references are provided as a guide for answering these questions. A complete answer key was provided to your instructor.

COMPLETION

Gallbladder Disease

Directions: Fill in the blanks to complete the statements.

1. The most frequent cause of cholecystitis is _____. *(691)*

2. _____ is the presence of gallstones within the gallbladder or in the biliary tract. *(690)*

3. The surgical procedure most often performed for treatment of cholelithiasis is _____ _____. *(692)*

4. Four types of people most at risk for developing cholelithiasis are those who: *(690)*

   a. _____

   b. _____

   c. _____

   d. _____

5. List four diagnostic tests that may be ordered to diagnose cholelithiasis or gallbladder disease. *(692)*

   a. _____

   b. _____

   c. _____

   d. _____

Diseases of the Liver and Pancreas

Directions: Fill in the blanks to complete the statements.

1. Ascites is the result of a condition in which there is _____ of the portal circulation. *(701)*

2. Medical treatment of ascites includes restriction of _____ and _____ and administration of _____. *(702)*

Copyright © 2013, 2009 by Saunders, an imprint of Elsevier Inc. All rights reserved.

3. The insertion of a large needle into the peritoneal cavity to remove ascitic fluid is called a(n) _____. *(702)*

4. A LaVeen shunt involves directing excess fluid in the peritoneal cavity from the _____ _____ to the _____. *(702)*

5. Neurologic changes that occur as a result of liver failure constitute a condition called _____ _____. *(698)*

6. Jaundice occurs when _____ flow out of the liver is blocked and _____ is entering the bloodstream. *(701-702)*

7. In liver failure, mental status changes that can progress to coma are due to excess _____ in the blood, which eventually reaches the brain cells and damages them. *(703)*

8. In an effort to minimize brain damage, a patient with neurologic symptoms due to advanced cirrhosis may be placed on a diet that is limited in _____. *(703)*

9. The most deadly of all complications of cirrhosis of the liver is _____ _____. *(704)*

10. Both hepatitis B and cirrhosis increase the risk of _____. *(694)*

11. If the tumor is confined to the liver, _____ is an option. *(708)*

12. The majority of cases of pancreatitis are caused by _____, _____, and _____. *(708)*

13. When powdered pancreatic enzymes are given with food, the powder should be mixed in _____; it should not be allowed to remain on the _____ because it will cause irritation. *(710)*

14. Cancer of the pancreas is twice as frequent among _____. *(710)*

REVIEW QUESTIONS FOR THE NCLEX® EXAMINATION

Directions: Choose the best answer(s) for the following questions.

1. The nurse is caring for a patient who is known to be infected with hepatitis A. Which infection control precautions should the nurse implement? *(Select all that apply.) (695, Table 31-2)*
   1. Wear a mask when entering the patient's room.
   2. Wear a gown when delivering the patient's meal tray.
   3. Wear a gown and gloves when bathing the patient.
   4. Wear latex gloves when emptying the bedpan after a bowel movement.
   5. Wear a face shield during dressing changes.
   6. Wear protective shoe covers when assisting patient with ambulation.

Copyright © 2013, 2009 by Saunders, an imprint of Elsevier Inc. All rights reserved.

2. The nurse is caring for a patient with acute pancreatitis. What is the priority nursing diagnosis? *(709)*
    1. Risk for infection
    2. Acute pain
    3. Impaired gas exchange
    4. Imbalanced nutrition, less than body requirements

3. The nurse is caring for several patients. The postcholecystectomy patient is requesting assistance with ambulation. The patient with pancreatitis is wanting medication for nausea. The cirrhosis patient has just noticed considerable blood in his stool. The patient with possible cancer of the liver is complaining of pain. Which patient should the nurse attend to *first*? *(692, 701, 708)*
    1. The postcholecystectomy patient
    2. The patient with cirrhosis of the liver
    3. The patient with pancreatitis
    4. The patient with possible cancer of the liver

4. Which medication is used to decrease ammonia levels in the patient with liver failure? *(703)*
    1. Vasopressin (Pitressin)
    2. Esomeprazole (Nexium)
    3. Furosemide (Lasix)
    4. Lactulose (Cephulac)

5. Hepatitis virus is transmitted by various routes. Which virus is transmitted by the gastrointestinal route? *(695, Table 31-2)*
    1. Hepatitis A
    2. Hepatitis B
    3. Hepatitis C
    4. Hepatitis D

6. If a patient presents with pain radiating to the back at the level of the shoulderblade, which problem often displays that symptom? *(690-691)*
    1. Cholelithiasis
    2. Cirrhosis of the liver
    3. Pancreatitis
    4. Cancer of the pancreas

7. When are the symptoms of cholecystitis usually the most noticeable? *(691)*
    1. After eating a fatty meal
    2. During exercising or exertion
    3. After drinking excessive alcohol
    4. Upon waking in the morning

8. The patient is diagnosed with liver failure and the ammonia level is elevated. Which nursing diagnosis would be most relevant? *(703)*
    1. Risk for acute confusion
    2. Risk for decreased cardiac perfusion
    3. Risk for infection
    4. Risk for shock

9. The *highest* priority of nursing care for the patient with pancreatitis would be: *(708-710)*
    1. providing supplemental enzymes for digestion of food.
    2. providing skin care to relieve pruritus.
    3. medicating for nausea whenever needed.
    4. providing adequate pain control.

Copyright © 2013, 2009 by Saunders, an imprint of Elsevier Inc. All rights reserved.

10. Important nursing actions for the patient with symptoms of hepatitis are: *(Select all that apply.)* *(694-695)*
    1. encourage as much rest as possible.
    2. encourage a high-protein diet.
    3. offer six small meals a day to counteract anorexia.
    4. reinforce teaching of hand hygiene.
    5. suggest diversional activities such as computer games

11. Which of these signs and symptoms could signal liver transplant rejection? *(707)*
    1. Change in color of stool or urine
    2. Depression and anxiety
    3. Right upper quadrant pain that is worse after eating
    4. Preference for fetal position to relieve pain

12. Which description of pain would the nurse expect to find when assessing a patient who is diagnosed with acute pancreatitis? *(709)*
    1. Acute, steady abdominal pain localized to the epigastrim
    2. Acute pain with abdominal rigidity below the umbilicus
    3. Generalized dull abdominal pain with marked ascites
    4. Right quadrant or flank pain with low-grade fever

13. What treatments are likely to be ordered for a patient who has acute pancreatitis? *(Select all that apply.)* *(709-710)*
    1. Pain control, often by PCA pump
    2. Clear liquid diet as tolerated
    3. Frequent vital signs
    4. Intravenous fluids
    5. Administration of pancreatic supplemental enzymes when oral feedings are resumed
    6. Nasogastric tube attached to suction

14. What are the main symptoms of pancreatic cancer? *(712)*
    1. Epigastric pain and weight loss
    2. Rectal bleeding and frequent diarrhea
    3. Increase in appetite and excessive thirst
    4. Intolerance to fatty foods with vomiting

15. The nurse is supervising a post-cholecystectomy patient who is selecting foods from a hospital menu. The nurse would intervene if the patient made which selection? *(692)*
    1. Oatmeal with skim milk
    2. Biscuits with gravy
    3. Toast with strawberry jam
    4. Coffee and orange juice

CRITICAL THINKING ACTIVITIES

Directions: Read the clinical scenario below and answer the questions that follow.

Scenario: Mr. Poe, age 29, is admitted to the hospital with possible viral hepatitis. He was in an automobile accident 6 weeks ago and had received two units of blood. One week ago, he returned from a vacation at the seashore where he had eaten a significant amount of shellfish. Within the past few days, he has felt very weak and tired and finally went to his doctor, who hospitalized him.

Copyright © 2013, 2009 by Saunders, an imprint of Elsevier Inc. All rights reserved.

1. What would you look for in Mr. Poe's health history that would be helpful to the health care provider in diagnosing his illness? *(694-695, Table 31-2)*

    a. _____

    b. _____

    c. _____

    d. _____

2. List subjective and objective data that would indicate inflammation or damage to Mr. Poe's liver. *(694-696, Table 31-2)*

    Subjective data: _____

    _____

    Objective data: _____

    _____

    _____

Within a few days of admission, Mr. Poe began to exhibit signs of severe jaundice. His diagnosis was type B viral hepatitis with liver damage.

3. List specific nursing actions that can be taken to help Mr. Poe with each of the following problems.

    a. Fatigue: *(698-701)*_____

    _____

    _____

    b. Bleeding tendency: *(698-701)*_____

    _____

    _____

    c. Nausea, vomiting, and anorexia: *(698-701)*_____

    _____

    _____

4. What special precautions to prevent the spread of infection would you expect to be necessary in the care of Mr. Poe? *(699)*

    _____

    _____

    _____

    _____

5. An IV infusion is ordered for Mr. Poe. The order reads D_5W 1000 mL at 100 mL/hr. The tubing set delivers 15 drops per mL. How many drops per minute should the IV run to infuse within the allotted time?

    _____

Copyright © 2013, 2009 by Saunders, an imprint of Elsevier Inc. All rights reserved.

6. What might be given to individuals who were in close contact with Mr. Poe to provide them with passive immunity against type B hepatitis? *(696-698)*

_____

_____

7. If Mr. Poe were to become a carrier of type B hepatitis, he would be at high risk for developing what conditions? *(701)*

a. _____

b. _____

c. _____

8. What should Mr. Poe know in order to avoid future liver damage from hepatotoxins? *(699, 701)*

_____

_____

_____

STEPS TOWARD BETTER COMMUNICATION

VOCABULARY BUILDING GLOSSARY

Term	Pronunciation	Definition
accessory	ek ses' ah ree	additional, supplemental
geared (to/for/toward)	geer' d	aimed, intended for, adapted for a particular situation
prevalent	prev'alent	common, often occurs, widespread
plugged up		stopped by a blockage

COMPLETION

Directions: Fill in each blank with the appropriate word from the Vocabulary Building Glossary.

1. Hepatitis is quite _____ among travelers.

2. The gallstone _____ the common duct, causing a backup of bile in the gallbladder and liver.

3. Much of the care of the patient with hepatitis A is _____ toward preventing the spread of infection.

4. The pancreas is a(n) _____ organ of the digestive system.

Copyright © 2013, 2009 by Saunders, an imprint of Elsevier Inc. All rights reserved.

PRONUNCIATION SKILLS

These words are somewhat difficult to pronounce:

cholelith'iasis (ko le li thy' ah sis)

cholan'giopan'creatog'raphy (ko lan' jee o pan' cree ah tog' rah fee)

phagocyte (fah' go syt)

phagocytic (fah' go sit' ic)

Directions: Practice pronouncing the above words with a peer partner.

Short "i" Sound

Short i (ĭ) is the sound of the letter "**i**" in the words it, is, infect, minute, and liver. It is usually written with the letter "i," but sometimes with the letter "y."

*Directions: Draw a line under the letters in the following words that have the sound of short "**i.**" Then practice pronouncing the words aloud.*

liver, filter, topic, digestive, insulin, lipid, sluggish, lipase, nutrition, cirrhosis, irritation, toxins, cholelithiasis, fluid deficit, bilirubin, Pitressin infusion, carcinogenic, phagocytic

WORD ATTACK SKILLS

Combining Forms

These combining forms are used frequently in Chapter 31:

chol/e	bile
lith/o	stone
-iasis	condition
-angi/o	vessel
pancreat/o	pancreas
-graphy	recording

Directions: Using vertical lines, break each word into its word elements (parts) and give the meaning of the word.

1. cholelithiasis: _____

2. cholangiopancreatography: _____

Copyright © 2013, 2009 by Saunders, an imprint of Elsevier Inc. All rights reserved.

GRAMMAR POINTS

When asking questions during assessment about things that happened *in the past over a period of time*, it is often necessary to use the verb construction *have* plus the past participle form of the verb (the present perfect tense). *Examples:*

Have you had any pain?
Have you had any injuries?
Have you had any problems with…?
Have you used cleaning agents containing carbon tetrachloride?
How long have you taken this medication?
Have you taken any other drugs?
Have you been exposed to pesticides or toxins?
Have you been exposed to hepatitis?
Have you been tired lately?
How long have you been drinking?

This is different from talking about something *that happened in the past and was completed*. These statements use the simple past form of the verb. *Examples:*

Did you see the doctor recently?

I saw him last week.

When did you have the accident?

I had it last year in February.

Copyright © 2013, 2009 by Saunders, an imprint of Elsevier Inc. All rights reserved.

The Musculoskeletal System

Answer Key: Textbook page references are provided as a guide for answering these questions. A complete answer key was provided to your instructor.

REVIEW OF ANATOMY AND PHYSIOLOGY

COMPLETION

Changes Occurring with Aging

Directions: Complete the following statements.

1. As we age, bone density decreases because of _____. *(718)*

2. Kyphosis in the elderly is because of thinning of the _____ and
   collapse of the _____. *(718)*

3. The bones of the elderly break more easily because they are _____ and _____
   _____. *(718)*

4. Stiffness and crepitation in the joints is a result of joint _____ and erosion
   from _____. *(718)*

5. Nighttime muscle cramping in the elderly is increased because of _____
   and accumulation of _____. *(718)*

SHORT ANSWER

Causes and Prevention of Musculoskeletal Disorders

Directions: Provide short answers to complete the following statements.

1. Poor nutrition can contribute to musculoskeletal problems because there may be _____
   _____. *(718-719)*

2. Malignant tumors can contribute to musculoskeletal disorders in two ways: *(718-719)*

   a. _____

   b. _____

Copyright © 2013, 2009 by Saunders, an imprint of Elsevier Inc. All rights reserved.

3. Five measures that can help prevent musculoskeletal disorders are: *(719)*

   a. _____

   b. _____

   c. _____

   d. _____

   e. _____

MATCHING

Diagnostic Tests

Directions: Match the procedure on the left with the most appropriate phrase on the right.

1. _____	Bone scan *(721, Table 32-2)*	a.	Measurement of range of motion of a joint
2. _____	Arthroscopy *(722, Table 32-2)*	b.	Apply ice or cold packs, support joint with pillows
		c.	Grading ranges from 0 (paralysis) to 5 (normal)
3. _____	Arthrocentesis *(722, Table 32-2)*	d.	After procedure, watch for signs of infection, hemarthrosis, swelling, and injury to joint or loss of feeling
4. _____	Synovial analysis *(722, Table 32-2)*	e.	Normal findings are clear, viscid fluid containing no or very few blood cells
5. _____	Culture *(722, Table 32-2)*	f.	After procedure, monitor site of venipuncture for signs of inflammation and hematoma
6. _____	Goniometry *(719)*		
7. _____	Muscle strength *(719)*	g.	Examination of bone tissue to identify infecting organism

APPLICATION OF THE NURSING PROCESS

Directions: Answer the questions that follow.

1. List three significant findings the nurse might record when taking a history during assessment of a patient with a disorder of the musculoskeletal system. *(723)*

   a. _____

   b. _____

   c. _____

2. List three observations that the nurse can make about a patient's ability to move and walk. *(724)*

   a. _____

   b. _____

   c. _____

Copyright © 2013, 2009 by Saunders, an imprint of Elsevier Inc. All rights reserved.

3. Three nursing diagnoses concerning physical aspects that would probably be found on the care plan for the patient who has severe rheumatoid arthritis affecting the hands, knees, and hips are: *(724-725, Table 32-3)*

    a. _____

    b. _____

    c. _____

4. Expected outcomes for the above nursing diagnoses might be: *(724-729, Table 32-3)*

    a. _____

    b. _____

    c. _____

COMPLETION

Directions: Fill in the blanks to complete the statements.

1. Joint mobility is maintained by regularly performing _____ exercises. *(719, 728)*

2. A patient who is immobilized for a long period of time loses _____ from his bones. *(719)*

3. Lengthy immobilization tends to cause muscle _____. *(728)*

4. If ankylosis of a joint is unavoidable, the joint is _____ so that the extremity will have maximum function. *(728)*

5. _____ exercise is helpful in preventing osteoporosis. *(719)*

6. Proper exercise and positioning of joints for an immobile patient is extremely important because a contracture can begin to occur within as little as _____. *(727-728)*

Copyright © 2013, 2009 by Saunders, an imprint of Elsevier Inc. All rights reserved.

PRIORITY SETTING

Directions: You are assigned to ambulate a 72-year-old female patient who is recovering after a pelvic fracture. She had been on bedrest and is still somewhat weak. Place the actions you would take into the order in which you would carry them out. She uses a cane to ambulate.

_____ a. Plan how far you will go with her as she will have to come back as well.

_____ b. Have her stand still to dispel any dizziness.

_____ c. Check the orders.

_____ d. Assist to sit in the chair.

_____ e. Assess her ability to move, stand, and ambulate.

_____ f. Attach the gait belt to her.

_____ g. Assist to the side of the bed.

_____ h. Identify the patient.

_____ i. Ambulate back to the room.

_____ j. Perform hand hygiene.

_____ k. Hand her the cane.

_____ l. Assist to stand.

_____ m. Ambulate the correct distance.

_____ n. Assist to sit on the side of the bed.

REVIEW QUESTIONS FOR THE NCLEX® EXAMINATION

Directions: Choose the best answer(s) to the following questions.

1. Magnetic resonance imaging is used to help diagnose a variety of musculoskeletal problems. What instructions would you give the patient who is to undergo an MRI? *(Select all that apply.)* **(721, Table 32-2)**
   1. A consent must be signed for this procedure.
   2. You must remove all metal from your body.
   3. You will be given a contrast medium to drink.
   4. You will need to remain perfectly still for 15–60 minutes.
   5. If you are claustrophobic, you may ask for a sedative beforehand.

2. When assessing whether crutches have been fitted to the patient properly, you know that when walking with them, the: *(Select all that apply.)* **(731)**
   1. axillary bar should be two finger-breadths below the axilla.
   2. elbow should be flexed at a 45-degree angle.
   3. elbow should be flexed at a 30-degree angle.
   4. crutches should be about 16 inches shorter than the patient's height.
   5. axillary pad should fit snugly into the axilla.

3. The patient is selecting foods from a menu to demonstrate knowledge of dietary calcium sources. Which selection indicates that the patient needs additional information about the absorption of calcium from food sources? **(719)**
   1. Green leafy vegetables
   2. Canned sardines
   3. Cheese and yogurt
   4. Milk

Copyright © 2013, 2009 by Saunders, an imprint of Elsevier Inc. All rights reserved.

4. The nurse is instructing the patient to do quadriceps and gluteal muscle exercises. Which instruction is correct? *(729)*
   1. Perform exercises 3-4 times a week for 20 minutes a day.
   2. Perform exercises 10-15 times hourly while awake.
   3. Instruct to stand erect and grasp a handrail while doing exercises.
   4. Instruct to do stretching and walking to warm up before exercises.

5. When checking the joints during a focused assessment, you should: *(Select all that apply.)* *(724)*
   1. palpate them for tenderness.
   2. position them to full extension and flexion.
   3. inspect them for swelling or deformity.
   4. assess for warmth over the joint.
   5. determine range of motion without pain.

6. The nurse is assigned to care for several orthopedic patients who just returned from diagnostic testing. In planning care, which patient is likely to need the most time for postprocedure care? *(720-723, Table 32-2)*
   1. Patient who had an electromyelography
   2. Patient who had an arthroscopy
   3. Patient who had a dual energy x-ray absorptiometry
   4. Patient who had a magnetic resonance imaging

7. When a walker is used for ambulation, it is important that it be appropriate height for the patient. Most walkers have adjustable legs. When walking with it, the walker height is correct when the patient's elbow is: *(731)*
   1. locked to sustain the weight of the upper body.
   2. bent at 15 to 30 degrees.
   3. at a 45-degree angle to swing the walker forward.
   4. just slightly bent.

8. Because the patient is immobilized, the physician has ordered Lovenox, low–molecular-weight heparin injections. The order reads: enoxaparin sodium 60 mg Subcut. per day in 2 divided doses. On hand is enoxaparin sodium 30 mg/mL. How much medication would you draw up for each injection? _____ mL

9. An elderly patient with arthritis has a nursing diagnosis of Functional incontinence. Which intervention should the nurse use? *(724, 726, Table 32-3)*
   1. Instruct the nursing assistant to report number of linen changes.
   2. Instruct the patient to call for assistance in getting to the toilet.
   3. Closely monitor the intake and output to observe for fluid balance.
   4. Suggest incontinence briefs until bladder control is achieved.

10. The nurse observes that an elderly patient has decreased strength, unsteady balance, slow reflexes, and a gait disturbance. What is the priority diagnosis? *(718, Table 32-2)*
    1. Risk for falls
    2. Impaired physical mobility
    3. Activity intolerance
    4. Self-care deficit

Copyright © 2013, 2009 by Saunders, an imprint of Elsevier Inc. All rights reserved.

CRITICAL THINKING ACTIVITIES

Scenario A: You are to teach a patient about proper and safe use of crutches. The patient cannot bear weight on the left leg. *(731)*

1. Describe how you would teach the patient to go up and down stairs.

2. What safety measures would you teach?

Scenario B: You are assigned a patient who has rheumatoid arthritis who is recovering from an appendectomy. You need to have the patient exercise her joints. *(728-729)*

1. How would you prepare the patient to do the exercises?

2. What would you do to prevent excessive pain during the exercise sessions?

STEPS TOWARD BETTER COMMUNICATION

VOCABULARY BUILDING GLOSSARY

Term	Pronunciation	Definition
deficit	def' ah sit	not enough, insufficient, less than required
distal		farthest away from, remote
dowager	dow' ah jer	an older woman, one who usually has money and owns property
initiate	in i' shee ayt	to start, begin, commence
flaccid	flas' id	limp, soft, hanging loose, drooping
trigger	trig' ger	initiate, cause to begin

Copyright © 2013, 2009 by Saunders, an imprint of Elsevier Inc. All rights reserved.

COMPLETION

Directions: Fill in the blanks with the correct words from the Vocabulary Building Glossary to complete the statements.

1. When an injury has occurred to an extremity, the nurse checks the pulse _____ to the area of trauma.

2. An abnormal finding on a musculoskeletal assessment would be _____ muscles in the right lower extremity.

3. Accidentally brushing against the weights of a traction device may _____ pain for the patient.

4. Osteoarthritis often causes a(n) _____ in joint motion.

5. Sometimes the nurse must _____ action to obtain heat or cold treatments for a patient who needs them.

6. The bent-forward position of the elderly lady showed that she had a(n) _____ hump.

COMMUNICATION EXERCISE

Directions: Here are some examples of what to say if a patient were to ask you the following questions.

1. What is the difference between a tendon and a ligament?

    Ligaments hold the joint together. Tendons anchor muscle to bone.

2. What is the purpose of cartilage?

    Cartilage provides a cushion between the bones of the joint.

3. What is the difference between a sprain and a strain?

    A sprain involves stretching or tearing of ligaments around a joint. A strain involves pulling and tearing of a muscle or a tendon or both.

WORD ATTACK SKILLS

Directions: Study the word parts and answer the related questions.

1. ankyl/o   crooked or bent

    Can you think of a joint whose name came from this word element? _____

2. ab-   from
    ad-   to, toward
    re-   gain, do again
    -sorb   to attract or retain substances

Directions: Write the meanings of the following words:

a. Absorb: _____

b. Adsorb: _____

c. Resorb: _____

Copyright © 2013, 2009 by Saunders, an imprint of Elsevier Inc. All rights reserved.

3. -esthesi/o   sensation

   If *anesthesia* means without pain and *paresthesia* means having numbness or tingling, what does *para-* mean? _____

Pronunciation

Directions: Practice pronouncing the following words with a peer.

throm'bophlebit'is (throm' bo flee by' tus)

ankylo'sis (ang' kee lo' sis)

kypho'sis (ki fo' sis)

crepi'ta'tion (KRĔP-ĭ-tā-shŭn)

Also practice pronouncing the terms given in the Focused Assessment box on pp. 723-724 of the textbook.

Descriptive Terms

Directions: Here are some terms commonly used to describe findings of physical assessment:

Posture: erect, slumped, rounded-shouldered, straight

Gait: normal, rolling, heel-toe, toe-heel, ataxic, ambling, slow, rapid, bouncy

Range of motion: full, limited, diminished, little, restricted

Spine: normal curve, S-shaped, abnormally curved, tender, rounded

Joints: normal, reddened, swollen, painful, deformed, immovable, contracted, freely movable

Skeletal muscles: good tone, well-developed, underdeveloped, tense, hard, soft, poor tone, atrophic, painful

COMMUNICATION EXERCISE

Assessment Questions: History-Taking

Using the Focused Assessment box on p. 724, practice asking and answering the questions with a peer. Answer either from your own experience or with imaginary answers. When you are the "patient," do not look in the book. Your responsibility is to listen and ask for repetition and clarification when you do not understand your partner, who is practicing the role of nurse.

Copyright © 2013, 2009 by Saunders, an imprint of Elsevier Inc. All rights reserved.

Care of Patients with Musculoskeletal and Connective Tissue Disorders

Answer Key: Textbook page references are provided as a guide for answering these questions. A complete answer key was provided to your instructor.

COMPLETION

Musculoskeletal and Connective Tissue Disorders

Directions: Fill in the blanks to complete the statements.

1. Subluxation is a partial dislocation that usually occurs from _____. *(735)*

2. Rest, exercise, analgesics, and _____ are the main treatments for osteoarthritis. *(745)*

3. The most common cause of below-the-knee amputation is _____. *(758)*

4. In addition to increasing calcium and vitamin D, one of the best ways for women to prevent osteoporosis is to perform _____. *(756)*

5. The most common cause of osteomyelitis is _____. *(741)*

6. The muscles most commonly afflicted with muscle strain are the _____, _____, and _____ muscles. *(735)*

SHORT ANSWER

Arthritis

Directions: Answer the following questions about arthritis in the spaces provided.

1. List four questions the nurse might ask when assessing the status of a patient with arthritis. *(753)*

   a. _____

   b. _____

   c. _____

   d. _____

2. What are some objective data the nurse might collect when assessing a patient with arthritis? *(746-747)*

   a. _____

   b. _____

   c. _____

Copyright © 2013, 2009 by Saunders, an imprint of Elsevier Inc. All rights reserved.

3. List some interventions for patient with arthritis and a nursing diagnosis of Activity intolerance. *(746-747, 753)*

   a. _____

   b. _____

   c. _____

   d. _____

   e. _____

4. Summarize important teaching points for applications of cold and heat for your patient with arthritis. *(754)*

   _____

   _____

   _____

   _____

LABELING

Fractures and Immobilization

Directions: Review the drawings below and identify each of the following types of fractures: comminuted, compound, greenstick, longitudinal, oblique, simple, spiral, and transverse. (737, Figure 33-1)

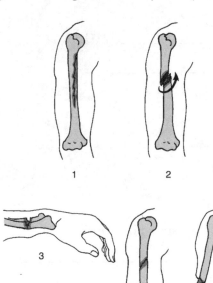
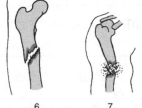

1. _____

2. _____

3. _____

4. _____

5. _____

6. _____

7. _____

8. _____

Copyright © 2013, 2009 by Saunders, an imprint of Elsevier Inc. All rights reserved.

APPLICATION OF THE NURSING PROCESS

Matching

Directions: Match the problem on the left with the appropriate nursing assessment or intervention on the right.

1. _____ Swelling and increased pressure within a fascial compartment *(743)*
2. _____ Inadequate immobilization *(741-742)*
3. _____ Cleaning of pin sites *(743)*
4. _____ Infection of a pin site or fracture site *(743)*
5. _____ Tachypnea, disorientation, crackles and wheezing, and rash with lesions that do not blanch with pressure *(741)*

a. Patient complains of grating sensation and unrelenting pain, especially with motion.
b. Notify the physician promptly; this is symptomatic of fat embolism. This is a rare but potentially fatal condition.
c. Presents as dull pain that becomes progressively worse, fever, purulent drainage, foul odor. Initiate wound and skin precautions.
d. Should be done daily with a 2 mg/mL chlorhexidine solution.
e. Test for sensation and do a capillary refill time test.

Short Answer

Directions: Provide a short answer to the following questions or provide the information requested.

1. The following nursing diagnoses might be on the nursing care plan for the patient who has had a joint replacement. For each nursing diagnosis, write an expected outcome. *(751-755)*

   a. Impaired mobility related to surgical procedure on knee

   _____

   b. Risk for ineffective tissue perfusion related to potential for thrombus formation

   _____

   c. Pain related to surgical procedure and rehabilitation exercises

   _____

2. Interventions to assist in improving mobility would include: *(751-755)* _____

   _____

   _____

3. Interventions to help prevent thrombus formation for this patient would include: *(752, Nursing Care Plan 33-1)*

   a. _____

   b. _____

   c. _____

   d. _____

Copyright © 2013, 2009 by Saunders, an imprint of Elsevier Inc. All rights reserved.

4. Other interventions besides analgesic administration to assist the patient with pain could include: *(751, 753-754, Nursing Care Plan 33-1)*

_____

_____

_____

5. What observations would indicate that expected outcomes are being met? *(751-755)*

_____

_____

PRIORITY SETTING

Scenario: You are assigned the following patients:
   a. Mr. Holmes who has just had a right knee replacement and is using a CPM machine.
   b. Ms. Tuttle who has been admitted for final tests before a left hip replacement.
   c. Mr. Conners who was in a motorcycle accident and has multiple injuries including a broken leg that is immobilized with balanced traction.
   d. Ms. Simpson who is 2 days postoperative for an amputation of her left foot. She is diabetic.

1. Indicate the priority order in which you would do your initial shift rounds. _____

2. Which patient requires the most thorough assessment at first visit? _____

3. All the call lights are on later in the morning. Mr. Holmes is asking for pain medication. Ms. Tuttle needs assistance to the bathroom. Mr. Connors says he doesn't feel well and sounds anxious. Ms. Simpson says her left foot is itching and would someone please help her. Which patient would you attend to first?

_____

Why? _____

_____

_____

_____

REVIEW QUESTIONS FOR THE NCLEX® EXAMINATION

Directions: Choose the best answer(s) for the following:

1. Mrs. C. is in her first postoperative day after a total hip replacement as treatment for degenerative arthritis. Mrs. C.'s operated limb must be kept in what position? *(750)*
   1. Adduction
   2. Externally rotated
   3. Internally rotated
   4. Abduction

Copyright © 2013, 2009 by Saunders, an imprint of Elsevier Inc. All rights reserved.

2. The nurse is caring for a patient who is immobilized after a recent hip fracture. What is the priority nursing diagnosis? *(750, 752)*
   1. Risk for self-care deficit related to restricted movement and pain
   2. Risk for infection, urinary tract, related to urinary stasis
   3. Risk for ineffective tissue perfusion related to deep vein thrombosis
   4. Risk for impaired mobility related to orthopedic appliance

3. When the patient with the new hip is being prepared for discharge, you should give which instructions to avoid dislocation of the prosthesis? *(Select all that apply.)* *(750)*
   1. Sit on straight chairs only.
   2. Use a raised toilet seat.
   3. Do not lie on your back in bed.
   4. Use a pillow between your knees when lying down.
   5. Do not cross your legs at the knee or ankle.
   6. Be careful not to bend at the hip more than 90 degrees.

4. A patient is discharged with a synthetic cast applied. What will he need to know to take care of himself and the cast? *(Select all that apply.)* *(739, 744)*
   1. How to assess the neurovascular status of the part encased in the cast
   2. How to dry the cast if it becomes wet
   3. Signs of infection under the cast
   4. Importance of reporting a broken or loose cast
   5. How to cut a window in the cast if there is pain or swelling
   6. Ways to safely scratch at the itching that will develop

5. The nurse is caring for several patients with hip or femur fractures on an orthopedic unit. Which patient should the nurse attend to *first*? *(736-741)*
   1. Patient complains of difficulty breathing, feeling very hot, and a fine red rash on the chest.
   2. Patient states that pain at the surgical site is unrelieved by medication or repositioning.
   3. Patient reports that there is an odor coming from the cast and the foot is red and swollen.
   4. Patient says that if no one comes to help her to the bathroom, she is going to call the supervisor.

6. The nurse is at a park and observes a workman who sustains an accidental amputation of a finger. The nurse would intervene if a bystander performs which action? *(758)*
   1. Rinses visible debris from the detached digit
   2. Wraps the digit in a clean dry cloth
   3. Immerses the digit in a cup of cold water
   4. Places the digit in a plastic bag and attaches a name tag

7. Whenever a patient has sustained a musculoskeletal injury, it is most important that you assess the patient's distal extremities for: *(735)*
   1. proper position and elevation.
   2. paresthesia, numbness, and decreased pulses.
   3. signs of deep vein thrombosis.
   4. edema, swelling, and soft tissue injury.

8. The patient who returns to the floor after a reduction and internal fixation of the right hip has an IV running. The order for the next IV reads: D_5NS 1000 mL at 150 mL/hr. The IV tubing has a drop factor of 10 gtts/mL. The IV should be set to run at _____ gtts/min.

Copyright © 2013, 2009 by Saunders, an imprint of Elsevier Inc. All rights reserved.

9. Rheumatoid arthritis patients who are receiving Enbrel or other biologic response modifiers must be watched for complications such as: *(Select all that apply.)* **(747-748)**
   1. hearing loss.
   2. serious infection.
   3. severe edema.
   4. blood dyscrasias.
   5. signs of demyelination.
   6. skin eruptions.

10. Disease-modifying antirheumatic drugs prevent joint and cartilage destruction by: **(747-748)**
    1. suppressing the immune system.
    2. stimulating cortisol production.
    3. providing collagen to the joints.
    4. blocking pain transmission.

11. The nurse is caring for a patient with a newly applied cast to the lower extremity. The patient continues to complain of pain despite medication and repositioning. What should the nurse do *first*? **(739, 744)**
    1. Call the physician to obtain an order for additional medication.
    2. Use distraction techniques, such as computer games or puzzle books.
    3. Assess the temperature of the toes, sensation to touch, and capillary refill.
    4. Tell the patient that the medication has not had enough time to work.

12. An elderly orthopedic patient refuses to perform the coughing and deep-breathing exercises because, "I have a broken hip, there is nothing wrong with my breathing." What should the nurse do *first*? **(Nursing Care Plan 33-1)**
    1. Document that the patient was instructed in the techniques but refused to do them.
    2. Obtain an incentive spirometer and ask the patient to try using it instead of the exercises.
    3. Use active listening and be supportive of the patient's right to refuse a therapy.
    4. Explain how immobility contributes to developing pneumonia or atelectasis.

CRITICAL THINKING ACTIVITIES

1. Your neighbor says she has an odd spot on her calf and asks you to look at it. She has a red spot that seems to have a reddish ring around it. What questions would you ask her? What advice will you give her after you collect the data?

2. Your older brother calls complaining of excruciating pain in his left big toe and asking for advice. What would you say to him?

3. What would you teach a patient about measures to prevent gout attacks?

4. Your neighbor sprains her ankle. What type of self-care remedies can you recommend while she is waiting to get a doctor's appointment?

5. Explain what happens when a bone heals and why it is important to establish and maintain a sturdy union of broken bone fragments.

Copyright © 2013, 2009 by Saunders, an imprint of Elsevier Inc. All rights reserved.

STEPS TOWARD BETTER COMMUNICATON

VOCABULARY BUILDING GLOSSARY

Term	Pronunciation	Definition
knit	nit	to grow together in small bits; to make clothing (sweaters) by connecting loops of yarn with long needles
impede'	im peed'	to slow, or get in the way of
imped'iment	im ped' ah ment	something that blocks or gets in the way of action
debris'	dah bree'	pieces left of something broken

COMPLETION

Directions: Fill in the blanks with the correct words from the Vocabulary Building Glossary to complete the statements.

1. Swelling under a cast may _____ blood flow.

2. Before a compound fracture is set, the surgeon cleans out any _____ in the wound.

3. A splint often causes less _____ to moving about than a cast.

4. If properly immobilized, the bone disrupted by a fracture will _____.

GRAMMAR POINTS

Giving Instructions

The words you use when talking to patients are critical to their understanding of what things are important and necessary for them to do. Here are some terms with the meanings they will have for the patient:

You can/you may indicate that the action is *optional*, the patient is responsible for choosing to do what he or she is capable of doing.

You should/you will indicate that the action is *recommended*, or is important to do.

Notice that using *should not* or *will not* (the negative) is usually stronger than the positive:

You can't/you shouldn't/you may not indicate the action is *required* or *necessary*.

You have to/you must/you mustn't/never indicate the action is *absolutely necessary*.

Here are some examples of each category.

Optional:
You can exercise your knee joint as many times a day as you can as long as it doesn't cause swelling.

You may apply ice packs to your back for the pain for 20 minutes of each hour.

If you like, **you can** use a heating pad for the discomfort.

Recommended:
Range-of-motion exercises **should** be done three or four times a day.

Copyright © 2013, 2009 by Saunders, an imprint of Elsevier Inc. All rights reserved.

You should keep a pillow wedged between your legs when you lie on your side after hip surgery.

You shouldn't cross your legs after hip surgery.

Required:

Don't poke anything down into the cast.

Be sure to keep your leg cast dry.

You may not smoke or have caffeine for 8 hours before the test.

You can't let the traction weights set down on the bed.

Absolutely necessary:

You have to keep your weight off your foot for at least 3 weeks.

You must lie perfectly still for the bone scan.

You mustn't have any metal on your body for the MRI test.

Never remove these screws.

Assume you are giving instructions to a patient with a new leg cast. Use some of the phrases above to give one instruction from each category.

1. Optional:_____

2. Recommended: _____

3. Required: _____

4. Absolutely necessary:_____

Other types of instruction statements:

Expectation or possibility statements:

Should can also mean *expectation* (The discomfort **should** be minimal, meaning that *you expect small discomfort*) or *possibility* (If there **should** be any pain, you can take aspirin, meaning that *if and when pain occurs…*). **Should** is also used to make a request more polite (I **should** think it would be good for you to exercise more often).

Consequence statements:

Consequence statements indicate cause and effect, and have the form of **If you…, then…**

If you get up and move around, **then** you will heal faster.

If you use heat treatments before you exercise, **then** your joint will not be as stiff.

If you get your cast wet, **then** it will have to be replaced.

Copyright © 2013, 2009 by Saunders, an imprint of Elsevier Inc. All rights reserved.

The Urinary System

chapter
34

Answer Key: Textbook page references are provided as a guide for answering these questions. A complete answer key was provided to your instructor.

REVIEW OF ANATOMY AND PHYSIOLOGY

Labeling

Anatomy of the Kidney

Directions: Label the following structures on the diagram of the kidney. **(765)**

renal artery

renal vein

fibrous capsule

renal pyramid

calyx

renal pelvis

renal papilla

medulla

cortex

renal column

ureter

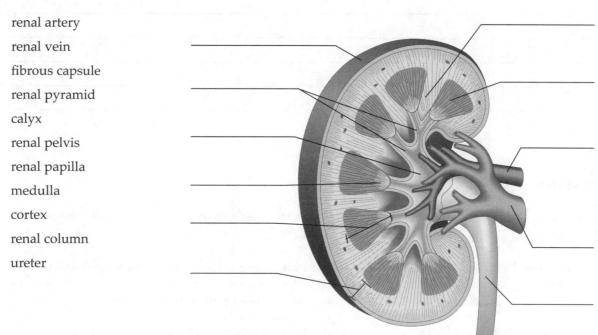

Copyright © 2013, 2009 by Saunders, an imprint of Elsevier Inc. All rights reserved.

SHORT ANSWER

Assessing the Urinary System

Directions: Read the clinical scenario and answer the questions that follow.

Scenario: You are caring for several patients who have actual or are at risk for urinary disorders. In your daily assessment of these patients, you should look for specific kinds of data.

1. List five questions that you might ask a patient who has or suspects urinary disorder. *(766-767, 768, 773)*

   a. _____

   b. _____

   c. _____

   d. _____

   e. _____

2. List five specific physical assessments that should be done on a patient with a urinary disorder. *(773-775)*

   a. _____

   b. _____

   c. _____

   d. _____

   e. _____

MATCHING

Diagnostic Testing

Directions: Match the diagnostic test (or test result) on the left with the most appropriate nursing action or assessment finding on the right.

1. _____	RBCs and WBCs in urine *(769, Table 34-2)*	a. Pink-tinged urine after test; increase fluid intake to minimize discomfort
2. _____	Hematuria *(773)*	b. Assess patient for signs of acidosis
3. _____	Urine pH below 4.5 *(769)*	c. Dilute urine
4. _____	Creatinine clearance *(769)*	d. Instruct patient in steps to follow to collect a clean-catch midstream urine specimen
5. _____	Ureteral and renal biopsy *(772)*	e. Assess patient for other signs of urinary tract infection
6. _____	Urine culture *(769)*	f. Try to determine at what point during urination blood first appears
7. _____	Specific gravity below 1.010 and urine osmolality below 100 mOsm/kg *(769)*	g. Obtain a 24-hour urine specimen and one blood sample during test
8. _____	Bladder scan *(772)*	h. Vital signs, popliteal and pedal pulses are checked every 15 minutes for the first hour
9. _____	Intravenous pyelogram (IVP) *(770)*	i. Verify BUN and creatinine results
10. _____	Renal angiography *(771)*	j. Palpate for the symphysis pubis and apply gel about 1 inch above

Copyright © 2013, 2009 by Saunders, an imprint of Elsevier Inc. All rights reserved.

COMPLETION

Urinary Disorders

Directions: Fill in the blanks to complete the statements.

1. An absence of urine is called _____, which rarely occurs, but may be associated with acute renal failure. *(775)*

2. Urination that occurs during the night is known as _____. *(775)*

3. _____ is voiding more often than every 2 hours because of inflammation, decreased bladder capacity, psychological disorders, or increased fluid intake. *(775)*

4. _____ is a delay in starting the stream of urine which may be related to partial obstruction. *(775)*

5. Emptying the bladder regularly prevents _____ and eliminates toxic substances. *(767)*

6. Long-term care residents and home care patients are continuously monitored for signs of urinary tract _____. *(766, 774)*

APPLICATION OF THE NURSING PROCESS

Caring for a Patient with Urinary Incontinence

Directions: Read the scenario and provide the answers to the following questions.

Scenario: Mr. Yakada is an elderly gentleman who was recently admitted to an extended-care facility. He has chronic urinary incontinence and currently he has an indwelling catheter. The family would like to have the catheter removed as soon as possible.

1. What factors could potentially contribute to Mr. Yakada's incontinence? *(777)*

    a. Health conditions: _____

    _____

    _____

    b. Medications: _____

    _____

2. List three things to assess when a patient has an indwelling catheter. *(776-777)*

    a. _____

    b. _____

    c. _____

Copyright © 2013, 2009 by Saunders, an imprint of Elsevier Inc. All rights reserved.

3. Write an expected outcome for the nursing diagnosis of Risk for infection related to indwelling catheter. *(776-777)*

   _____

   _____

4. List five nursing interventions to prevent infection for a patient with an indwelling catheter. *(776-777)*

   a. _____

   b. _____

   c. _____

   d. _____

   e. _____

5. The physician writes an order to encourage fluids without restriction. At the end of the shift, the I & O sheet indicates that Mr. Yakada had 8 ounces of water at 8:00 AM, 300 mL of juice for breakfast, 12 ounces of coffee for lunch, 10 ounces of milk for dinner and 800 mL is gone from his 1000 mL bedside water pitcher. How many mL total do you record for intake for this shift? _____ mL

6. List five alternatives (nonsurgical) to an indwelling catheter for patients such as Mr. Yakada. *(781-782)*

   a. _____

   b. _____

   c. _____

   d. _____

   e. _____

7. Which urinalysis results indicate that the expected outcome (free from infection) is being met? *(769, Table 34-2)*
   a. Color: amber yellow
   b. Odor: aromatic
   c. Specific gravity: 1.030
   d. White blood cells: 0–4 (per low power field)

PRIORITY SETTING

Directions: Read the scenario and prioritize the nursing actions as appropriate.

Scenario A: You are caring for Mrs. Popovitch on a rehabilitation unit. She has been doing well and is frequently ambulating off the unit with her family. She tells you that she is having urinary frequency, but currently denies any other symptoms.

1. What is your priority action?
   a. Measure and record urinary output every hour.
   b. Check to see if fluid intake is higher than usual.
   c. Obtain an order for a urinalysis.
   d. Notify the physician or RN.

Copyright © 2013, 2009 by Saunders, an imprint of Elsevier Inc. All rights reserved.

Scenario B: You are working with a new nursing assistant who disconnects the catheter from the drainage bag tubing "in order to collect a fresh urine specimen."

1. What is your priority action?
   a. Report the incident to the nurse manager.
   b. Allow her to continue and later talk to her in private.
   c. Do everything that assists her to maintain asepsis.
   d. Immediately stop her and do the procedure yourself.

Scenario C: The nurse is caring for a patient who is currently en route to have diagnostic testing to include a intravenous pyelogram (IVP) and blood cultures. Which abnormal laboratory result should the nurse deal with first?
   a. Call primary care physician to report protein in the urine
   b. Call nephrologist to report uric acid greater than 750 mg/24 hours
   c. Call urologist to report a postvoid residual volume of 250 mL
   d. Call radiologist to report a blood urea nitrogen of 30 mg/dL

REVIEW QUESTIONS FOR THE NCLEX® EXAMINATION

Directions: Choose the correct answer(s) for the following questions.

1. The patient reports having a color change in the urine. What question should the nurse ask first, in order to collect more information about this symptom? *(768, 773)*
   1. "Do you have any history of kidney problems?"
   2. "What color is the urine?"
   3. "Are you having any pain with urination?"
   4. "When did you first notice this?"

2. The patient is diagnosed with urinary retention. Which characteristic is least likely to be associated with this disorder? *(782)*
   1. Dribbling of urine or passing only the overflow
   2. Inability to void after removal of an indwelling catheter
   3. Residual urine of greater than 100 mL
   4. Passing urine when laughing, sneezing, or coughing

3. A major cause of end-stage kidney disease is: *(767)*
   1. hypertension.
   2. hyperthyroidism.
   3. prostate enlargement.
   4. kidney stones.

4. The patient is scheduled to have an retrograde pyelogram. Which laboratory results should be reported to the radiologist before the patient has the procedure? *(770, Table 34-2)*
   1. An elevated WBC
   2. An elevated BUN
   3. A decreased RBC
   4. Urinalysis positive for nitrates

5. The nurse is explaining the procedure for a cystoscopy. After the procedure, the patient should expect which set of circumstances ? *(771, Table 34-2)*
   1. NPO status for several hours after the procedure
   2. Burning, frequency, and pink-tinged urine
   3. Bedrest with bathroom privileges for 24 hours
   4. Indwelling catheter in place to measure output

Copyright © 2013, 2009 by Saunders, an imprint of Elsevier Inc. All rights reserved.

6. The patient has returned from diagnostic testing. The physician's orders indicate to check vital signs, popliteal and pedal pulses q 15 min for the first hour, then q 2 hours x 2. This postprocedure care is appropriate for which test? *(771, Table 34-2)*
   1. Radionuclide renal scan
   2. Renal ultrasound
   3. Renal angiography
   4. Renal biopsy

7. The nurse hears in report that the patient is having oliguria, but the etiology is currently unknown. Which intervention is the nurse most likely to incorporate into the plan of care? *(775)*
   1. Measure and record the output every hour.
   2. Provide extra time and assistance in going to the bathroom.
   3. Obtain an order for urine culture and sensitivity.
   4. Encourage the patient to take extra fluids.

8. The nurse must check the residual urine on a patient who reports urinary frequency. Which instruction should the nurse give to the patient? *(782)*
   1. Advise the patient to avoid eating or drinking after midnight.
   2. Instruct the patient to void and empty bladder as much as possible prior to the test.
   3. Have the patient drink 2 or 3 glasses of fluid prior to the test.
   4. Ensure that the patient understands the bowel preparation procedure.

9. The patient had a Foley catheter removed 4 hours ago, but reports inability to void with a subjective sensation of needing to urinate. Which action should the nurse perform *first*? *(774, 782)*
   1. Notify the RN or the physician.
   2. Initiate hourly intake and output.
   3. Gently palpate the bladder for fullness.
   4. Put the patient on the toilet and turn on the water.

10. The nurse is looking at the urine results for several patients. Which patient is the nurse most immediately concerned about? *(773-774, Table 34-3)*
   1. Pregnant woman has bright yellow urine
   2. A diabetic patient has very pale urine
   3. A young male athlete with brownish-red urine
   4. A patient taking amitriptyline (Elavil) with bluish-green urine

CRITICAL THINKING ACTIVITIES

Scenario: You are caring for Mr. Whipple who is scheduled for a renal biopsy. He is very apprehensive. This is his first biopsy, and he admits that he does not know anything about it; however, he fears the worst about the procedure and the results.

1. List two purposes of a renal biopsy. *(772, Box 34-2)*

   a. _____

   b. _____

Copyright © 2013, 2009 by Saunders, an imprint of Elsevier Inc. All rights reserved.

2. Write a very brief explanation of how the procedure is done and what Mr. Whipple will experience. *(772, Box 34-2)*

   _____

   _____

   _____

   _____

3. What two interventions could you use to help Mr. Whipple decrease his anxiety? *(768)*

   a. _____

   b. _____

4. What is the most serious immediate postprocedure complication of a renal biopsy? *(768, 772, Box 34-2)*
   a. Vomiting related to anesthesia
   b. Frank bleeding and hemorrhage
   c. Infection and inflammation
   d. Decreased urinary output

5. Mr. Whipple expresses fear and anxiety while waiting for the results. "I just can't stand this waiting. Call the doctor right now, or I am leaving the hospital!" What is the best response? *(768, 772)*
   a. "It's too dangerous for you to leave. You just had the procedure."
   b. "I'll call the doctor if you agree to calm down and wait."
   c. "You can leave if you want to; it is your right to do as you wish."
   d. "I see that you are anxious. Let me check on the status of the report."

STEPS TOWARD BETTER COMMUNICATION

VOCABULARY BUILDING GLOSSARY

Term	Definition
hy poth' e size	to suggest an answer that explains a group of phenomena
pa' tent	open, unobstructed
pa' ten cy	the condition of being open

PRONUNCIATION SKILLS

Directions: Pronounce the following words.

Lithotripsy (lith'o trip' sy)	crushing stones in an organ such as the kidney
Plasmapheresis (plas'ma fer ee'sis)	removal of plasma from withdrawn blood and retransfusion in a different form into the donor
Oliguria (ol i gu' ree a)	diminished urine secretion in relation to fluid intake
Polyuria (pol i u'ree a)	excessive secretion of urine
Suprapubic (su' pra pew' bik)	above the pubes
Extracorporeal (ex' tra kor po'ree al)	situated or occurring outside the body

Copyright © 2013, 2009 by Saunders, an imprint of Elsevier Inc. All rights reserved.

COMPLETION

Directions: Fill in the blank with the correct word from the Vocabulary Building Glossary and Pronunciation Skills.

1. Make sure the tube is _____ before you use it.

2. We _____ that the infection is bacterial, but we will need to check it.

3. The physician will perform a(n) _____ on the patient with kidney stones.

WORD ATTACK SKILLS

Directions: Write the meaning of the word element.

1. Olig(o)-: _____

2. Poly-: _____

3. Supra-: _____

4. Extra-: _____

5. Hypo-: _____

COMMUNICATION EXERCISE

1. With a peer, practice performing a urologic assessment and history-taking. Use the Focused Assessment box on p. 773 in the textbook. Each partner should listen for clear pronunciation and may ask for an explanation of a word or procedure.

2. Write a dialogue you could use to ask a patient questions about drug history.

GRAMMAR POINTS

When you are trying to establish a history from a patient, it is very important to use the correct past or present tense. You want to clearly determine what has happened in the past, such as what medications he/she has taken, as opposed to what medications are being used now. Use *tag phrases* or *time words*, to be clear.

Examples:
Have you had frequency of urination *in the past*?
Do you have frequency of urination *now*?

CULTURAL POINTS

There are many commonly used terms for urination, many which are nonmedical and were learned in childhood but are still used by adults. You may need to know these when talking with your patients. For example, I need to *urinate, void, pee, make pee-pee, go pee, make water, take a leak, piss, use the urinal, go to the toilet/ bathroom*, etc. With your classmates, make a list of as many medical and nonmedical terms you can think of.

Copyright © 2013, 2009 by Saunders, an imprint of Elsevier Inc. All rights reserved.

Care of Patients with Disorders of the Urinary System

Answer Key: Textbook page references are provided as a guide for answering these questions. A complete answer key was provided to your instructor.

COMPLETION

Directions: Fill in the blanks to complete the statements.

1. _____ is the accumulation of nitrogenous products, which is signaled by an increase in BUN and serum creatinine. *(802)*

2. The patient complaining of burning is experiencing the symptom called _____ _____. *(795, see also Chapter 34)*

3. You assess an arteriovenous shunt by feeling for a(n) _____ over the shunt. *(806)*

4. Having to get up at night more than once to urinate is called _____. *(see Chapter 34)*

5. _____ commonly occurs about 2 to 3 weeks after a group A beta-hemolytic strepto-coccal infection. *(789)*

6. When the normal flow of urine is obstructed, urine can back up into the urinary tract and fill the kidney pelvis. This is called _____. *(790)*

SHORT ANSWER

Cancers of the Urinary System

Directions: Provide answers for the following questions.

1. Often the only sign of cancer of the bladder is _____. *(795)*

2. What are four risk factors for cancer of the bladder? *(795)*

   a. _____

   b. _____

   c. _____

   d. _____

Copyright © 2013, 2009 by Saunders, an imprint of Elsevier Inc. All rights reserved.

3. What are three diagnostic tests that are used to confirm bladder cancer? *(795)*

   a. _____

   b. _____

   c. _____

4. How does photodynamic therapy for bladder cancer work? *(795)*_____

   _____

   _____

5. The primary treatment for cancer of the kidney is _____ before metastasis has occurred. *(798)*

Urinary Diversion

Directions: Read the scenario and provide the answers to the following questions.

Scenario: You are caring for several patients who have urinary diversions. You recognize that while there are various surgical procedures that the physician may perform, there are some commonalities in the nursing care such as I & O and ostomy care.

1. An ileal conduit provides for evacuation of _____. *(797)*

2. A cutaneous ureterostomy produces _____ urine. *(796)*

3. The problem with a sigmoid conduit is that _____ frequently occurs. *(797)*

4. The immediate postoperative nursing care plan of a patient with diversion of urinary flow should include the following nursing actions: *(797-798)*

   a. Measurement of: _____

   b. Observation of: _____

5. Write a short-term goal for the nursing diagnosis Body image disturbance related to ostomy. *(798)*

   _____

   _____

   _____

6. List three common causes of periostomal skin problems *other than* seepage of urinary waste around the stoma. *(797)*

   a. _____

   b. _____

   c. _____

Copyright © 2013, 2009 by Saunders, an imprint of Elsevier Inc. All rights reserved.

7. List five nursing interventions that could help a patient prevent or overcome odor from an ureterostomy. *(798)*

   a. _____

   b. _____

   c. _____

   d. _____

   e. _____

LABELING

Different Types of Urinary Diversions

Directions: Label the drawings below with the correct name of the procedure depicted using the following list. (796)

ureterosigmoidostomy (sigmoid conduit)
ileal reservoir (Kock's pouch)
cutaneous ureterostomy
ileal conduit

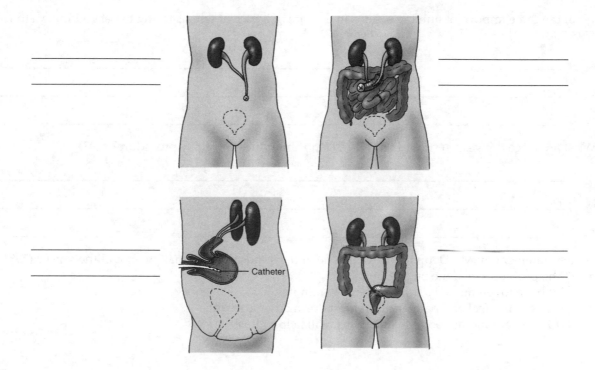

Copyright © 2013, 2009 by Saunders, an imprint of Elsevier Inc. All rights reserved.

APPLICATION OF THE NURSING PROCESS

Caring for a Patient with a Kidney Stone

Directions: Read the scenario and provide the answers to the following questions.

Scenario: You are working in a clinic and Mr. Depp arrives in acute distress and complains of severe left lower back pain. He is restless and pacing and unable to focus on your questions. His wife tells you that he "is peeing small amounts of bloody urine."

1. List at least four risk factors for kidney stones. *(792, Table 35-2)*

   a. _____

   b. _____

   c. _____

   d. _____

2. Which nursing diagnosis is the priority for Mr. Depp? *(793)*
   a. Risk for alteration in urinary elimination related to obstruction of flow
   b. Pain related to ureteral spasm and probable movement of kidney stone
   c. Risk of urinary tract infection related to urinary stasis
   d. Communication, impaired related to discomfort

3. What are three important nursing actions in the care of a patient who is trying to pass a kidney stone? *(793-794)*

   a. _____

   b. _____

   c. _____

4. What are three things you should teach Mr. Depp about the lithotripsy procedure? *(793)*

   a. _____

   b. _____

   c. _____

5. Which statement by Mr. Depp indicates that he understands the information about lithotripsy? *(793)*
   a. "The procedure is done on a x-ray table."
   b. "I'll have to remain very still for about 10 minutes."
   c. "I should not feel any pain or discomfort during the procedure."
   d. "If I walk around as soon as I am able, it will help to flush stones."

Copyright © 2013, 2009 by Saunders, an imprint of Elsevier Inc. All rights reserved.

PRIORITY SETTING

Directions: Read the scenario and prioritize as appropriate.

Scenario: Mr. Wyaksit is postoperative from a kidney transplant and was transferred 5 days ago from the ICU to the general medical-surgical unit. He appeared to be recovering quickly and was independently ambulating. Last night, he tripped and fell to the floor, but appeared uninjured and told the nurse, "no damage done." This morning he is reluctant to get out of bed. Which set of assessment findings is the most critical?
   a. Pulse 110/min, BP 120/60, Hct 30%
   b. Fever 101° F, redness at the incision site
   c. Urinary output of 40 mL/hr, rising BUN
   d. Pain over the iliac fossa transplant area
   e. Bruise and swelling with decreased pulse over right wrist
   f. Decreased appetite with subjective dry mouth

REVIEW QUESTIONS FOR THE NCLEX® EXAMINATION

Directions: Choose the correct answer(s) for the following questions.

1. The nurse is teaching a patient at risk for stone formation how to avoid developing kidney stones. What information should the nurse give the patient? *(792)*
    1. Drink enough liquids to produce at least 3500 mL of urine every 24 hours.
    2. Fluid intake should approximate urine output every 24 hours.
    3. Eat a well-balanced diet with high-quality protein and fruit and vegetables.
    4. Try to exercise at least 4 times a week and sleep 8 hours a night.

2. The patient is diagnosed with a bladder infection. Which characteristic is least likely associated with this disorder? *(786)*
    1. Burning upon urination
    2. Foul-smelling urine
    3. Decreased urinary output
    4. Elevated temperature

3. Hemodialysis is performed for the end-stage kidney disease patient. Data that indicate effectiveness would be: *(803, 809, 811)*
    1. a rise in hemoglobin and hematocrit.
    2. a fall in glucose and sodium levels.
    3. a fall in potassium, creatinine, and urea levels.
    4. an increased alertness and a sense of well-being.

4. Other than taking baseline vital signs, an important nursing intervention to perform the morning of dialysis is: *(806)*
    1. keeping the patient NPO until after the dialysis.
    2. administering 1 liter of normal saline to prevent shock.
    3. giving subcutaneous heparin to prevent blood clotting during dialysis.
    4. withholding blood pressure medications until the pressure has stabilized after dialysis.

5. When planning nursing care for the patient who has renal failure, the nurse encourages a diet that is: *(810)*
    1. high in calories but low in protein and potassium.
    2. high in protein, moderate in calories, and low in sodium.
    3. high in fat and protein but low in potassium and sodium.
    4. high in fiber, with mainly fruits and vegetables and some grains.

Copyright © 2013, 2009 by Saunders, an imprint of Elsevier Inc. All rights reserved.

6. A nursing intervention for the patient who has just returned from surgery with a new arteriovenous shunt is to: *(806)*
   1. maintain a heparin drip to prevent clotting in the shunt.
   2. release the elevated extremity and perform range-of-motion exercises every 2 hours.
   3. assess the shunt site for hematoma and check for bruit every 2–4 hours.
   4. assess the shunt for visual signs of clotting every 2–4 hours.

7. The nurse is looking at abnormal results of a urinalysis. Which finding is more specific to chronic glomerulonephritis, and is less likely to be present if the patient has an acute cystitis? *(789)*
   1. Glucose
   2. Red blood cells
   3. Urinary casts
   4. White blood cells

8. Planning nursing care for the patient with cystitis who is experiencing considerable discomfort includes: *(786-788)*
   1. decrease fluid intake to prevent discomfort of voiding.
   2. hot sitz baths to increase circulation and decrease discomfort.
   3. continuous intravenous fluid administration.
   4. obtain a urine specimen for culture and sensitivity.

9. Sulfamethoxazole-trimethoprim (Bactrim) is prescribed for the patient's cystitis. When doing discharge teaching, the nurse would be sure to instruct the patient to: *(786, Table 35-1)*
   1. take the medication between meals to enhance absorption.
   2. take 3000–4000 mL of fluid per day to prevent crystallization.
   3. be aware that this medication might turn the urine orange or red.
   4. watch for signs of jaundice associated with liver toxicity.

10. What changes in the urinary system occur with aging that predispose elderly women to urinary frequency and infection? *(786)*
    1. Decreased fluid intake to prevent incontinence
    2. An increased glomerular filtration rate
    3. Estrogen depletion that results in structural atrophy
    4. An increased bladder capacity due to loss of tone

11. Which signs and symptoms are associated with nephrotic syndrome? *(790)*
    1. Proteinuria, hyperlipidemia, hypoalbuminemia, and severe edema
    2. Hematuria, frequent and urgent urination, and low back pain
    3. Burning, itching, frequency in voiding, and dysuria
    4. Unilateral flank pain that radiates into the genitalia and inner thigh

12. A patient has acute renal failure and is in the diuretic phase. With an increased output, there is a danger of: *(790)*
    1. hyponatremia.
    2. hyperkalemia.
    3. fluid overload.
    4. catabolism.

13. A patient with chronic renal failure is receiving epoietin alpha (Epogen). The purpose of this medication is to: *(806, Table 35-4)*
    1. increase urinary output.
    2. bind phosphate; given with meals.
    3. prevent problems of calcium loss.
    4. treat anemia; promotes RBC formation.

Copyright © 2013, 2009 by Saunders, an imprint of Elsevier Inc. All rights reserved.

14. One of the relevant nursing diagnoses in caring for a patient with renal failure is Activity intolerance related to metabolic changes. Which intervention would be appropriate in helping the patient accomplish ADLs? *(801)*
    1. Tell the patient to do as much as he can and then return later to help him finish.
    2. Instruct the nursing assistant to watch him do ADLs and report back on his progress.
    3. Instruct the nursing assistant to do everything for him unless he tells her that he can do it himself.
    4. Assess his energy level in the AM and then direct the nursing assistant to do specific tasks for him.

15. What is characteristic of stage 1 chronic renal failure? *(802)*
    1. BUN and serum creatinine levels begin to rise.
    2. Glomerular filtration rate falls and oliguria and edema occur.
    3. Urine concentration is decreased and polyuria and nocturia occur.
    4. Electrolyte and fluid imbalances are serious; wastes accumulate.

16. Which patient needs counseling about contacting all sexual partners for follow-up care? *(788)*
    1. Patient diagnosed with chronic glomerulonephritis
    2. Patient diagnosed with hydronephrosis
    3. Patient diagnosed with nephrotic syndrome
    4. Patient diagnosed with urethritis

17. The nurse is caring for a patient with acute glomerulonephritis and observes obvious edema. What is the best rationale for frequent auscultation of the lung fields for this patient? *(789)*
    1. Assessing the lungs is the standard of care for any acutely ill patient.
    2. The patient is on continuous bedrest and will suffer the effects of immobility.
    3. Observable edema on the body surface suggests congestion in the internal organs.
    4. The patient is likely to have had a preexisting throat infection.

18. The nurse is supervising a nursing student who is preparing to irrigate a nephrostomy tube. Which action would the nurse advise the student to perform *first*? *(791)*
    1. Talk to the patient and explain the procedure.
    2. Read the physician's order to clarify the instructions.
    3. Check the chart and make sure informed consent was signed.
    4. Obtain all the equipment and mentally review the procedure.

19. The physician orders a Foley catheter for a patient involved in a serious car accident. The nurse notes that there is bleeding at the urethral meatus. What is the priority action? *(794-795)*
    1. Obtain extra supplies to cleanse the meatus.
    2. Get a bedpan and ask the patient to void.
    3. Insert the Foley and closely monitor for hematuria.
    4. Notify the physician, because there may be a tear.

20. Which patient has the greatest risk for acute renal failure? *(798-801)*
    1. Trauma patient with an episode of prolonged hypovolemia
    2. Chronic renal failure patient who is noncompliant with dietary restrictions
    3. Patient with frequent kidney stones undergoing nephrolithotomy
    4. Patient with bladder tumor and painless hematuria

Copyright © 2013, 2009 by Saunders, an imprint of Elsevier Inc. All rights reserved.

CRITICAL THINKING ACTIVITIES

Scenario: Mr. Sounds has chronic renal failure. His physician has decided that Mr. Sounds is a good candidate for peritoneal dialysis. This is a new therapy for Mr. Sounds, but he is eager to learn and cooperate.

1. Prepare a brief description of the purpose of peritoneal dialysis and the principle by which it works to help Mr. Sounds understand this new therapy. *(800, 806-808)*

   _____

   _____

   _____

2. List five nursing actions specific to the care of Mr. Sounds for his peritoneal dialysis. *(808)*

   a. _____

   b. _____

   c. _____

   d. _____

   e. _____

3. When administering peritoneal dialysis to Mr. Sounds, you would evaluate him each day. What is the most common complication? *(807)*
   a. Peritonitis
   b. Clotting of the catheter
   c. Hemorrhage from heparin in the solution
   d. Retention of in-flow solution within the abdomen

STEPS TOWARD BETTER COMMUNICATION

VOCABULARY BUILDING GLOSSARY

Term	Pronunciation	Definition
urgency	er' jen see	a need for immediate action, hurry
linked	link'd	connected, joined
intermittent	in ter mit' ent	happening with stops and starts; periodic
pertinent	per' tin ent	pertaining to or related to; important to know in relation to a subject
flank	flaynk	the side of the body between the ribs and ilium
void	voyd	to expel urine from the bladder; to make invalid

Copyright © 2013, 2009 by Saunders, an imprint of Elsevier Inc. All rights reserved.

COMPLETION

Directions: Fill in each blank with the correct word from the Vocabulary Building Glossary.

1. A sign of kidney infection is pain in the _____ area.

2. The nurse asks the patient to _____ into a specimen container for a urinalysis.

3. If the patient states that there has been blood in the urine, it is a very _____ piece of information.

4. The patient with cystitis experiences dysuria, but may also have urinary _____.

5. Smoking has been _____ as a risk factor in cancer of the bladder.

6. The male with benign prostatic hypertrophy (BPH) may experience a(n) _____ stream when he urinates.

WORD ATTACK SKILLS

Combining Forms

nephr/o-	kidney
glomerul/o-	network of capillaries
ur/o-	urine, urinary tract
ren/o-	kidney
oli/olig/o-	little, few, scanty
poly-	many, much

Directions: Using slash marks, break these words into their word elements or parts. Write the meaning of each word part, then give the meaning of the word.

1. Glomerulonephritis: _____

   _____

   _____

2. Hypoalbuminemia: _____

   _____

   _____

3. Nephrolithotomy: _____

   _____

   _____

4. Pyelonephrolithotomy: _____

   _____

   _____

5. Ureterosigmoidostomy: _____

   _____

   _____

Copyright © 2013, 2009 by Saunders, an imprint of Elsevier Inc. All rights reserved.

PRONUNCIATION SKILLS

Directions: Pronounce these abbreviations and write their meanings.

1. ARF: _____

2. CRF: _____

3. GFR: _____

4. ATN: _____

5. UTI: _____

6. NSU: _____

7. ESRD: _____

8. ESWL: _____

9. TURP: _____

10. AV: _____

11. CAPD: _____

Pronunciation Pairs Exercise

Many words are pronounced the same except for the last letter that creates the final sound. It is important that this final sound be pronounced correctly so that the listener will understand the meaning of what is being said. Many of these sounds are difficult for the second language speaker to hear and pronounce.

Pronunciation

Directions: With a study partner, take turns pronouncing the word pairs listed below while the other listens without looking at the list. The listener should write down the words heard. Take turns speaking and then listening. Check to see that the words written by the listener are correct. (For extra practice, write the word pairs on small cards and mix up the order. Do the exercise frequently.)

life	live	barf	bark	duct	duck
of	up	ureter	urethra	tape	take
have	had	loop	lose	waste	wake
can	can't	lose	loose	help	health
out	ouch	tube	tooth	holds	holes
track	tract	gland	clamp	stones	stomas
putting	pudding	car	cart	lab	lap

Copyright © 2013, 2009 by Saunders, an imprint of Elsevier Inc. All rights reserved.

The Endocrine System

chapter

36

Answer Key: Textbook page references are provided as a guide for answering these questions. A complete answer key was provided to your instructor.

COMPLETION

Directions: Fill in the blanks to complete the statements.

1. The _____ is often referred to as the "master gland" of the body. *(822)*

2. Parathormone acts on the renal tubules to increase the excretion of _____ in the urine and the reabsorption of _____. *(821)*

3. Parathormone raises the serum calcium level by stimulating _____ and increasing calcium absorption in the _____ tract. *(819, 821, Table 36-1)*

4. A hormone produced by the adrenal cortex, which influences sodium and water balance, is _____. *(819, Table 36-1)*

5. The adrenal medulla secretes _____ and _____ _____. *(821)*

6. The adrenal cortex secretes mainly _____ and _____ _____. *(821)*

7. The mineralocorticoids affect the balance of _____. *(821)*

8. The glucocorticoids are essential for proper utilization of _____, _____, and _____. *(821)*

9. The primary glucocorticoid is _____. *(821)*

10. Primary actions of cortisol are to increase _____ levels and to _____ the inflammatory response. *(821)*

Copyright © 2013, 2009 by Saunders, an imprint of Elsevier Inc. All rights reserved.

TABLE ACTIVITY

Hormone Changes that Occur with Aging

Directions: Complete the table below. Add the hormones that increase, decrease, or essentially remain unchanged with aging. The first block is done for you. (822)

Hormones that usually decrease with age	aldosterone, renin, calcitonin, and growth hormone; in the older female, estrogen and prolactin; and in the older male, testosterone
Hormones that may increase with age	
Hormones that remain unchanged or are slightly decreased	

SHORT ANSWER

Hypothyroidism

Directions: Read the clinical scenario and answer the questions that follow.

Scenario: You are working in an endocrinology clinic. Mrs. Venucha is an older woman who has been referred by her family doctor for a possible thyroid disorder. Mrs. Venucha tells you that she has been slowing down lately and has felt "mildly bloated, sluggish, and constipated." She agreed to have some diagnostic testing done, but she feels she needs some general information about the thyroid and the diagnostic testing.

1. List five effects of thyroid hormones. *(819, 821)*

   a. _____

   b. _____

   c. _____

   d. _____

   e. _____

2. Name four serum tests that are done to evaluate thyroid function. *(825, 827, Table 32-2)*

   a. _____

   b. _____

   c. _____

   d. _____

Copyright © 2013, 2009 by Saunders, an imprint of Elsevier Inc. All rights reserved.

3. List four commonly used drugs that can alter the results of thyroid tests. *(825)*

   a. _____

   b. _____

   c. _____

   d. _____

4. List at least three teaching points to include for a patient who needs a radioactive iodine uptake exam to assess thyroid function. *(826)*

   a. _____

   b. _____

   c. _____

5. Briefly describe how aging affects the thyroid gland and thyroid hormone levels. *(822)*

   a. _____

      _____

   b. _____

      _____

   c. _____

      _____

   d. _____

      _____

APPLICATION OF THE NURSING PROCESS

Caring for Patients at Risk for Type 2 Diabetes

Directions: Read the scenario and provide the answers to the following questions.

Scenario: You are working in an ambulatory clinic. Mr. Bob, a middle-aged gentleman, comes in for a check-up and he reports having mild fatigue and some gradual but progressive weight gain over the past 6 months. He suspects he may have diabetes, "because my father had it."

1. List five or six questions to ask a patient who is suspected of having an endocrine disorder. *(829)*

   _____

   _____

   _____

   _____

   _____

Copyright © 2013, 2009 by Saunders, an imprint of Elsevier Inc. All rights reserved.

2. Write an example of an appropriate outcome for the nursing diagnosis Imbalanced nutrition, more than body requirements, related to altered glucose metabolism. *(829-831, Table 36-5)*

_____

_____

3. List three general nursing interventions that will help a diabetic patient who has Imbalanced nutrition, more than body requirements to maintain a normal body weight. *(829-830, Table 36-5)*

   a. _____

   b. _____

   c. _____

4. Write an example of evaluation outcome for the following goal: Patient will verbalize beginning under-standing of diagnostic testing for diabetes at the end of teaching session. *(830, Table 36-5)*

   _____

   _____

   _____

   _____

   _____

   _____

5. Mr. Bob currently weighs 225 lbs. The doctor has suggested that he should gradually lose weight to achieve a target goal of 85 kg. Mr. Bob asks you help him with some calculations.

   a. How long will it take him to achieve the target goal if he can lose 2 pounds/month? _____

   b. How long will it take him to achieve the target goal if he can lose 5 pounds/month? _____

   c. How long will it take him to achieve the target goal if he can lose 8 pounds/month? _____

PRIORITY SETTING

Directions: Read the scenario and prioritize as appropriate.

Scenario: You are the only nurse standing in the nurse's station and the unit secretary hands you computer printouts of several laboratory values.

1. Which patient needs priority attention? *(825, 828, Table 36-2, Table 36-3)*
   a. Mr. Jez has positive ketone bodies in the urine.
   b. Ms. Lukic has serum T_4 of 10 mg/dL.
   c. Mr. Doig has a 2-hour postprandial glucose of 150 mg/dL.
   d. Mrs. Kost has a fasting blood glucose of 20 mg/dL.

Copyright © 2013, 2009 by Saunders, an imprint of Elsevier Inc. All rights reserved.

2. You recognize that one of the patients needs immediate attention; however, Mr. Jez, Mr. Doig, and Mrs. Kost have been assigned to other nurses. Of the four patients, Ms. Lukic is the only patient that has been assigned to you. What is your priority action? *(825, 828, Table 36-2, Table 36-3)*
   a. Check on Ms. Lukic.
   b. Find the nurse assigned to the critical patient.
   c. Inform the charge nurse about the lab values.
   d. Check on the most critical patient.

REVIEW QUESTIONS FOR THE NCLEX® EXAMINATION

Directions: Choose the correct answer(s) for the following questions.

1. The patient is experiencing fatigue with loss of energy and is currently undergoing multiple diagnostic tests to diagnose a possible endocrine disorder. She states, "I just want to know what is going on. I'm so tired of these tests." What is the most therapeutic response?
   1. "Did you talk to your doctor about the test results?"
   2. "Let me go look at your chart and find the results."
   3. "You sound really frustrated about the diagnostic testing."
   4. "I'd be tired too, if I had to deal with everything you have."

2. A patient is diagnosed with a thyroid disorder. The nurse anticipates that the patient is mostly likely to have problems with: *(819)*
   1. metabolic rate.
   2. water reabsorption.
   3. bone fragility.
   4. increased blood glucose.

3. Which patient is most likely to have a nursing diagnosis of Imbalanced nutrition: less than body requirements? *(822-824)*
   1. Patient with hyperthyroidism
   2. Patient with decreased estrogen production
   3. Patient who has type 2 diabetes
   4. Patient with hypothyroidism

4. The patient is undergoing a hypertonic saline test to detect diabetes insipidus. One of the nursing responsibilities is to teach the patient to: *(827, Table 36-2)*
   1. produce a urine specimen using a clean-catch technique.
   2. produce a urine specimen in the marked container each hour.
   3. void in the early AM and discard the first urine specimen.
   4. produce a urine specimen at the end of the test period.

5. The doctor orders a dexamethasone suppression test to assist in the diagnosis of Cushing's disease. An appropriate nursing action would be to: *(826, Table 36-2)*
   1. collect a clean-catch urine specimen.
   2. note the start and end time on the laboratory slip.
   3. check orders for drugs to be withheld.
   4. administer vasopressin SC as ordered.

6. A patient is being tested to determine the degree of diabetic control of blood sugar over the preceding 6–8 weeks. What is the correct test to make this determination? *(328, Table 36-3)*
   1. Fasting blood glucose
   2. 2-hour postprandial blood glucose
   3. Glucose tolerance test
   4. Hemoglobin A_{1C}

Copyright © 2013, 2009 by Saunders, an imprint of Elsevier Inc. All rights reserved.

7. Which patient has the greatest risk for injury related to bone fracture? *(821)*
   1. Patient with a thyroid disorder
   2. Patient with a parathyroid disorder
   3. Patient with a pancreatic disorder
   4. Patient with a testicular disorder

8. The doctor orders laboratory tests for several serum electrolytes. Which set of electrolytes would most likely reflect the parathyroid function? *(821)*
   1. Calcium and phosphorus
   2. Sodium and magnesium
   3. Potassium and chloride
   4. Sodium and potassium

9. The patient needs several diagnostic tests to rule out endocrine disorders. Which task would be appropriate to assign to the nursing assistant? *(825-828)*
   1. Note medications that the patient takes on laboratory slip.
   2. Ask the patient if he has any questions or needs anything.
   3. Instruct the patient on how to obtain a clean-catch specimen.
   4. Deliver the urine specimen to the laboratory.

10. The physician orders an aldosterone urine test for a patient. No one on the unit, including the charge nurse, is familiar with this test. What should the nurse do? *(827, Table 36-2)*
    1. Collect a clean-catch urine specimen and send it to the laboratory.
    2. Call the physician and ask for clarification of the order and procedure.
    3. Check the laboratory policy and procedure manual.
    4. Ask the patient not to void until after the procedure is clarified.

CRITICAL THINKING ACTIVITIES

Scenario A: Your neighbor tells you that she is thinking about taking synthroid to lose weight because a relative has been taking synthroid that was obtained "through the Internet" and that person lost about 15 pounds very easily.

1. How would you respond to your neighbor? *(819, 821)* _____

   _____

   _____

   _____

2. One of the functions of the thyroid hormones is to affect tissue response to epinephrine and norepinephrine. Briefly describe to your neighbor the potential effects on blood pressure and heart rate. *(819, 821, Table 36-1)*

   _____

   _____

Copyright © 2013, 2009 by Saunders, an imprint of Elsevier Inc. All rights reserved.

3. Discuss some of the problems that might occur as people try to save money by using the Internet as a health care resource.

_____

_____

_____

_____

_____

Scenario B: Your cousin tells you that she thinks she has hypoglycemia. She wants your opinion about whether she might have diabetes. Her doctor has reassured her that she does not have diabetes, but she doesn't believe him.

1. Write a brief statement that you could use to redirect your cousin back to her doctor. *(827-830, Table 36-3)*

_____

_____

_____

_____

_____

2. List at least five questions that your cousin could ask her doctor. *(827-830, Table 36-3)*

    a. _____

    b. _____

    c. _____

    d. _____

    e. _____

3. Would you feel comfortable giving her an opinion about the diabetes? Why or why not?

_____

_____

_____

_____

Copyright © 2013, 2009 by Saunders, an imprint of Elsevier Inc. All rights reserved.

STEPS TOWARD BETTER COMMUNICATION

VOCABULARY BUILDING GLOSSARY

Term	Pronunciation	Definition
alter	al'ter	to change, to make different
aspect	as'pect	area, or part of a surface
assay	ass'ay	a test for purity
elicit	e lis'it	to gather or solicit information from someone
lability	lay bil'ity	instability, likely to change, easily altered
negative feedback	neg' ah tiv feed' bak	a response to a message which is intended to change or stop the message
postprandial	post pran' dee al	after dinner, or after any other meal
render	ren'der	to cause a change
sluggish	slug'gish	slow-moving, inactive
stalk	stawk	1. (noun) a stem or support of a plant or organ. 2. (verb) to follow pursue secretly.
synthesis	sin'the sis	combining of parts to make a whole

COMPLETION

Directions: Fill in the blanks with the appropriate words from the Vocabulary Building Glossary to complete the statements.

1. The person who has hypothyroidism usually feels _____.

2. A patient should be instructed not to _____ their medication regimen without first consulting a physician.

3. When there is too much circulating cortisol in a person's system, he often displays emotional _____.

4. Pituitary problems may _____ a female infertile.

5. When checking for thyroid disease, the examiner pays particular attention to the frontal _____ _____ of the neck.

6. Fructosamine _____ is another test to monitor control of glucose over time.

7. The word *parathormone* is a(n) _____ of the two words *parathyroid* and *hormone*.

8. The patient gave _____ in response to the questionnaire about the new hospital menus.

9. She cut the _____ of the flower so that it would fit the vase.

10. A nap is often the favorite _____ activity of many people.

11. A good history-taking will _____ a lot of information from the patient.

Copyright © 2013, 2009 by Saunders, an imprint of Elsevier Inc. All rights reserved.

WORD ATTACK SKILLS

hyper-	over, more
hypo-	under, less
endo-	internal
exo-	external
para-	beside, next to; near

PRONUNCIATION SKILLS

Directions: Take turns practicing with a peer the pronunciation of these words to increase your ability to speak English clearly.

adenohypophysis (ad noh hi po' fi sis)	anterior pituitary
adrenocorticotropic (ah dree'no kor'tih ko tro'pik)	a hormone acting on the adrenal cortex
verbalization (ver'bal iz a' shun)	putting into words
antiinflammatory (an' tee in flam'ah tor y)	preventing inflammation
hypopituitary (hi' po pih too' ih tar y)	decreased secretions from the pituitary gland

Copyright © 2013, 2009 by Saunders, an imprint of Elsevier Inc. All rights reserved.

Care of Patients with Pituitary, Thyroid, Parathyroid, and Adrenal Disorders

chapter
37

Answer Key: Textbook page references are provided as a guide for answering these questions. A complete answer key was provided to your instructor.

COMPLETION

Directions: Fill in the blanks to complete the statements.

1. Simple goiter causes problems when it enlarges to the point of placing _____
   _____. *(838-839)*

2. Graves' disease is another name given to _____. *(839)*

3. The danger in an Addisonian crisis is severe _____ and possible shock. *(848)*

4. Patients with Cushing's syndrome may have weakness due to abnormal protein catabolism and have
   loss of _____. *(852)*

5. The syndrome of inappropriate antidiuretic hormone (SIADH) secretion causes
   _____ of fluid. *(837-838)*

6. Pheochromocytoma is a rare tumor of the _____ which secretes catechol-
   amines. *(847)*

APPLICATION OF THE NURSING PROCESS

Care of Patients with Hyperthyroidism

Directions: Read the clinical scenario and answer the questions that follow.

Scenario: You are caring for a middle-aged woman, Mrs. Riata, who has been admitted for treatment of her hyperthyroidism. Mrs. Riata has been living with this diagnosis for a period of time; however, she has not had success with conservative therapy, so she is being admitted for a partial thyroidectomy. Although she is knowledgeable about the disease and the impending surgery, she is emotionally labile and appears exhausted.

1. The physical signs and symptoms of hyperthyroidism include: *(839)*_____

   _____

   _____

Copyright © 2013, 2009 by Saunders, an imprint of Elsevier Inc. All rights reserved.

2. Psychological or emotional symptoms of hyperthyroidism include episodes of: *(839)*_____

_____

_____

_____

3. Which diagnosis is likely to be included in the care plan for Mrs. Riata? *(839)*
   a. Self-care deficit related to lethargy
   b. Altered nutrition, more than body requirements, related to decreased metabolic rate
   c. Self-esteem disturbance related to facial puffiness and swelling
   d. Constipation related to decreased gastrointestinal motility
   e. Anxiety related to agitation and difficulty concentrating

4. List three nursing actions that should be included in the postoperative nursing care plan of a patient after partial thyroidectomy. *(840-843)*

   a. _____

   _____

   b. _____

   _____

   c. _____

   _____

5. Write an example of an evaluation outcome for the following patient goal. Patient will rest at least 7 hours per night and take frequent rest breaks during the day while in the hospital. *(840-843)*

   _____

   _____

   _____

   _____

   _____

PRIORITY SETTING

Directions: Read the clinical scenario and prioritize nursing actions as appropriate. Also identify tasks that can be performed by various members of the health care team.

Scenario: You arrive for your shift at the hospital. Before you can even get your coat off, the day shift RN says, "Quick! Come and help me! I have a patient who is going down the tubes!" You run to the room and recognize Mrs. Dredge who has hypothyroidism. The RN says, "The doctor has just diagnosed her with myxedema coma and wrote these orders. Will you help me and the nursing assistant so that we can take care of this lady quickly?" *(844-845)*

1. Prioritize the top five interventions that need to be accomplished first.

2. Identify which tasks (if any) could be assigned to the nursing assistant or the unit secretary.

Copyright © 2013, 2009 by Saunders, an imprint of Elsevier Inc. All rights reserved.

3. Identify which tasks (if any) should be done only by the RN.

_____ a. Assess response to external warming blanket

_____ b. O$_2$ at 3 L per N/C

_____ c. Vital signs q 2 hours and notify physician for BP <100/60 or > 160/90

_____ d. Blood glucose STAT

_____ e. Levothyroxine sodium now 0.5 mg IV push over 5 minutes

_____ f. IV access X 2 (Saline lock X 1)

_____ g. IV bolus 250 mL X 1 over 30 minutes STAT

_____ h. Place on cardiac monitor

_____ i. Place continuous pulse oximeter

_____ j. Maintenance IV D$_5$.45 NS 150 mL/hour

_____ k. Call for EKG now

_____ l. Give 1/2 amp D$_{10}$ IV push for BS < 60

REVIEW QUESTIONS FOR THE NCLEX® EXAMINATION

Directions: Choose the correct answer(s) for the following questions.

1. A patient is admitted for a minor elective surgery. He also has a diagnosis of Cushing's syndrome. Which physical assessment findings are associated with Cushing's syndrome and are likely to be documented in the patient's record? *(852)*
   1. Dry, scaly skin and brittle nails.
   2. Abnormal protrusion of the eyeballs
   3. Enlarged thyroid gland
   4. Buffalo hump and moon face

2. A patient is diagnosed with diabetes insipidus. Which finding is characteristic of this disorder? *(836)*
   1. Excessive dilute urine
   2. An increased blood pressure
   3. Tachycardia
   4. Exertional dyspnea

3. The nurse is caring for a patient who has SIADH. Which nursing intervention is appropriate for the care of this patient? *(838)*
   1. Giving hypotonic enemas as ordered
   2. Restricting fluids to 500–1000 mL/day as ordered
   3. Administering somatropin via subcutaneous injection as ordered
   4. Administering IV calcium gluconate as ordered

4. The nurse is caring for a patient who is receiving large doses of radioactive iodine. The care plan should include which precaution? *(840)*
   1. No special precautions beyond standard precautions
   2. Wearing lead aprons when delivering nursing care
   3. Isolation of the patient for 8 days (half-life of drug)
   4. Having the patient wear a radiation detection badge

Copyright © 2013, 2009 by Saunders, an imprint of Elsevier Inc. All rights reserved.

5. The patient is diagnosed with a rare tumor of the adrenal gland (pheochromocytoma). The nurse recognizes that the priority vital sign to monitor frequently is: *(847)*
   1. respiratory rate.
   2. temperature.
   3. blood pressure.
   4. pulse.

6. The nurse is caring for a postoperative patient who has had a hypophysectomy. Which nursing intervention(s) would be appropriate in the care of this patient? *(Select all that apply.) (834)*
   1. Keep the patient flat in bed.
   2. Note and report change in mental status.
   3. Change nasal drip pad as needed.
   4. Instruct patient to cough deeply.
   5. Assist the patient with mouth rinses.

7. The nurse is assessing a patient with simple goiter. What is the first sign usually noticed in this condition? *(838)*
   1. Difficulty swallowing
   2. Difficulty breathing
   3. Enlargement in the front of the neck
   4. Abnormal protrusion of the eyeballs

8. The nurse is administering an iodine preparation to a patient. What is a nursing implication in administering this drug? *(839)*
   1. Monitoring the vital signs, especially the blood pressure
   2. Diluting and administering through a straw to prevent staining teeth
   3. Administering the drug SQ in the abdominal area
   4. Monitoring the lab results for hyponatremia or hyperkalemia

9. Which statement by the patient indicates a need for additional teaching about the treatment plan for hyperthyroidism? *(840)*
   1. "I could be treated with antithyroid drugs and ablation therapy."
   2. "Ablation therapy could possibly cause hypothyroidism."
   3. "I'll have a thyroidectomy first and then get ablation therapy."
   4. "I could get ablation therapy on an outpatient basis."

10. The nurse is administering antithyroid drugs to the patient. Which dangerous adverse effects are a concern with antithyroid drugs? *(840)*
    1. Agranulocytosis and hepatotoxicity
    2. Hypoglycemia and neurotoxicity
    3. Hyponatremia and renal toxicity
    4. Seizures and ototoxicity

11. The nurse is carefully assessing a postoperative patient who had a thyroidectomy. Which assessment finding is most likely to be associated with one of the potential complications of this surgery? *(840-841, 843)*
    1. Blindness
    2. Tetany
    3. Profound diuresis
    4. Hypertensive crisis

12. The nursing student is reinforcing dietary and medication teaching with a patient who is taking parathormone replacement therapy. What is an inappropriate piece of information to give this patient? *(846)*
    1. You will be taking extra-large doses of vitamin D.
    2. The goal of medications and diet is to increase your serum calcium level.
    3. You should eat generous amounts of milk, yogurt, and processed cheese.
    4. The medication and dietary modifications are lifelong therapies.

Copyright © 2013, 2009 by Saunders, an imprint of Elsevier Inc. All rights reserved.

13. Which therapies and medication is the physician likely to order for a patient who is experiencing an Addisonian crisis? *(848)*
    1. Fluid restriction and prazosin (Minipress)
    2. IV glucose and levothyroxine sodium (Synthroid)
    3. Isotonic sodium chloride and calcitonin (Caltin)
    4. Fluid bolus and IV hydrocortisone (Solu-Cortef)

14. When planning care for a patient with hypothyroidism, what would the nurse do? *(844)*
    1. Provide extra snacks and encourage the patient to eat frequently.
    2. Place the patient in a cool room to avoid overheating.
    3. Provide extra time to avoid rushing the patient.
    4. Provide a calm, quiet atmosphere for episodes of emotional outbursts.

15. Which endocrine disorder is most likely to mimic the symptoms of a cardiac disease? *(839)*
    1. Hyperthyroidism
    2. Myxedema
    3. Sheehan's syndrome
    4. Diabetes insipidus

16. The nurse is caring for a patient with hyperparathyroidism. Which set of laboratory values is the primary concern? *(846)*
    1. Calcium and phosphorus
    2. Glucose and potassium
    3. White blood cell count
    4. Urinalysis and blood urea nitrogen

17. A patient has recently had a thyroidectomy. The nurse notes that the patient demonstrates sudden onset of muscular twitching and spasms. What is the priority intervention? *(841, 843)*
    1. Initiate seizure precautions.
    2. Check the patency of the IV site.
    3. Obtain the emergency airway equipment.
    4. Check the patient's temperature.

18. Which patient has the greatest risk for developing Cushing's syndrome? *(852)*
    1. Patient who recently had a subtotal parathyroidectomy
    2. Patient who has diabetes insipidus
    3. Patient on long-term steroid therapy
    4. Patient with a low serum calcium

19. The nurse is caring for a patient with diabetes insipidus. Which pattern of urinary output would be the most typical of this disorder? *(836)*
    1. Usually more than 2.5 L/day
    2. 30 mL/hour
    3. Output will approximate intake
    4. Urine cortisol level will be high

20. The nurse is caring for several patients with endocrine disorders. Which patient is most likely to have Desmopressin acetate (DDAVP) ordered as part of the therapy? *(837)*
    1. Patient with hypoparathyroidism
    2. Patient with Graves' disease
    3. Patient with hyperthyroidism
    4. Patient with diabetes insipidus

Copyright © 2013, 2009 by Saunders, an imprint of Elsevier Inc. All rights reserved.

21. What are signs and symptoms of hypothyroidism? (*Select all that apply.*) *(844)*
    1. Decreased appetite but increased weight
    2. Bagginess under eyes and swelling of face
    3. Feeling overheated
    4. Pressured speech
    5. Sluggish mental activity, impaired memory, depression
    6. Constipation, abdominal distention, flatulence
    7. Husky voice, thinning eyebrows, hair loss

22. What are signs and symptoms of adrenal cortical insufficiency (Addison's disease)? (*Select all that apply.*) *(847-848)*
    1. Generalized malaise
    2. Muscle weakness, muscle pain
    3. Orthostatic hypotension, and vulnerability to cardiac dysrhythmias
    4. Anorexia, nausea and vomiting, flatulence, and diarrhea
    5. Anxiety, depression, and loss of mental acuity
    6. Hyperglycemia

23. The physician orders IV normal saline to infuse 500 mL over 6 hours. What is the pump setting?

    _____

CRITICAL THINKING ACTIVITIES

Scenario: Your patient is diagnosed with pheochromocytoma. This is a rare condition that can be fatal. The patient was just admitted and the night nurse is not able to give you much information about pheochromocytoma; however, "the patient is stable and did not have any problems for me."

1. What is the most likely complication of this tumor if it is not treated? *(847)* _____

   _____

2. What are the signs and symptoms that you might see with this condition? *(847)* _____

   _____

   _____

3. Identify at least three actions (with rationale) that you should immediately take if this patient shows signs of a hypertensive crisis. *(847)*

   _____

   _____

   _____

4. When you are working on the unit and encounter patient conditions that are unfamiliar to you (and maybe unfamiliar to the rest of the staff), how can you quickly access the necessary information that you need to care for the patient?

   _____

   _____

   _____

   _____

Copyright © 2013, 2009 by Saunders, an imprint of Elsevier Inc. All rights reserved.

STEPS TOWARD BETTER COMMUNICATION

VOCABULARY BUILDING GLOSSARY

Term	Pronunciation	Definition
bulge	bulj	to extend outward, stick out, protrude
fidget	fi' djet	to move nervously, especially the hands
hence	hens	for this reason, therefore
husky	hus'ky	low-sounding, rough; sturdy
idiopathic	id' ee o path' ik	the cause is not known
inertia	in er' shah	lack of movement, resisting change
lethargic	lah thar' jik	tired, inactive
moody	moo' dee	changing emotions frequently; often sad
slurred	slur'd	not clear, words run together
taper off	tap'er off	to gradually become smaller or less
tetany	tet' ah nee	muscle cramps or twitching
"think straight"		think clearly and normally
undue	un dew'	excessive, too much
wringing	ring' ing	to twist or squeeze (hands or soft material)

COMPLETION

Directions: Fill in the blanks with the appropriate words from the Vocabulary Building Glossary to complete the statements.

1. If the parathyroid glands are accidentally removed during a thyroidectomy, the patient will experience
   _____.

2. When cortisone is prescribed to treat a nonhormonal illness, it is important that the patient
   _____ the dosage gradually to prevent a hormone imbalance.

3. The patient with Addison's disease becomes very fatigued and may seem to be in a state of
   _____.

4. The patient the thyroid condition was irritable and _____.

5. Hypoparathyroidism can be caused by a(n) _____ atrophy of the glands.

6. While the patient was still groggy from the anesthetic, her words were _____
   _____.

7. Cushing's disease is from a(n) _____ amount of cortisol circulating in the blood.

8. The nurse could tell that the patient was nervous because she kept _____ her
   hands.

9. There was a big _____ in the man's hip pocket where he kept his wallet.

10. Mr. Johnson was confused and kept saying, "I can't _____."

Copyright © 2013, 2009 by Saunders, an imprint of Elsevier Inc. All rights reserved.

11. The child was restless and she began to _____ in the chair.

12. After I ate that huge meal, I felt sleepy and _____.

WORD ATTACK SKILLS

myx/o-   mucus

-crine, -crin/o   secrete

PRONUNCIATION SKILLS

Directions: Take turns practicing with a peer pronouncing these words to increase your ability to speak English clearly.

ac'romeg'aly (ak' ro meg' ah lee)   thickening of lips and nose, enlargement of extremities (hyperpituitarism)

ex'ophthal'mos (ek' sof thal' mos)   abnormal protrusion of the eye; eyes bulge or stand out in the face

myx'ede'ma (mik' sah dee' mah)   a condition resulting from low thyroid production

phe'ochromocytoma (fe' o kro'mo si' to ma) a small tumor of the adrenal glands

CULTURAL POINT

Some people think that Americans, especially American women, are too concerned about their body images. Do you think this is true? If you are from a different country, is this different in your native country? What is the ideal body image there? Is there a relationship between body image and health?

_____

_____

_____

Copyright © 2013, 2009 by Saunders, an imprint of Elsevier Inc. All rights reserved.

Care of Patients with Diabetes and Hypoglycemia

Answer Key: Textbook page references are provided as a guide for answering these questions. A complete answer key was provided to your instructor.

COMPLETION

Directions: Fill in the blanks to complete the statements.

1. The long-term consequences of diabetes mellitus are chiefly the result of damage to the large and small _____. *(874)*

2. It is known that the risk of having some form of diabetes increases in proportion to the _____ of relatives who are affected, the _____ of the relatives, and the severity of their disease. *(858)*

3. Weight loss in patients with type 1 diabetes occurs partly because of the loss of _____ and partly because in the absence of sufficient _____, the body begins to metabolize its own proteins and stored fat. *(859)*

4. People with poor control over their diabetes are prone to infection because of decreased function of _____ and abnormal phagocyte function. *(859)*

5. The older diabetic is at risk of developing hypoglycemia up to _____ hours after exercising if the exercise is too strenuous. *(860)*

6. Diabetic _____ occurs directly from changes in the renal blood circulation. *(860)*

7. When insulin is not present in adequate amounts to meet metabolic needs, the body breaks down _____ and _____ for energy. *(873)*

8. An abundance of the byproducts of fat metabolism results in potent organic acids called _____. *(873)*

9. The Dawn phenomenon is the reason why most people with diabetes do not tolerate _____ well in the morning. *(874)*

10. Two out of three people with diabetes die prematurely from _____ or _____. *(875)*

Copyright © 2013, 2009 by Saunders, an imprint of Elsevier Inc. All rights reserved.

SHORT ANSWER

Type 2 Diabetes

Directions: Read the clinical scenarios and answer the questions that follow.

Scenario: Mr. Eick is an elderly widower with type 2 diabetes. He has been managing his own diabetic condition for the past 15 years; however, he recently moved in with his eldest daughter because he has been increasingly lonely and forgetful. Mr. Eick's daughter also has diabetes and has a good general knowledge of diabetes, but she asks you for some information specific to diabetes in the elderly.

1. Why is "tight control" not advised for elderly type 2 diabetic patients? *(860)* _____

    _____

2. Why is weight loss not a priority goal for an elderly diabetic patient? *(860)* _____

    _____

    _____

    _____

    _____

3. What are two problems concerning exercise for older diabetic patients? *(861)* _____

    _____

    _____

    _____

    _____

4. Which exercise activities are considered the safest for older diabetic patients? *(861)* _____

    _____

5. For older patients who are taking oral hypoglycemic agents, list two relevant facts related to aging. *(862, Table 38-2)*

    a. _____

        _____

    b. _____

        _____

SHORT ANSWER

Medications for Diabetes

Directions: Answer the following questions related to insulin injection preparation.

1. When regular insulin and long-acting insulin are to be mixed together for an injection, which insulin is drawn up first? _____ *(864)*

Copyright © 2013, 2009 by Saunders, an imprint of Elsevier Inc. All rights reserved.

2. How are NPH and lente insulin "mixed" before being drawn up with the syringe? *(864)*_____

_____

3. Why is insulin never given orally? *(864)*_____

_____

4. What is the proper way to warm chilled insulin? *(864)* _____

_____

5. The patient is to receive 3 units of regular insulin and 11 units of NPH. After both medications are drawn up, how many total units will be in the syringe? _____ units

6. Every patient on insulin should be monitored for _____ after insulin injections. *(866, 871)*

Directions: Answer the following questions related to oral hypoglycemic agents.

7. If a patient is allergic to sulfonamide antibiotics, which group of antihypoglycemic agents could cause a similar allergic reaction? *(863)*

_____

8. What are the two most common side effects of the second-generation oral hypoglycemic agents? *(863)*

_____

_____

9. How is metformin (Glucophage) thought to work? *(862, Table 38-2)* _____

_____

10. What disease or condition would be a contraindication for the drug acarbose (Precose)? *(862, Table 38-2)*

_____

11. Why must you always check for drug interactions when a patient is taking an oral hypoglycemic? *(862-863)*

_____

_____

_____

APPLICATION OF THE NURSING PROCESS

Caring for Patients with Diabetic Ketoacidosis (DKA)

Directions: Read the scenario and provide the answers to the following questions.

Scenario: Jason, age 16, is on the school track team and he was able to maintain a B average in his studies. Jason's mother reports that within the past several months he has lost about 20 lbs., lost interest in his classes at school, and complains of being too tired to study or participate in any sports at school or at home. He began running a fever several days ago with flulike symptoms and now presents to the emergency department

Copyright © 2013, 2009 by Saunders, an imprint of Elsevier Inc. All rights reserved.

with nausea and vomiting. He is listless, flushed, and dehydrated. The emergency department physician makes a medical diagnosis of diabetic ketoacidosis (DKA).

1. What are possible causes of DKA? *(873)*

   a. _____

   b. _____

   c. _____

   d. _____

2. List at least six physical assessment findings that are likely to be seen with DKA. *(873)*

   a. _____

   b. _____

   c. _____

   d. _____

   e. _____

   f. _____

3. List four general treatment goals for patients with DKA. *(873)*

   a. _____

   b. _____

   c. _____

   d. _____

4. Write an expected outcome for the nursing diagnosis Fluid volume deficit related to hyperosmolar state. *(874)*

   _____

   _____

5. List three nursing interventions (including assessments) that are appropriate to restore fluid balance. *(873)*

   a. _____

   b. _____

   c. _____

6. List at least two laboratory tests that would be used to evaluate treatment outcomes for a patient in DKA. *(873-874)*

   a. _____

   b. _____

Copyright © 2013, 2009 by Saunders, an imprint of Elsevier Inc. All rights reserved.

7. Which task would be appropriate to assign to the nursing assistant? *(870)*
   a. Assist Jason to don a patient gown.
   b. Take the initial set of vital signs.
   c. Gather emergency equipment.
   d. Inform Jason's mother about wait time.

PRIORITY SETTING

Directions: Read the scenario and prioritize nursing actions.

Scenario: You are working in an extended-care facility. You walk into Mr. Jipnak's room and the nursing assistant tells you that Mr. Jipnak refused his breakfast this morning and went out for a brisk walk. He appears pale, diaphoretic, and is too lethargic to swallow. His blood sugar is 30 mg/dL. You have standing orders to treat hypoglycemia with 1 mg Glucagon IM if the patient is unable to swallow. *(874)*

Directions: Prioritize the nursing actions below to assist Mr. Jipnak during this hypoglycemic episode.

_____ a. Turn the patient on his side.

_____ b. Give a fast-acting source of sugar and a longer-acting source, such as crackers and cheese or a meat sandwich if alert enough to swallow.

_____ c. Administer 1 mg of Glucagon by injection after mixing the solution in the bottle until it is clear.

_____ d. If the patient does not awaken within 15 minutes, give another dose of Glucagon and inform a physician of the situation immediately.

_____ e. Assess ability to swallow after second dose of Glucagon.

_____ f. Assess level of consciousness and ability to swallow.

REVIEW QUESTIONS FOR THE NCLEX® EXAMINATION

Directions: Choose the correct answer(s) for the following questions.

1. The patient is a type 1 diabetic who has been admitted for ketoacidosis and influenza. Which assessment findings are most likely to be documented in this patient's record? *(871)*
   1. Headache, thirst, and anorexia
   2. Weight gain, polyuria, and dizziness
   3. Diaphoresis, headache, and nervousness
   4. Weakness, stomach pain, and sweating

2. A patient is recently diagnosed with latent autoimmune diabetes (LADA). According to evidence-based management, which medication is the physician mostly likely to prescribe in the early phase? *(858)*
   1. Metformin (Glucophage)
   2. Glyburide (DiaBeta)
   3. Glipizide (Glucotrol)
   4. NovoLog insulin

3. What is an important safety intervention for type 1 diabetes patients? *(866, 871)*
   1. Provide an 1800-calorie ADA diet.
   2. Assess for signs of hypoglycemia after insulin is given.
   3. Monitor intake and output carefully.
   4. Do not allow ambulation without assistance.

Copyright © 2013, 2009 by Saunders, an imprint of Elsevier Inc. All rights reserved.

4. Evaluation of correct balance of food, exercise, and insulin for a diabetic patient would be to: *(871)*
   1. assess trends of blood sugar levels.
   2. assess daily weight trends.
   3. determine what the blood pH is now.
   4. determine if electrolytes are in balance.

5. An infection such as influenza can be a cause of diabetic ketoacidosis because: *(858, 874)*
   1. patients continue insulin but do not eat properly.
   2. use of over-the-counter decongestants interferes with insulin.
   3. infection causes an increased metabolic rate and release of extra glucose.
   4. the patient does not rest well or sleep because of cough and discomfort.

6. Which diagnostic test would be ordered to evaluate the response to therapy at a 6-month follow-up appointment? *(858, 871)*
   1. Glucose tolerance test
   2. Fasting blood sugar test
   3. 2-hour postprandial blood sugar test
   4. Hemoglobin A_{1C}

7. The reason a patient with uncontrolled type 2 diabetes tends to gain weight is because: *(860)*
   1. he has a big appetite and experiences polyphagia.
   2. of insulin resistance; the food he eats is not fully metabolized.
   3. the excess glucose in his body makes him retain excess water.
   4. he tends to become very sedentary because of little energy.

8. Whenever a type 1 diabetic patient knows that he is going to exercise heavily, he should: *(861)*
   1. skip his insulin dose both before and after the exercise.
   2. drink a large quantity of water.
   3. eat an extra high-protein snack to prevent hypoglycemia.
   4. take extra insulin to compensate for that used during the exercise.

9. The diabetic patient undergoing surgery experiences considerable stress, which alters his blood sugar levels. For this reason, he is usually given: *(866)*
   1. an extra allotment of calories before surgery.
   2. intravenous insulin during surgery.
   3. twice as much IV fluid as the usual patient receives.
   4. a large dose of long-acting insulin prior to surgery.

10. One problem that occurs fairly often in elderly type 2 diabetes patients is hyperglycemic hyperosmolar nonketotic syndrome (HHNKS). It occurs most often after: *(874)*
    1. abdominal surgery and nasogastric suction.
    2. fractures that cause immobility.
    3. multiple diagnostic tests during which patients have been NPO.
    4. a febrile illness or gastrointestinal flu.

11. For type I diabetes, what is most likely to be included in the treatment plan ? *(857)*
    1. Usually responds to diet and exercise only
    2. Must receive exogenous insulin
    3. Can be managed with oral hypoglycemics
    4. Islet cell transplantation

Copyright © 2013, 2009 by Saunders, an imprint of Elsevier Inc. All rights reserved.

12. Why are diabetics more prone to infection? (*Select all that apply.*) *(859)*
    1. Poor control of diabetes
    2. Increased function of leukocytes and phagocyte function
    3. Decreased blood supply to the tissues related to atherosclerosis of blood vessels
    4. Chronic neurologic and vascular changes allow organisms to enter tissues
    5. Diabetic patients are overweight and have poor hygiene

13. The American Diabetes Association (ADA) recommends screening all adults, especially if overweight, for type 2 diabetes: *(858)*
    1. starting at age 21, to be repeated every 5 years.
    2. starting at age 45, to be repeated every 3 years.
    3. starting at age 50, to be repeated every year.
    4. starting at age 60 to be repeated every 2 years.

14. Which statement by a patient most strongly indicates a need for further assessment and possible diagnostic testing to screen for diabetes? *(859)*
    1. "Typically, I urinate a moderate amount just before I go to bed."
    2. "I seem to be really thirsty, but I guess it could be the heat."
    3. "I like to have a snack after I exercise, but I try to watch my calories."
    4. "I probably have diabetes; most of my friends have it."

15. Which statement by a patient's family member indicates an understanding of the signs and symptoms of hypoglycemia? *(859)*
    1. "He could refuse to eat because he is angry."
    2. "He could be flushed and look dehydrated."
    3. "He could be irritable because his sugar is low."
    4. "He will urinate a lot and be very thirsty."

16. Which viral agent is thought to attack the beta cells of the pancreas causing an onset of insulin-dependent diabetes mellitus (type 1)? *(858)*
    1. Herpes simplex
    2. *Staphylococcus aureus*
    3. Cytomegalovirus
    4. Coxsackievirus

17. The patient is admitted with a diagnosis of HHNKS. The nurse recognizes that because of the extremely high blood glucose levels associated with this disorder, the priority nursing diagnosis is: *(874)*
    1. Imbalanced nutrition, more than body requirements, related to alteration in glucose utilization by cells
    2. Risk for infection related to elevated blood glucose level
    3. Fluid volume deficit related to hyperosmolar state
    4. Nausea related to gastrointestinal distress

18. Which statement by the patient indicates a need for additional teaching on diabetic foot care? *(875)*
    1. "I should check both feet daily for cracks, blisters, or abrasions."
    2. "I should cut the nails straight across and smooth with an emery board."
    3. "I should elevate my feet whenever possible to improve circulation."
    4. "I should soak my feet in hot water every day and use mild soap."

19. The nurse is teaching the patient how to manage his diabetes during times of minor illness, such as during mild gastrointestinal upset. What is appropriate information to tell the patient? *(872)*
    1. Discontinue your insulin if you are vomiting.
    2. Take at least 1 cup of water or calorie-free, caffeine-free liquid each hour.
    3. Test your blood sugar once or twice a day.
    4. If taking an oral hypoglycemic agent, increase the dose for 2–3 days while ill.

Copyright © 2013, 2009 by Saunders, an imprint of Elsevier Inc. All rights reserved.

20. The nurse is interviewing a patient to establish a database. The patient has reported being excessively thirsty, but has never been diagnosed with diabetes. Which questions would be appropriate to ask the patient during this initial interview? *(Select all that apply.)* **(867)**
    1. Have you had any recent weight loss?
    2. Have you become increasingly hungry over the past few months?
    3. Are you having any trouble sticking to your dietary plan?
    4. Do you have to urinate (go to the toilet) more than you used to?
    5. Have you noticed that you are more tired than you were 6 months ago?
    6. Have you made any plans on how to cope with a chronic illness?
    7. Has anyone in your family ever been told he or she has diabetes?

CRITICAL THINKING ACTIVITIES

Scenario: Mrs. Thomas, age 62, has been diagnosed as a type 2 diabetic. She is 50 pounds overweight and leads a very sedentary life. She worked as a secretary until 3 months ago, when she began to feel weak and "tired all the time." Her physician has prescribed diet and exercise and Glucophage for the management of her diabetes. Mrs. Thomas is reluctant about engaging in an exercise program and has many questions about it. How would you answer the following questions? *(859-862)*

1. "What does exercise do for a person with diabetes?" _____

   _____

   _____

   _____

2. "What kind of exercise do I have to do?" _____

   _____

   _____

   _____

3. "Do I have to keep a record of exercise, too?" _____

   _____

   _____

   _____

Copyright © 2013, 2009 by Saunders, an imprint of Elsevier Inc. All rights reserved.

STEPS TOWARD BETTER COMMUNICATION

VOCABULARY BUILDING GLOSSARY

Term	Pronunciation	Definition
sequelae	se kwe' lay	(plural) consequences
brittle	brit' el	easily broken; (referring to diabetes: hard to control, with wide daily variations in glucose level)
postprandial	post' pran' dee al	after a meal
first generation	first' jen er ay' shun	original in a line of creation or descent: families (e.g., *first-generation* American); objects or inventions (e.g., original is *first generation,* further development is *second generation*)
tight control	tyt' kun trol'	control within a narrow range; carefully regulated control
unmask	un mask'	uncover something hidden
basement membrane	bays' ment mem' brayn	a delicate membrane in the secreting glands
susceptible	su sep' ti bul	likely or liable to develop; to be affected by

COMPLETION

Directions: Fill in each blank with the appropriate word from the Vocabulary Building Glossary to complete the statement.

1. The child's glucose level was difficult to keep within normal limits because his diabetes mellitus was very _____.

2. Diabinese is a(n) _____ hypoglycemic agent.

3. The physician was trying to _____ what was causing the patient's symptoms of extreme shakiness and headaches that occurred periodically.

4. Blindness and renal failure are _____ of long-term uncontrolled blood glucose levels.

5. Older adults who are obese seem to be more _____ to diabetes mellitus.

6. When screening for diabetes mellitus, the physician may order a(n) _____ blood sugar level drawn.

7. The best way to avoid complications of diabetes mellitus is to maintain _____ of blood glucose.

Copyright © 2013, 2009 by Saunders, an imprint of Elsevier Inc. All rights reserved.

WORD ATTACK SKILLS

Directions: Sometimes words that you find in daily speech are used in a different way in the hospital or medical setting. Can you give the two meanings for each?

1. Brittle

    a. Medical usage: _____

    b. Everyday usage: _____

2. Basement

    a. Medical usage: _____

    b. Everyday usage: _____

PRONUNCIATION SKILLS

melli'tus (mel eye' tus **or** mel ee' tus) (may vary depending on the part of the country where you live)

Somo'gyi (so mo' gee)

Directions: Practice pronouncing the following terms:

HHNK: hyperosmolar hyperglycemic nonketotic

DKA: diabetic ketoacidosis

CULTURAL POINT

Young people in the United States are very sensitive to the opinions of others, especially their peers, about body image, their attractiveness, friends, and capabilities in school and sports. They do not want to appear different. For example, they like to wear the same style of clothing and hair, and eat the same kinds of food. This can make it very difficult for a young person who is diabetic and must eat differently, perform blood sugar checks often, and self-administer insulin.

You must work with the patient and family to help the patient lead as normal a life as possible. Encouraging sports with guidelines for blood sugar checks, extra snacks, and insulin adjustments promotes safe participation. When the patient wishes to sleep over at a friend's house, appropriate snacks can be sent along and the friend's parents can be made aware of the patient's requirements of blood sugar checks, insulin, and meals. You can teach the patient how to make smart food choices when out with friends at restaurants or fast-food places.

COMMUNICATION EXERCISE

When working with diabetic patients, you must assess for problems relating to compliance with prescribed treatment. Trust between you and the patient must be developed before the patient will be open and honest discussing problems related to the diet, exercise program, blood glucose monitoring, and medication schedule. There are certain ways of approaching these topics that seem to work better than others.

Copyright © 2013, 2009 by Saunders, an imprint of Elsevier Inc. All rights reserved.

The following are questions nurses often ask diabetic patients; there is an example in italics of a better way to obtain the desired explanation, in each case.

"Are you sticking to your meal plan?"

"Tell me about any problems you are having with your meals."

"How much are you exercising now?"

"Are you able to exercise as much as you thought you could?"

"Are you checking your blood sugar before meals?"

"Tell me how your blood sugar checks with the glucometer are going."

"Are you taking your insulin at the times it is scheduled?"

"What kind of problems, if any, are you having in giving yourself the insulin at the designated times?"

"Are you checking your feet for problems each day?"

"Tell me, when have you have managed to work checking your feet into your daily routine?"

"Are you remembering to take your oral medication each day?"

"How are things going with taking your oral medication?"

This rephrasing allows patients, especially teens, to perceive themselves in charge of the situation and avoid what they see as accusatory questions.

Copyright © 2013, 2009 by Saunders, an imprint of Elsevier Inc. All rights reserved.

Care of Women with Reproductive Disorders

Answer Key: Textbook page references are provided as a guide for answering these questions. A complete answer key was provided to your instructor.

COMPLETION

Health Promotion and Self-Examination

Directions: Fill in the blanks to complete the statements.

1. Lifestyle changes to reduce the incontinence symptoms associated with pelvic relaxation syndrome include increased _____ and a(n) _____ diet to avoid constipation, and maintaining optimum _____. *(903)*

2. The amount of blood loss with normal menstruation is _____ to _____ mL. *(883)*

3. Patients at risk for osteoporosis should be advised to stop smoking and to avoid excessive _____, _____, _____, or soft drink intake. *(890, Box 39-3)*

4. _____ measures are designed to decrease the probability of becoming ill. Examples include maintaining a health or nutrition history and providing immunizations. *(892)*

5. The only means to prevent conception 100% is _____. *(884, Table 39-1)*

6. Some medication for emergency contraception can be effective when taken up to _____ days after unprotected sex. *(888)*

7. Breast self-examination should be done monthly, about _____ after menstruation begins, or on a specific date each month after menopause. *(892)*

8. Vulvar self-examination should be performed _____. *(894)*

Medical Examination and Diagnostic Testing

Directions: Fill in the blanks to complete the statements.

1. A test that is performed for postmenopausal bleeding is a(n) _____. *(895, Table 39-2)*

2. Regular scheduled mammograms after age _____ are recommended by the American College of Obstetricians and Gynecologists. *(910)*

Copyright © 2013, 2009 by Saunders, an imprint of Elsevier Inc. All rights reserved.

3. A(n) _____ is to used evaluate abnormal cells and lesions, particularly after a positive Pap smear. *(895, Table 39-2)*

4. A vaginal ultrasound may be done to detect the _____ of the uterine lining, _____ of the uterus, the presence of _____, the size of ovaries and the presence of cysts or tumors. *(896, Table 39-2)*

5. Dilation and evacuation can be performed to find the cause of _____ bleeding; removal of hypertrophied _____ lining, retained placenta, or tissue remaining from incomplete _____. *(895, Table 39-2)*

6. You should inform the patient who is having an endometrial biopsy that severe _____ may occur during the procedure. *(895)*

Menopause

Directions: Read the scenario and answer the questions that follow.

Scenario: Mrs. Stahl, age 52, has begun having menstrual irregularity, alternating between a scanty flow and heavy bleeding, and often missing periods. Her gynecologist assures her that she is entering the climacteric and there are no signs of abnormalities of her uterus. Mrs. Stahl is an engineer and she works mostly with men at her office. She asks you for more information.

1. Menopause is described as cessation of menses for a(n) _____-month period due to decreased estrogen production. *(882, 890)*

2. Because of atrophy of the vaginal walls and dryness, the postmenopausal woman may experience _____. *(890)*

3. One of the biggest complaints as women go through menopause is _____. *(890)*

4. Women may be prescribed vaginal creams containing estrogen to restore _____ and _____ to vaginal tissues. *(890)*

5. In addition to menstrual irregularity, list at least seven other psychologic and physiologic symptoms that sometimes accompany menopause. *(890)*

   a. _____

   b. _____

   c. _____

   d. _____

   e. _____

   f. _____

   g. _____

Copyright © 2013, 2009 by Saunders, an imprint of Elsevier Inc. All rights reserved.

6. The first sign of osteoporosis is loss of height, back pain, and the development of a(n) _____ _____ in which vertebrae fail to support the upper body in an upright position. *(891)*

7. Because of all of the potential side effects of hormone therapy, the recommendation for its use is that the patient be _____, _____, and the lowest effective dose used. *(891)*

8. Postmenopausal women are at increased risk for coronary heart disease due to changes in _____ metabolism and a rise in total _____. *(891)*

9. What are some foods that you could recommend to Mrs. Stahl for nutritional therapy related to menopause? *(892)*

   a. _____

   b. _____

   c. _____

   d. _____

COMPLETION

Disorders of the Reproductive System

Directions: Fill in the blanks to complete the statements.

1. A diet high in _____ helps decrease the symptoms of _____ _____. *(902)*

2. Uterine bleeding may be considered abnormal if the interval between menstruations is less than _____ days or more than _____ days; the duration of menstrual flow is more than _____ days or the amount of blood loss exceeds _____ mL. *(904)*

3. A recommendation to decrease the cramping from menstruation is the use of _____. *(902)*

4. Common symptoms of leiomyoma include backache, a sense of lower _____ pressure, constipation, urinary _____ or _____, and abnormal uterine bleeding. *(905)*

5. Continuous hormonal contraceptive therapy for endometriosis includes drugs such as _____ or _____, which suppress growth of the endometrial tissue. *(906)*

6. Toxic shock syndrome (TSS) is a rare and potentially fatal disorder caused by strains of _____ _____ that produce toxins that cause shock, coagulation defects, and tissue damage if they enter the bloodstream. *(906-907)*

Copyright © 2013, 2009 by Saunders, an imprint of Elsevier Inc. All rights reserved.

7. If removal of a tumor from the uterine wall is needed, a(n) _____ is performed. *(908)*

8. The patient with endometriosis often experiences _____ and excessive _____ with menstruation. *(906)*

SHORT ANSWER

Nursing Assessment of the Reproductive System

Directions: Read the scenario and answer the following questions about nursing assessment of a patient's gynecologic health status.

Scenario: You are working in a gynecology clinic. Jean Simmons is a new patient who comes in for a routine pelvic examination and her annual Pap smear. You are collecting information that will contribute to identifying problems and educational needs.

1. Why is the female patient's age relevant to a nursing assessment? *(897)*

   _____

   _____

   _____

2. Why would you be interested in Jean's sexual activities; for example, at what age she became sexually active and how many partners she has had? *(892)*

   _____

   _____

3. List information that would be included in the patient's menstrual history. *(897)*

   a. _____

   b. _____

   c. _____

   d. _____

   e. _____

4. List some subjective and objective data that would be useful in assessment of a patient with a gynecologic disorder. *(892-894, 897)*

   Subjective data:

   a. _____

   b. _____

   c. _____

   d. _____

   e. _____

Copyright © 2013, 2009 by Saunders, an imprint of Elsevier Inc. All rights reserved.

Objective data:

a. _____

b. _____

c. _____

d. _____

Hysterectomy

Directions: Read the scenario and answer the questions that follow.

Scenario: Ms. Toliver, age 49, has been divorced from her husband for 5 years. She has been told by her gynecologist that she needs to have a hysterectomy, but she does not want to have this surgery. She is currently dating a man she eventually hopes to marry and is afraid the surgery will make her less attractive to him.

1. List three clinical indications for hysterectomy. *(903-907)*

a. _____

b. _____

c. _____

2. List two other factors that should be considered in the decision to have or refuse this type of surgery. *(897)*

a. _____

b. _____

3. Ms. Toliver eventually decided to have the recommended hysterectomy after obtaining a second opinion from another gynecologist. List the kinds of information that should be included in the plan for her discharge after the hysterectomy. *(898-900, 905)*

a. _____

b. _____

c. _____

Cancers of the Reproductive System

Directions: Read the scenario and answer the questions that follow.

Scenario: You have been asked to do a community presentation that includes some basic information about gynecologic cancers. You want to share information about the risk factors and signs and symptoms that women should watch for.

1. The most common malignant tumor of the female reproductive tract is _____ cancer. *(907)*

Copyright © 2013, 2009 by Saunders, an imprint of Elsevier Inc. All rights reserved.

2. List six risk factors for cervical cancer. *(907)*

   a. _____

   b. _____

   c. _____

   d. _____

   e. _____

   f. _____

3. List three risk factors for ovarian cancer. *(908)*

   a. _____

   b. _____

   c. _____

4. What are the signs and symptoms of vulvar intraepithelial neoplasia (VIN)? *(907)* _____

   _____

5. Explain in your own words why ovarian cancer is known as the "silent cancer." *(908)* _____

   _____

   _____

   _____

6. Regular pelvic examinations and Pap smears may enable early diagnosis of _____
   and provide opportunity for early and more successful intervention. *(907)*

7. The _____ vaccine given to girls at or before puberty may prevent the type of HPV infection that causes cervical cancer. *(907)*

PRIORITY SETTING

Directions: Read the scenario and prioritize the steps of assisting with a pelvic exam.

Scenario: Ms. Gian has come in for a pelvic exam and a Pap smear. You are preparing her for examination
and will assist the doctor during the procedure. *(894-895, 897, Table 39-2)*

_____ a. Assemble clean gloves and supplies.

_____ b. Encourage Ms. Gian to void because a full bladder will make the exam more uncomfortable.

_____ c. Stay with Ms. Gian, encourage her, and give information.

_____ d. Orient Ms. Gian to the equipment and the purpose of the exam.

_____ e. Position Ms. Gian appropriately (i.e., lithotomy position).

_____ f. The unit should provide privacy and good lighting.

Copyright © 2013, 2009 by Saunders, an imprint of Elsevier Inc. All rights reserved.

APPLICATION OF THE NURSING PROCESS

Care of the Patient with Breast Cancer

Directions: Read the scenario and provide the answers to the following questions.

Scenario: Mrs. Donner has been diagnosed with breast cancer and is admitted for a lumpectomy. She has had some preoperative teaching prior to being admitted to the hospital. The RN completed the admission assessment and history.

1. In evaluating preoperative teaching with Ms. Donner, which of the following statements by the patient indicates that she understands what is happening during the procedure of lumpectomy? *(910)*
   a. The doctor removes only the tumor.
   b. The doctor removes the entire breast and axillary lymph nodes.
   c. The doctor removes the tumor and a portion of the surrounding breast tissue and axillary lymph nodes.
   d. The doctor removes the breast, axillary lymph nodes, and chest wall muscles under the breast.

2. Ms. Donner's maintenance IV is dextrose 5% with normal saline 1000 mL to infuse over 8 hours. What is the pump setting? _____

3. What is your first concern for Mrs. Donner when she returns from the operating room? *(910-912)*
   a. Risk for depression
   b. Risk for bleeding
   c. Risk for infection
   d. Risk for falls

4. List four specific nursing measures that would be included in the nursing care plan for Ms. Donner immediately after lumpectomy. *(913)*

   a. _____

   b. _____

   c. _____

   d. _____

5. Which of the following tasks would be appropriate to assign to the nursing assistant? *(913)*
   a. Assist Ms. Donner to use the spirometer correctly.
   b. Do bilateral pulse checks on the upper extremities.
   c. Teach Ms. Donner that no blood pressures are taken on affected side.
   d. Assist Ms. Donner to ambulate in the hall.

6. List information that would be helpful to Ms. Donner in planning her discharge after lumpectomy. *(913)*

   a. _____

   b. _____

   c. _____

   d. _____

Copyright © 2013, 2009 by Saunders, an imprint of Elsevier Inc. All rights reserved.

REVIEW QUESTIONS FOR THE NCLEX® EXAMINATION

Directions: Choose the best answer(s) for the following questions.

1. Which statement by a patient indicates a need for additional teaching about the "morning after pill"? *(886-888, Table 39-1)*
   1. "It has to be taken 72 hours after unprotected sex."
   2. "It works by preventing ovulation, implantation, or fertilization."
   3. "It may cause nausea and vomiting, so I should take an antiemetic."
   4. "It can be used to terminate a first trimester pregnancy."

2. An intrauterine medication to treat dysmenorrhea is: *(903, Table 39-4)*
   1. an intrauterine device.
   2. levonorgestel-releasing system.
   3. mefenamic acid.
   4. COX-2 inhibitor.

3. When should a female start having routine pelvic exams and Pap smears? *(894)*
   1. As soon as she becomes sexually active or at age 20
   2. At age 16, if she has family history of cervical cancer
   3. When her family doctor or pediatrician directs her to do so
   4. Whenever she starts her menstrual periods

4. The nurse is assessing a patient for risk factors for breast cancer. The nurse includes questions about: *(Select all that apply.)* *(909, Box 39-5)*
   1. family history of relative with breast cancer.
   2. early menarche, late menopause.
   3. late first pregnancy or no children.
   4. abnormal cells in previous breast biopsy.
   5. history of being less than ideal body weight.

5. When teaching a patient who has premenstrual stress to control her symptoms, the nurse should encourage her to: *(902)*
   1. eat a high-protein diet.
   2. take vitamin C and iron supplements.
   3. avoid salty and high-sodium foods.
   4. sleep 9–10 hours night.

6. Pelvic relaxation syndrome may lead to: *(903)*
   1. abdominal pain.
   2. cervical dysplasia.
   3. metrorrhagia.
   4. a cystocele.

7. The nurse is assessing the sexual health of an elderly woman. Which is the most likely physical symptom that an elderly woman would report? *(890)*
   1. Does not feel attractive any more.
   2. Is always too tired for sex.
   3. Has no sexual desire.
   4. Has decreased vaginal lubrication.

8. The patient is pregnant. Which would the nurse expect to find documented in this patient's chart? *(904)*
   1. Metrorrhagia
   2. Amenorrhea
   3. Oligomenorrhea
   4. Menorrhagia

Copyright © 2013, 2009 by Saunders, an imprint of Elsevier Inc. All rights reserved.

9. In an elderly woman, vaginal bleeding is a possible sign of: *(905)*
   1. hormone imbalance.
   2. cervical or uterine cancer.
   3. breast cancer.
   4. vaginal-rectal fistula.

10. Measures that may decrease the discomfort of dysmenorrhea include: *(Select all that apply.) (902-903)*
    1. doing aerobic exercises when the discomfort first starts.
    2. avoiding foods such as asparagus and watermelon.
    3. using a heating pad and doing pelvic rock exercises.
    4. avoiding use of tampons and douching.

11. Motrin, Anaprox, and Advil are examples of drugs used for dysmenorrhea because they inhibit: *(902)*
    1. the transmission of pain along nerve pathways.
    2. salt and water retention.
    3. smooth muscle spasm in the uterus.
    4. production of prostaglandins.

12. Two measures that have been found to decrease the discomfort of fibrocystic breast changes are: *(908)*
    1. taking vitamin C and getting sufficient exercise.
    2. decreasing fat and protein in the diet.
    3. controlled weight loss and wearing a support bra.
    4. taking vitamin E and decreasing caffeine intake.

CRITICAL THINKING ACTIVITIES

Scenario: You are talking to several neighbors about sexual activity and the use of birth control among teenagers and young adults. There are various opinions among the parents and you can tell that it is a very controversial topic. Several of the parents want to know your opinion about the how to deal with their sexually active teens and what they should tell them about birth control.

1. What factors are involved in selecting a method of contraception? *(883)* _____

   _____

   _____

2. What are the advantages and disadvantages of using a condom? *(885, Table 39-1)* _____

   _____

3. What other types of contraception should be taught? *(883-888)* _____

   _____

   _____

4. What is the female condom? Why is it generally not widely used? *(884, Table 39-1)* _____

   _____

   _____

   _____

   _____

Copyright © 2013, 2009 by Saunders, an imprint of Elsevier Inc. All rights reserved.

STEPS TOWARD BETTER COMMUNICATION

VOCABULARY BUILDING GLOSSARY

Term	Pronunciation	Definition
slough, slough off	sluf	(verb) separating and dropping off of dead tissue; to shed
period	pir' ee ud	a woman's monthly menstrual flow
"the change of life"		psychologic response to menopause

COMPLETION

Directions: Fill in the blank with the correct word from the Vocabulary Building Glossary to complete the sentence.

1. During menstruation, the uterine lining will _____.

2. When calculating the due date for pregnancy, the doctor asks the date of the woman's last _____ _____.

3. With family support and an optimistic outlook for the future, a woman can view _____ as a new transitional period.

PRONUNCIATION SKILLS

This exercise gives you practice in speaking and listening for pronunciation of final consonants.

Directions: With a partner, take turns saying the words below. The speaker chooses and pronounces one word in each line, marking the word pronounced. The listener numbers a sheet of paper from 1 to 11 and writes the words heard (or circles the words in the book). Check for listening accuracy. Switch roles and do the exercise again. Take special care to pronounce the end of each word fully and clearly.

1. birth   burn   bird
2. risk   wrist
3. weight   weighed   wake   wait
4. pain   pale   pay   paid
5. take   tape
6. cost   cot
7. age   aids
8. sigh   sign   sight   side
9. team   teen   teeth   teach
10. you   use   used   youth
11. not   nod

Copyright © 2013, 2009 by Saunders, an imprint of Elsevier Inc. All rights reserved.

WORD ATTACK SKILLS

Directions: Using the word elements listed below, give the meaning of each word.

a-   lack, none, not, without

dys-   bad, difficult, wrongly

men/o-   month

meta/o-   after, beyond, above

-rrhea   flow, discharge

-rrage   excessive bleeding

-rrhagia   hemorrhage

1. Menorrhea:_____

2. Amenorrhea: _____

3. Dysmenorrhea: _____

4. Metrorrhagia:_____

5. Menorrhagia: _____

ABBREVIATIONS

Directions: Write in the meaning for each abbreviation.

1. ART: _____

2. BSE: _____

3. VSE:_____

4. PCOS: _____

5. IUD:_____

6. D&E: _____

7. PMS: _____

8. BBT: _____

9. ORWH: _____

10. HRT: _____

Copyright © 2013, 2009 by Saunders, an imprint of Elsevier Inc. All rights reserved.

CULTURAL POINTS

Confidentiality

Confidentiality is a nursing responsibility in all patient situations. When discussing matters of very personal nature such as reproductive problems, it is particularly important to offer the patient reassurance that any information given will remain private. Such information must not be discussed even with other nurses, unless these others are directly involved in the patient's care.

Culture and Tradition

Culture and tradition influence attitudes and values toward sex and sexuality. Some cultures are very open about sexual matters, while others are very close-mouthed and such issues are not discussed with others. Many cultures have attitudes that lie somewhere in between openness and extreme privacy. In any culture, there are accepted and unacceptable modes of behavior, and there are people who follow the traditions and people who do not.

Think about the traditions you grew up with and what you learned about how to feel toward sexual behavior. How is your attitude toward sexuality different from the traditions you see around you today? How do you feel about these differences? How will such a difference affect your behavior as a nurse? Can you be nonjudgmental about sexuality?

Copyright © 2013, 2009 by Saunders, an imprint of Elsevier Inc. All rights reserved.

Care of Men with Reproductive Disorders

Answer Key: Textbook page references are provided as a guide for answering these questions. A complete answer key was provided to your instructor.

COMPLETION

Directions: Fill in the blanks to complete the statements.

1. With aging, the decrease in _____ may affect erectile function. *(920)*

2. Erectile dysfunction has both _____ and organic causes. *(923)*

3. Whenever examining the genital area, _____ and providing _____ are essential to prevent embarrassment. *(921-923)*

4. The reliability of condoms is reduced if _____ is also used. *(920)*

5. Follow-up care for vasectomy includes a second sperm count that should be done _____ later to verify that the vas deferens is not intact. *(920-921)*

6. Inflammatory epididymitis is most likely to result after an infection of _____, _____. *(932)*

7. Hydrocele causes enlargement of the _____ and is usually _____ _____. *(925)*

8. When a patient has BPH, the appropriate nursing diagnosis is _____. *(927)*

9. The patient with epididymitis complains of _____ pain plus _____ and pain in the scrotum. *(932)*

10. Testicular torsion is commonly caused by _____ levels in young adult males but can also be the result of _____ trauma. *(926)*

11. _____ is a condition which results in the inability to have a uniform erection of the penis. *(927)*

12. Men who have had an undescended or partially descended testicle are most at risk for _____ cancer. *(933)*

13. A man is more likely to experience erectile dysfunction if he has been _____ _____ for some time. *(924)*

Copyright © 2013, 2009 by Saunders, an imprint of Elsevier Inc. All rights reserved.

14. _____ is the gold standard of treatment for benign prostatic hypertrophy (BPH) and is performed under spinal anesthesia. *(929, Table 40-3)*

15. An enlarged prostate may eventually cause _____. *(927)*

16. BPH produces no symptoms until the growth becomes large enough to press against the _____. *(927)*

17. Because hemorrhage always is a danger after prostate surgery, vital signs are taken every _____ hours initially, then every _____ hours. *(928)*

18. After prostate surgery, a high-fiber diet and stool softeners may be prescribed to prevent straining, which increases _____ pressure and can cause further bleeding. *(928)*

19. If a postprostatectomy patient reports severe pain in the bladder region, you should check for an obstruction in the _____ or the _____ before administering an analgesic. *(929)*

20. Bilateral orchitis is serious and very often causes _____. *(932)*

21. _____ usually is given to lessen the severity of mumps orchitis. *(932)*

22. Cancer of the penis is rare, occurring mostly in males with _____ infections or males who were not _____. *(933)*

23. Dilation and clumping of the tributary vessels of the spermatic vein creates a(n) _____. *(926)*

24. All males between the ages of _____ should practice testicular self-examination regularly on a monthly basis. *(933)*

25. Men over the age of _____ should have an annual digital rectal exam and prostate-specific antigen (PSA) test to help reduce the death rate from _____. *(934)*

26. For postoperative self-care, the physician instructs the patient to drink 12–14 glasses (8 ounces/glass) of water each day. Convert the range of intake/day into mL. _____

APPLICATION OF THE NURSING PROCESS

Care of the Patient with Epididymitis

Directions: Read the scenario and provide the answers to the following questions.

Scenario: You are working at the university student health center. Roy Jefferson comes in and tells you he would like to see a physician because he thinks he might have an infection. He is reluctant to disclose information to any female nurses or physicians and would "rather talk to a guy."

Copyright © 2013, 2009 by Saunders, an imprint of Elsevier Inc. All rights reserved.

1. Identify four strategies that you can use to help patients of the opposite gender to feel more comfortable in talking about sexual health. *(921, 923)*

    a. _____

    b. _____

    c. _____

    d. _____

2. List subjective and objective data that should be included in the nursing assessment of a patient with a disorder of the male reproductive system. *(921-923)*

    Subjective data:

    a. _____

    b. _____

    c. _____

    Objective data:

    a. _____

    b. _____

    c. _____

    d. _____

3. The physician tells Mr. Jefferson that he has epididymitis. What is the treatment for this disorder? *(932)*

    a. _____

    b. _____

    c. _____

    d. _____

    e. _____

4. Which of the following nursing diagnoses would be the priority to help Mr. Jefferson to prevent future problems with reproductive organs and maintain good sexual health? *(932)*
    a. Knowledge deficit related to self-care and safe sex practices
    b. Risk for sexual dysfunction related to impotence
    c. Anxiety related to health care interview
    d. Risk for infection related to poor hygiene

5. Which statement by Mr. Jefferson indicates a need for additional patient teaching about the treatment and prevention of epididymitis? *(932)*
    a. "My sexual partners should be treated for HPV infection."
    b. "My other testicle could become infected."
    c. "Treatment includes antibiotics and analgesics."
    d. "The scrotum is elevated and I can use an ice pack."

Copyright © 2013, 2009 by Saunders, an imprint of Elsevier Inc. All rights reserved.

SHORT ANSWER

Care of the Patient with Benign Prostatic Hypertrophy

Directions: Read the clinical scenario and answer the questions that follow.

Scenario: Mr. O'Grady is an older man who has always enjoyed good health. He reports some dribbling after urination and also nocturia that has slowly but progressively become more annoying. The physician informs him that he has BPH. *(927-928)*

1. Signs and symptoms of BPH include:

   a. _____

   b. _____

   c. _____

   d. _____

   e. _____

2. What are the drug therapies that are used to treat BPH?

   a. _____

   b. _____

3. What are some dietary modifications that you could review with Mr. O'Grady?

   a. _____

   b. _____

CRITICAL THINKING ACTIVITIES

Promoting Men's Reproductive and Sexual Health

Directions: Read the clinical scenario and answer the questions that follow.

Scenario: You are participating in a men's health fair. You have been asked to collect information about various topics regarding men's sexual health and disorders of the reproductive system.

1. What are three ways in which disorders of the male reproductive organs might be prevented? *(935-936)*

   a. _____

   b. _____

   c. _____

2. Describe when, how, and why a testicular self-examination should be done. *(933, 935)*

   a. When:_____

   b. How: _____

   c. Why:_____

Copyright © 2013, 2009 by Saunders, an imprint of Elsevier Inc. All rights reserved.

3. Name four ways that you can be instrumental in the community in promoting male reproductive and sexual health. *(935-936)*

a. _____

b. _____

c. _____

d. _____

PRIORITY SETTING

Directions: Read the scenario and prioritize appropriately.

Scenario: You are working in an emergency department. It is a busy night. Several of the following patients are very uncomfortable and all are anxious to receive care and attention.

1. Which of the following male patients has the condition with the highest priority for attention? *(926)*
   a. The patient with a testicular torsion
   b. The patient with urinary retention secondary to BPH
   c. The patient with orchitis
   d. The patient with Klinefelter's syndrome

REVIEW QUESTIONS FOR THE NCLEX® EXAMINATION

Directions: Choose the best answer(s) for the following questions.

1. When discussing prostate cancer with a patient who has a strong family history of the disorder and BPH, the nurse tells him that _____ is a medication used to help prevent prostate cancer. *(928)*
   1. Finasteride
   2. Doxazosin
   3. Terazosin
   4. Tamsulosin

2. When assessing a patient's history, the nurse looks for risk factors for testicular cancer. She therefore questions him about a: *(933)*
   1. history of an undescended testicle.
   2. family history of cancer.
   3. history of urinary tract infections.
   4. history of exposure to toxic inhalants at work.

3. The patient tells the nurse that he has decided to have a vasectomy. He asks if could have children after a few years. The nurse reinforces to the patient that this sometimes can be successfully _____. *(920-921)*

4. A patient asks the nurse for information about prostate cancer and how it develops. The nurse answers: *(934)*
   1. "It is a quick-growing cancer and the nodule is small."
   2. "Prostate cancer is a very slow-growing cancer."
   3. "It is a cancer that is related to sexually transmitted viruses."
   4. "This type of cancer is embryonic and continues to grow slowly after birth."

Copyright © 2013, 2009 by Saunders, an imprint of Elsevier Inc. All rights reserved.

5. After a transurethral resection of the prostate (TURP), a priority nursing diagnosis in the immediate postoperative period is: *(928-929)*
   1. Activity intolerance related to required bedrest.
   2. Pain related to bladder spasms.
   3. Risk for bleeding related to surgery.
   4. Anxiety related to sexual function after surgery.

6. Which diagnostic test would most likely be performed on an elderly patient who has a PSA result of 7.2? *(934)*
   1. Another blood sample for PSA
   2. CT scan of the pelvis
   3. Voiding urethrogram
   4. Prostate needle biopsy

7. A patient returns to the physician. He states that for the past month he has been restricting fluids in the late afternoon and evening, but this has not helped to control nocturia. The physician is likely to prescribe a(n): *(927)*
   1. beta-blocker.
   2. diuretic.
   3. adrenergic blocker.
   4. anti-estrogen agent.

8. Terazosin (Hytrin) is prescribed, and the nurse explains to the patient that it: *(927)*
   1. lowers testosterone levels.
   2. lowers PSA levels.
   3. decreases the prostate size by 50%.
   4. promotes relaxation of smooth muscle.

9. The nurse teaches a patient that a potential side effect of terazosin (Hytrin) is postural hypotension and that he should: *(927)*
   1. take his blood pressure each day.
   2. change positions slowly to prevent dizziness.
   3. call the office if he starts having headaches.
   4. rest for half an hour each afternoon.

10. Which instruction(s) would be appropriate to teach a patient regarding self-care following a TURP? *(Select all that apply.) (928-931, 935)*
    1. Drink 3–4 glasses of water during the day.
    2. Avoid bladder stimulants such as alcohol and spicy foods.
    3. Avoid strenuous exercise for 2–3 weeks after surgery.
    4. Keep follow-up appointments.
    5. Catheterize self as needed to prevent urinary retention.

11. The elderly patient is unable to pass urine. He is diagnosed with BPH and the physician has ordered the insertion of a Foley catheter. Which task would be appropriate to assign to the nursing assistant? *(927-930)*
    1. Insert the Foley catheter using surgical technique.
    2. Clean the Foley catheter and provide perineal care.
    3. Observe the meatus for skin breakdown during hygienic care.
    4. Evaluate the patient's response to the Foley insertion.

Copyright © 2013, 2009 by Saunders, an imprint of Elsevier Inc. All rights reserved.

CRITICAL THINKING ACTIVITIES

Scenario: Your neighbor confides that she and her husband have been trying to have a baby for several years without success. They suspect that he may have some infertility problems, because she had a successful and uneventful pregnancy when she was a teenager and ultimately the baby was adopted. Your neighbor tells you that they are having trouble talking about it, because "Jason doesn't think he is infertile and he is having some trouble with the idea that I was pregnant before. What can I do to get Jason to get checked out? Is there anything that you know that we should or should not be doing?" *(924-925)*

1. Would you feel comfortable giving advice to this neighbor? If so, what would you say? _____

   _____

   _____

   _____

   _____

   _____

2. How is male fertility assessed? *(924)*

   a. _____

   b. _____

   c. _____

   d. _____

   e. _____

3. What are some of the environmental factors that can affect fertility in males? What are some teaching points that address these factors? *(925)*

   a. _____

   _____

   b. _____

   _____

   c. _____

   _____

Copyright © 2013, 2009 by Saunders, an imprint of Elsevier Inc. All rights reserved.

STEPS TOWARD BETTER COMMUNICATION

VOCABULARY BUILDING GLOSSARY

Term	Pronunciation	Definition
cessation	ses sa' shun	stopping, ceasing
open-ended questions		questions that cannot be answered by "yes," "no," or by a short answer; open-ended questions begin with "Why?" or "How?" or "What can you tell me about..." and open-ended questions do not expect a specific response
gonads	go' nads	sex glands; the testes and ovaries

COMPLETION

Directions: Fill in the blanks with the appropriate words from the Vocabulary Building Glossary to complete the statements.

1. Suppressing secretion of testosterone by the _____ is a method of treating prostate cancer.

2. After a TURP, if a clot occludes the urinary catheter, there is a(n) _____ of urine drainage.

3. Using _____ when assessing for sexual dysfunction often elicits the most information.

ABBREVIATIONS

Directions: Write the meaning of each abbreviation. Pronounce each abbreviation.

1. BPH: _____

2. PSA: _____

3. TSE: _____

4. TURP: _____

WORD ATTACK SKILLS

-cele   tumor; hernia

Copyright © 2013, 2009 by Saunders, an imprint of Elsevier Inc. All rights reserved.

GRAMMAR POINTS

When taking medical histories and performing assessments, use the following phrases to obtain time-specific information from the patient.

Occurring now	Occurred in the past	Continues to occur
Do you feel	Have you felt	Have you been feeling
Do you have	Have you had	Have you been having
Have you noticed	Have you ever had	What have you been noticing
What do you take	What did you take	Have you been taking
Do you use	Did you use	Have you been using
Are you using	Have you used	
Would you describe	Is there a history	
Do you perform	Did you perform	Have you been performing
How much do you drink/eat/sleep		

PRONUNCIATION SKILLS

Directions: Practice saying these words aloud, giving special attention and emphasis to the syllables with accent marks (') and extra emphasis to the syllables in **boldface***.*

epididymitis (ep′ i did′ i **my′** tis)

cryptorchidism (krip **tor′** ki dizm)

suprapubic prostatectomy (su′ prah **pew′** bic pro′ sta **tek′** tow mee)

transure′thral resection of the prostate (trans you **ree′** thral ree sek′ shun of the pro stayt′) (TURP)

COMMUNICATION EXERCISE

Practice Assessment

With a male partner, practice performing an assessment by asking the questions in the Focused Assessment box on p. 921 of the textbook. The partner should listen for clear pronunciation of the questions and should answer clearly. He may ask for an explanation of a question or procedure.

Popular Slang Terminology

There are other terms your patients may use to name sex organs and functions. Proper medical terms are given below in **boldface**. Nonmedical but polite terms are in parentheses ( ). The others are not medical terms and are not polite, but they are words you should understand when you hear them.

genitals, (private parts), privates, down below

penis, dick, cock, dong, shlong, prick

testes, (testicles), gonads, scrotum, balls, nuts

sexual intercourse, (have sex, make love), do it, fuck, screw, make it, bonk, bang

ejaculate, come, have it off, jack, jack-off

Copyright © 2013, 2009 by Saunders, an imprint of Elsevier Inc. All rights reserved.

Care of Patients with Sexually Transmitted Infections

Answer Key: Textbook page references are provided as a guide for answering these questions. A complete answer key was provided to your instructor.

COMPLETION

Directions: Fill in the blanks to complete the statements.

1. _____ have an increased risk of sexually transmitted infection (STI) spread by intimate physical contact. *(939)*

2. The largest population groups affected by STIs are _____ and _____ _____. *(938)*

3. _____ and _____ associated with STIs increases the risk of developing human immunodeficiency virus (HIV) infection that can result in AIDS. *(938)*

4. There is an increase in STIs among single women over 60. Often they mistakenly assume that because they cannot get pregnant, they do not need to use _____ when having intercourse. *(938)*

5. In men, _____ associated with sexual activity may be the first sign of STI. *(939-940)*

6. The Centers for Disease Control (CDC) Advisory Committee on Immunization Practices has recommended routine human papillomavirus (HPV) vaccinations for all _____-year-old females. *(940)*

7. Symptoms of PID include _____, _____, and _____ _____ . *(939)*

8. Chlamydia is a danger to women because it can cause _____. *(939)*

9. STIs are primarily passed through intimate contact with _____. *(938)*

10. The _____ virus can cause _____ in the female. *(940, 942, Table 41-1)*

11. Discharge from the skin lesions of a patient with syphilis is contagious in the primary stage until _____. *(947, Table 41-1)*

12. A mother with hepatitis B (HBV) transmits the disease to her fetus via the blood traveling through the _____. *(940, 945)*

13. STIs are to be reported to the _____. *(940-941)*

14. The female patient should be advised not to _____ before a vaginal examination. *(941)*

Copyright © 2013, 2009 by Saunders, an imprint of Elsevier Inc. All rights reserved.

SHORT ANSWER

Care of the Patient with Syphilis

Directions: Read the clinical scenario and answer the questions that follow.

Scenario: You are working in a downtown STI clinic. Mr. Delmonico, a young man, tells you that he had sexual relations several weeks ago and suspects that he may have contracted an STI. The doctor orders a Venereal Disease Research Laboratory (VDRL).

1. List at least four questions that you would ask Mr. Delmonico to collect data regarding his risk for STI. *(941, 948)*

   a. _____

   _____

   b. _____

   _____

   c. _____

   _____

   d. _____

   _____

2. What are the symptoms of primary syphilis? *(947, Table 41-1)*_____

   _____

   _____

   _____

3. What is the treatment for syphilis? *(947, Table 41-1)*_____

   _____

   _____

4. The doctor orders a STAT dose of benzathine penicillin 1.8 g (2.4 million units) IM. The pharmacy delivers benzathine penicillin 600,000 units/mL. How many mL should you give? _____ mL

5. What follow-up information related specifically to syphilis would be appropriate for Mr. Delmonico? *(947, Table 41-1)*

   a. _____

   b. _____

   c. _____

   d. _____

Copyright © 2013, 2009 by Saunders, an imprint of Elsevier Inc. All rights reserved.

PRIORITY SETTING

Directions: Read the scenario and prioritize as appropriate.

Scenario: You are caring for several patients with STIs. Prioritize the order in which you will attend to the needs of these patients. *(938-950)*

_____ a. Jill Jones needs information about STIs for a school project.

_____ b. Leandra Rodriguez needs her first dose of IV antibiotics for acute pelvic inflammatory disease (PID).

_____ c. Joe Kowolski needs reinforcement of follow-up procedure for syphilis.

_____ d. Bill Sakai needs an IM dose of ceftriaxone for gonorrhea.

_____ e. Loki Hantu needs encouragement to identify multiple sexual partners.

APPLICATION OF THE NURSING PROCESS

Care of the Patient with Pelvic Inflammatory Disease

Directions: Read the scenario and provide the answers to the following questions.

Scenario: Ms. Tesoro is admitted for acute PID. She is a young woman and she appears to be very ill and suffering with pain. She tells you that she has been treated for an STI in the recent past.

1. What are two possible causes of PID? *(939)*

   a. _____

   b. _____

2. Which of the following signs and symptoms would you expect to find in the documentation of a patient with acute PID? *(939)*
   a. Severe abdominal and pelvic pain and fever
   b. Clear, copious, mucus-like vaginal discharge
   c. Multiple open lesions on the labia and vulva
   d. Back pain and heavy menstrual periods

3. Review the procedure for assessing the abdomen and abdominal pain. *(see Chapter 28)* _____

   _____

   _____

   _____

   _____

   _____

4. Write a sample outcome for the nursing diagnosis Abdominal pain related to inflammation. *(see Chapter 28)*

   _____

   _____

Copyright © 2013, 2009 by Saunders, an imprint of Elsevier Inc. All rights reserved.

Ms. Tesoro feels much better after 2 days of IV antibiotics. She tells you that she has had STIs several times, "but I always bounce back from it after the antibiotics."

5. List four or five education points that you could review with Ms. Tesoro. *(948, 950)*

   a. _____

   b. _____

   c. _____

   d. _____

   e. _____

6. Write a sample evaluation statement for the following nursing diagnosis and patient goal: Knowledge deficit of self-care to prevent recurrence or other STI; Patient will verbalize three ways to prevent recurrence of STIs after patient teaching sessions. *(950)*

   _____

   _____

   _____

REVIEW QUESTIONS FOR THE NCLEX® EXAMINATION

Directions: Choose the best answer(s) for the following questions.

1. When teaching a patient who is being treated for *Chlamydia trachomatis,* the nurse should stress that: *(939, 942, 950, Table 41-1)*
   1. medication must be taken every day for a month.
   2. partner(s) must be treated concurrently.
   3. swimming and hot-tubbing are contraindicated while under treatment.
   4. lesions must be kept clean and dry to prevent secondary infections.

2. Doxycycline is prescribed for the patient with a chlamydia infection. The order would most likely say to administer the medication _____ for _____ days. *(942, Table 41-1)*

3. When the nurse teaches about "safer sex" practices, it should be stated that proper use of condoms includes using: *(950)*
   1. petroleum jelly as a lubricant.
   2. saliva as a lubricant.
   3. a spermicide containing nonoxynol-9.
   4. lambskin condoms.

4. A patient has come to the clinic after having been notified of exposure to gonorrhea. He states that his exposure occurred 11 days ago. If he is infected, signs and symptoms that would be expected are: *(944, Table 41-1)*
   1. headache, rash, stiff neck, irritability, and joint pain and stiffness.
   2. urinary frequency and burning with purulent discharge from the urethra.
   3. nausea, diarrhea, fever, and urinary frequency and urgency.
   4. burning sensation of the penis and swollen lymph nodes in the groin.

Copyright © 2013, 2009 by Saunders, an imprint of Elsevier Inc. All rights reserved.

5. When teaching about the HPV vaccine (Gardasil), include which fact? *(940)*
   1. Only one dose is required.
   2. Should not be given to girls under 14 years old.
   3. Is effective in preventing genital warts.
   4. Is effective in preventing STIs.

6. Chlamydia is tested for in the female by: *(942, Table 41-1)*
   1. low vaginal swab for culture and identification.
   2. blood test for VDRL.
   3. Pap smear.
   4. Vaginal swab for gram stain.

7. Which nursing responsibilities are related to collecting specimens for diagnosis of STIs? *(Select all that apply.) (941)*
   1. If antimicrobials have been started, note this on the lab slip.
   2. Provide appropriate draping and privacy.
   3. Female patients should douche before vaginal cultures or smears.
   4. Document medication history.
   5. Cultures and smears usually are obtained with a clean swab.
   6. Label specimens and deliver to the lab with the corresponding lab slips.

8. The patient is reluctant to talk about his sexual history. Which statement by the nurse would be the most appropriate to complete the task of obtaining a sexual history, while considering the psychological comfort of the patient? *(941, 948)*
   1. "This will only take a few minutes to complete these questions."
   2. "Let's take a short break; then we can continue."
   3. "Don't be embarrassed. I ask everybody these same questions."
   4. "Let's start with your kidneys. Are you having trouble with urination?"

9. A new nursing assistant expresses fear in caring for patients with HIV/AIDS. Later, the nurse observes this assistant helping a hepatitis B patient who is menstruating with toileting. She is not wearing gloves. Which statement(s) would help the nursing assistant to understand infection control precautions in caring for patients with STIs? *(939-940)*
   1. "Use Standard Precautions for all patients, especially when body fluids are involved."
   2. "Good hand hygiene is adequate when caring for patients with STIs."
   3. "Hepatitis patients and HIV/AIDS patients deserve equal care and attention."
   4. "Hepatitis virus is actually more virulent than HIV/AIDS, so you should be more afraid of hepatitis patients."

10. Which statement(s) made by a patient indicates an understanding of the information and teaching about genital herpes? *(943, Table 41-1)*
    1. "It is highly contagious, but it is only transmitted by sexual contact."
    2. "I am cured once vesicles in the genital area crust over and resolve."
    3. "Numbness and tingling may occur 24 hours before lesions appear."
    4. "If lesions are present, it is best to use a condom and spermicide."

Copyright © 2013, 2009 by Saunders, an imprint of Elsevier Inc. All rights reserved.

CRITICAL THINKING ACTIVITIES

Scenario: You are talking to a group of young female commercial sex workers at a local community health drop-in center. Most of them report using condoms and they claim awareness of the potential for STIs; however, you decide to take advantage of this teachable moment to reinforce STI information.

1. Explain in your own words why having a treatable STI such as gonorrhea still puts one at higher risk for an untreatable STI such as HIV/AIDS. *(944, Table 41-1)*

    _____

    _____

2. Explain in your own words why young women are at an increased risk for STIs. *(939)* _____

    _____

    _____

    _____

    _____

    _____

    _____

3. Explain in your own words the advantage of a single-dose antibiotic treatment for a group such as the commercial sex workers. *(Table 41-1)*

    _____

    _____

    _____

    _____

Copyright © 2013, 2009 by Saunders, an imprint of Elsevier Inc. All rights reserved.

STEPS TOWARD BETTER COMMUNICATION

VOCABULARY BUILDING GLOSSARY

Term	Pronunciation	Definition
genital	jen'ah tal	pertaining to the reproductive organs
monogamous	mon og' ah mus	a relationship with only one other person
heterosexual	het' ah ro sek' shoo al	prefers sexual relationships with the opposite sex
homosexual	ho' mo sek' shoo al	prefers sexual relationships with the same sex
draping	dray'ping	covering with a sheet or towel to provide privacy and prevent embarrassment
reluctant	re luk' tant	hesitant; not wanting to do something
assurance	ah shur' ans	self-confidence; certainty
nonjudgmental attitude	non judj men'tal at'ti tood	indicating by words, facial expressions, and body language that you have no opinion, good or bad, about what a person has done or what is happening

COMPLETION

Directions: Fill in the blanks with the appropriate words from the Vocabulary Building Glossary to complete the statements.

1.   One way to practice "safer sex" is to be _____.

2.   A person diagnosed with an STI is often _____ to tell his or her partner.

3.   A male-female sexual relationship is called a(n) _____ relationship.

4.   _____ relationships in our society often meet with community condemnation in this country.

5.   It takes practice to perform an assessment for sexually transmitted infection with _____ _____.

6.   You should provide appropriate _____ for all examinations and procedures that involve the genital area.

7.   You must present a(n) _____ when caring for a patient with an STI.

Copyright © 2013, 2009 by Saunders, an imprint of Elsevier Inc. All rights reserved.

ABBREVIATIONS

Directions: Write out the meaning for the following abbreviations.

1. OC: _____

2. STI: _____

3. HBIG: _____

4. HPV: _____

5. PID: _____

6. HBV: _____

COMMUNICATION EXERCISE

Obtaining a history of sexual activity requires tact, sensitivity, and an objective attitude to make the history-taking easier for you and the patient. Here are some phrases you could use.

"I know this is a sensitive area, but we need to have this information to help you."

"This information is necessary to protect your baby." *(For a pregnant woman or expectant father)*

"Are you willing to give me the names of your former sex partners so they can get the health care they need?"

"I am legally required to ask you about your sex partners, for their protection."

Here is some body language you could use.

Introduce yourself and shake hands when you meet.

Smile, but be businesslike rather than overly friendly.

Sit in an alert but relaxed position. Try to seem at ease yourself. Keep a neutral facial expression.

Do not be apologetic; this is necessary business.

Look the person in the eye when you are talking, but not constantly. You may look at your history form some of the time when listening.

Careful, quiet, nonjudgmental listening is helpful.

Maintain an appropriate distance. Getting too close may make the patient uncomfortable; too much distance indicates distaste, formality, or coldness.

A touch on the shoulder or arm at an appropriate time may be reassuring.

Allow sufficient time for the interview, so you are not rushed.

Be attentive and quiet; do not fidget.

Offering a tissue to a person who becomes tearful is considerate and shows awareness of the person's feelings.

Use illustrations and models for teaching purposes to help maintain objectivity.

Respect confidentiality and privacy.

Ensure privacy for dressing and undressing; drape the patient for exams.

Knock—and pause—before entering the room.

Interview in a space where others cannot hear.

Copyright © 2013, 2009 by Saunders, an imprint of Elsevier Inc. All rights reserved.

The Integumentary System

Answer Key: Textbook page references are provided as a guide for answering these questions. A complete answer key was provided to your instructor.

REVIEW OF ANATOMY AND PHYSIOLOGY

Terminology

Directions: Match the term on the left with the correct definition, function, or statement on the right. **(952-953)**

1. _____	Dermis	a.	Act to excrete water and salt
2. _____	Epidermis	b.	Produce new cells to heal skin
3. _____	Subcutaneous tissue	c.	Skin becomes thinner and more transparent
4. _____	Stratum corneum	d.	Corium
5. _____	Melanocytes	e.	Contain keratin
6. _____	Fibroblasts	f.	Provides a barrier to bacteria
7. _____	Glands	g.	Consists of squamous epithelium
8. _____	Nails	h.	Contribute color to skin
9. _____	Skin	i.	Attaches skin to underlying structures
10. _____	Ultraviolet light	j.	Transmit feelings of heat, cold, pain, touch, and pressure
11. _____	Melanin	k.	Absorbs light and protects tissue from ultraviolet light
12. _____	Nerve receptors	l.	Cells die and slough off
13. _____	Hair follicles	m.	Sebaceous, sweat, or ceruminous
14. _____	Sweat glands	n.	Skin molecules convert it to vitamin D
15. _____	Change that occurs	o.	Produce hair with aging

COMPLETION

Age-Related Changes in the Skin

Directions: Fill in the blank with the correct word or phrase.

1. Wrinkling and sagging of skin as we age occurs because the _____

   decreases and _____ tissue diminishes. **(953)**

2. The elderly person's skin is more _____ and slower to heal because there is a loss of

   _____. **(953, 955)**

Copyright © 2013, 2009 by Saunders, an imprint of Elsevier Inc. All rights reserved.

3. Skin of the elderly becomes drier and may itch due to reduced _____
   _____. *(953)*

4. Because of changes in the skin with aging, the elderly are more susceptible to _____ and
   _____. *(954)*

5. Hair thins as we age because the hair growth rate declines and the number of _____
   decreases. *(954)*

6. Nail characteristics change as we age and this makes the nails more susceptible to _____
   _____. *(954)*

7. Melanocyte production changes make the elderly more susceptible to _____ and
   causes the appearance of _____. *(954)*

8. Seborrheic keratoses in the elderly appear as _____
   _____ on the trunk, arms, and face. *(958)*

SHORT ANSWER

Causes and Prevention of Skin Problems

Directions: Write brief statements to answer the questions.

1. List four distinct functions of the skin. *(953)*

   a. _____

   b. _____

   c. _____

   d. _____

2. What are three ways that a person can help prevent skin problems? *(954-956)*

   a. _____

   b. _____

   c. _____

3. What are four ways to protect yourself against damage caused by ultraviolet rays of the sun? *(955)*

   a. _____

   b. _____

   c. _____

   d. _____

Copyright © 2013, 2009 by Saunders, an imprint of Elsevier Inc. All rights reserved.

APPLICATION OF THE NURSING PROCESS

Caring for a Patient with Fragile Skin Who Is at Risk for Skin Tears

Scenario: You are making home visits to Mrs. Nutrim, an elderly woman who is recovering from surgery. Currently she requires assistance with ADLs and moving from bed to chair. She is living with her daughter until she recovers enough to return to her own home. The patient tells you that she takes "quite a few medications for my heart and breathing problems."

1. Skin tears frequently occur in the elderly when they are _____ or _____ from bed to chair by nursing personnel. *(956)*

2. Skin tears are usually the result of the forces of _____ or _____ _____. *(956)*

3. Skin tears are very common among the elderly, cause considerable discomfort, are sometimes difficult to heal, and are mostly _____. *(956)*

4. Describe how you can determine skin turgor for Mrs. Nutrim. *(960)* _____

_____

_____

5. List five risk factors for skin tears for Mrs. Nutrim. *(956, Box 42-1)*

   a. _____

   b. _____

   c. _____

   d. _____

   e. _____

6. List six measures that could be used to prevent skin tears. *(956, Box 42-2)*

   a. _____

   b. _____

   c. _____

   d. _____

   e. _____

   f. _____

7. While reviewing Mrs. Nutrim's discharge summary from the hospital, you see that a category I skin tear was identified using the Payne-Martin classification system. Which intervention is most appropriate for this wound? *(956)*
   a. Cover with a transparent adhesive dressing.
   b. Remove the moist skin flap with sterile scissors.
   c. Gently cleanse the skin tear with normal saline.
   d. Apply a pressure dressing to areas of bleeding.

Copyright © 2013, 2009 by Saunders, an imprint of Elsevier Inc. All rights reserved.

8. Despite all precautions and patient teaching, Mrs. Nutrim accidentally causes a small skin tear on her right forearm as she is reaching for an item on her food tray. List four things that should be included in the documentation of this new skin tear. *(956-957)*

    a. _____

    b. _____

    c. _____

    d. _____

SHORT ANSWER

Directions: Provide a brief answer for each of the following questions.

1. A thorough medication history is important in diagnosing skin disorders because _____
    _____. *(958)*

2. The two most common complaints of patients with skin disorders are _____
    and _____. *(958)*

3. Adequate intake of _____ and _____ is essential for healthy skin. *(954)*

4. Black-skinned people need special hair care because _____
    _____. *(958)*

Copyright © 2013, 2009 by Saunders, an imprint of Elsevier Inc. All rights reserved.

TABLE ACTIVITY

Skin Lesions

Directions: In the table below, write down examples of disorders or conditions where you might see each type of lesion.

Types of Skin Lesions

Lesion	Description
Macule	Circumscribed, flat area with a change in skin color; <1 cm in diameter *Examples:*
Papule	Elevated, solid lesion; <1 cm in diameter *Examples:*
Vesicle	Circumscribed, superficial collection of serous fluid; <1 cm in diameter *Examples:*
Plaque	Circumscribed, elevated, superficial, solid lesion; >1 cm in diameter *Examples:*
Wheal	Firm, edematous, irregularly shaped area; diameter variable *Examples:*
Pustule	Elevated, superficial lesion filled with purulent fluid *Examples:*

REVIEW QUESTIONS FOR THE NCLEX® EXAMINATION

Directions: Choose the best answer(s) for the following questions.

1. The nurse is reviewing the documentation of a patient's skin assessment. Which piece of data causes the most immediate concern? *(959-960)*
   1. Presence of patches of senile purpura
   2. Skin stays tented after several seconds
   3. Some seborrheic keratoses on the face
   4. Formation of a keloid over a surgical site

Copyright © 2013, 2009 by Saunders, an imprint of Elsevier Inc. All rights reserved.

2. The physician is preparing to examine the patient for a probable fungus infection. The nurse should assist by obtaining what type of equipment? *(957)*
   1. Wood's lamp
   2. Local anesthetic
   3. Glass slide
   4. Culture tube

3. Environmental factors that could be responsible for a skin disorder include: *(Select all that apply.)* *(955-956)*
   1. cold weather.
   2. tropical climates.
   3. exposure to chemicals and other irritants.
   4. exposure to malignant lesions.
   5. ultraviolet light exposure.

4. Significant subjective data in the assessment of a patient with a skin disorder include: *(958-960)*
   1. appearance of skin adjacent to the lesions.
   2. having difficulty eating meals, especially breakfast.
   3. localized or generalized edema of the skin.
   4. complaints of itching sensation in the affected area.

5. Health teaching for the prevention of skin disorders should include: *(960)*
   1. precautions to avoid gamma radiation.
   2. dietary restrictions to prevent acne.
   3. avoidance of soap products when bathing.
   4. proper way to clean the skin and preserve natural oils.

6. When itching is a problem, the physician might ask the nurse to give the patient which type of bath? *(962)*
   1. Oatmeal
   2. Oil
   3. Tar
   4. Calamine

7. The physician tells the nurse that the patient had positive reaction to a skin patch test. Which manifestation would the nurse expect to observe? *(957)*
   1. Patient has mild shortness of breath.
   2. Patient has a generalized rash.
   3. Patient has a wheal at the test site.
   4. Patient has localized exudate.

8. Which diagnostic test would be used to differentiate benign versus malignant skin lesions? *(957)*
   1. Culture and sensitivity test
   2. Cold light examination
   3. Diascopy
   4. Skin biopsy

9. The nurse advises the patient that tanning salons are not recommend. The patient states, "I have talked to a bunch of people who have been using a tanning salon for years without any problems." What is the best response? *(955)*
   1. "They may not be having problems now, but there will be consequences in the future."
   2. "Professional dermatologists are convinced that tanning has adverse long-term effects."
   3. "It seems like you are interested in talking to people. Let me get you some additional resources."
   4. "I can tell that you don't believe me, but I would like you to talk to some patients with skin cancer."

Copyright © 2013, 2009 by Saunders, an imprint of Elsevier Inc. All rights reserved.

10. Your patient is suffering from poison ivy and the physician has prescribed a steroid injection. The order reads: methylprednisolone (SoluMedrol) 35 mg with dexamethasone (Decadron) 2 mg IM. On hand are SoluMedrol 25 mg/mL and Decadron 4 mg/mL. You will give one combined injection of _____ mL.

CRITICAL THINKING ACTIVITIES

Scenario: Ms. Paula Weiskoff, age 86, is visiting the clinic for a blood pressure check. She has areas of excoriation on her arm and when you ask her about them, she says that her skin itches and the excoriation is from scratching.

1. What would you teach this patient about skin care? *(954-955, 960, 962)*

2. What would you recommend she do to prevent excoriating the skin? *(954-955, 960, 962)*

3. Should you advise this patient to see a physician for this problem? Discuss your rationale for the advice that you decide to give.

STEPS TOWARD BETTER COMMUNICATION

VOCABULARY BUILDING GLOSSARY

Term	Pronunciation	Definition
exasperating	eg zas' pah ray ting	frustrating, psychologically irritating, making one lose patience
trauma	traw' mah	a physical wound or emotional shock

COMPLETION

Directions: Fill in each blank with the correct word from the Vocabulary Building Glossary to complete the statement.

1. A bad burn causes emotional as well as physical _____.

2. A skin problem that does not clear up easily can be very _____ for a patient.

Copyright © 2013, 2009 by Saunders, an imprint of Elsevier Inc. All rights reserved.

WORD ATTACK SKILLS

Word Roots

Root words in English can have several meanings and can be used in many forms. You may need to think about which meaning is being used. It may be a new meaning for you, or it may be a new way to use a word you know. One example from this chapter is the word *compromise* (kom' pro miz). *Compromise* is a verb with two meanings:

1. Take an action that endangers health: *Inadequate fluid replacement may compromise the patient's recovery.*

2. Make a decision by mutual consent where both sides get something they want but neither side gets everything: *The family compromised on the hours they would assist with their father's care.*

Compromise is also a noun, meaning "the decision that is made by this method": *The compromise called for fewer hours but less pay for the nurses.*

Compromised is an adjective from the first verb meaning and means "endangered" (it is also the past tense form of the verb): *The patient's health was compromised by the nurse's action.*

PRONUNCIATION SKILLS

wheal (hweel)	itchy, raised, skin area
psori'asis (so ri' ah sis)	skin disorder with patchy areas of silvery scales
es'char (es' kar)	leathery layer of dead tissue resulting from a full-thickness burn or within a pressure ulcer

CULTURAL POINT

In some time periods and cultures, fair, pale, untanned skin implied wealth and leisure, with no need to be out in the sun working. Today in the United States, it is the opposite. Pale skin to some people indicates the pallor of ill health, or the necessity of working inside. Tanned skin means the person has leisure time and money to be outside at the beach, tennis court, or golf course. A tan is looked upon as more "healthy." Therefore, many people want to look tanned. How can you teach people that tanning can be dangerous to their health?

_____

_____

_____

_____

Copyright © 2013, 2009 by Saunders, an imprint of Elsevier Inc. All rights reserved.

Care of Patients with Integumentary Disorders and Burns

Answer Key: Textbook page references are provided as a guide for answering these questions. A complete answer key was provided to your instructor.

SHORT ANSWER

Integumentary Disorders

Directions: Supply a brief answer or fill in the blank(s).

1.   An infection with _____ appears as lesions on the lips and nares that are commonly called *cold sores* or *fever blisters*. *(970-971)*

2.   Herpes virus infection can be spread from one area of the body to another by _____
_____. *(970)*

3.   Herpes zoster is caused by _____ and is transmissible from one person to another. *(971)*

4.   Fungal infections of the skin can be prevented by _____
_____. *(972)*

5.   Scabies mites burrow under the top layers of the skin and cause _____. *(974)*

6.   Lice are acquired by contact with infested people or their _____ and _____
_____ have also been known to carry lice and the scabies mite. *(974)*

7.   The treatments most often used for persistent psoriasis are _____

_____

_____ . *(969)*

8.   The best preventive measure for skin cancer is _____
_____. *(975)*

9.   A common skin change in the elderly that can precede cancerous skin lesions is _____
_____. *(975)*

Copyright © 2013, 2009 by Saunders, an imprint of Elsevier Inc. All rights reserved.

SHORT ANSWERS

Caring for a Patient with Acne

1. Acne is thought to be due to _____, _____,

   _____, and _____. *(967-968)*

2. Recommended basic care for teenage facial skin problems includes: *(968)*_____

   _____

   _____

   _____

   _____

3. Discuss some of the issues related to the use of the drug Accutane for cystic acne which has been especially effective in controlling cases that are resistant to other forms of treatment. *(968)* _____

   _____

   _____

   _____

   _____

   _____

Copyright © 2013, 2009 by Saunders, an imprint of Elsevier Inc. All rights reserved.

MATCHING

Skin Cancers

Directions: Match the type of skin cancer on the left with the characteristics on the right that best describe it. (975-976, Table 43-1)

1. _____ Basal cell epithelioma

2. _____ Squamous cell epithelioma

3. _____ Malignant melanoma: superficial, spreading

4. _____ Malignant melanoma: nodular

5. _____ Malignant melanoma

a. Arises from a lesion that resembles a large, flat freckle

b. Accounts for 70% of all skin cancers

c. Occurs mainly on head, neck, and hands

d. Horizontal growth can continue for years, vertical growth worsens prognosis

e. Rarely spreads; easily treated

f. Small tumor nodules may ulcerate and bleed

g. Crusted or ulcerated center has a pearly border

h. Itching, oozing, and bleeding may be present

i. Can appear in a variety of colors

j. Has an irregular surface and notched border

k. Is uniformly blackish-grayish color; resembles a blackberry

l. Is somewhat rare

m. Spreads rapidly

COMPLETION

Directions: Fill in the blanks to complete the statements.

1. Is there an age group in which skin cancer is more common? *(975)*_____

2. What is the method of diagnosis for a suspected skin cancer? *(975-977)*_____

    _____

3. What is included in the treatment for melanoma? *(975)*_____

    _____

    _____

    _____

Copyright © 2013, 2009 by Saunders, an imprint of Elsevier Inc. All rights reserved.

TABLE ACTIVITY

Burn Care

Directions: Complete the following table correlating the pathophysiology and clinical management of a major burn.
(983-991)

Pathophysiology	Medical Management	Nursing Interventions
Dilatation of capillaries and small vessels in area; increase in capillary permeability; plasma seeps out; edema		
Fluid loss; hemoconcentration; reduced efficiency of circulation		
Fall in blood pressure; hypovolemic shock; cellular dehydration		
Sloughing of dead tissue; large open wounds; infection		
Pulmonary and respiratory changes due to inhalation injury, pulmonary edema, obstructed airway		
Pain in response to injury		
Emotional shock due to pain, long-term therapy, changed body image; depression, boredom		

Copyright © 2013, 2009 by Saunders, an imprint of Elsevier Inc. All rights reserved.

APPLICATION OF NURSING PROCESS

Caring for a Patient with Poison Ivy

Directions: Answer the following questions in the spaces provided.

1. An appropriate nursing diagnosis for the patient who has contracted poison ivy on his arms would be: *(966-967)*

   _____

   _____

2. An expected outcome for the above nursing diagnosis for this patient might be: *(967)* _____

   _____

3. Appropriate nursing measures for the patient who is experiencing poison ivy and considerable itching are: *(967)*

   a. _____

   b. _____

   c. _____

   d. _____

   e. _____

CARING FOR PATIENTS WITH PRESSURE ULCERS

Table Activity

Directions: Complete the following table and describe the characteristics of pressure ulcer stages. (978, 980)

Stage	Characteristics
Suspected deep tissue injury:	
Stage I	
Stage II	
Stage III	
Stage IV	
Unstageable	

Copyright © 2013, 2009 by Saunders, an imprint of Elsevier Inc. All rights reserved.

SHORT ANSWERS

1. The use of a lifting device, a lift sheet, or a trapeze bar to reposition is beneficial to prevent skin damage from _____. *(977)*

2. Patients with limited mobility need to utilize a(n) _____ device on the bed or in the wheelchair. *(978)*

3. Whenever a patient is turned, the _____ that were against the bed should be assessed. *(978)*

4. The way to tell if a reddened area on the skin is a beginning pressure ulcer is _____ _____. *(978)*

5. List at least five measures to use that would help in the prevention of pressure ulcers. *(977-979)*

   a. _____

   b. _____

   c. _____

   d. _____

   e. _____

6. An expected outcome for the nursing diagnosis of Impaired skin integrity related to presence of a pressure ulcer would be: *(977-981)*

   _____

   _____

7. What data would you use to evaluate whether the above expected outcome is being met? *(977-981)*

   _____

   _____

REVIEW QUESTIONS FOR THE NCLEX® EXAMINATION

Directions: Choose the best answer(s) for the following questions.

1. Contact dermatitis can be caused by any number of substances. When considering whether a skin problem is contact dermatitis, you would look for which sign(s) and/or symptom(s) indicating that disorder? *(Select all that apply.) (966-967)*
   1. Erythema and swelling
   2. Ulcerated lesions
   3. Scaling
   4. Pruritus
   5. Vesicular lesions

Copyright © 2013, 2009 by Saunders, an imprint of Elsevier Inc. All rights reserved.

2. Stevens-Johnson syndrome may occur around 14 days after beginning drug therapy. The most common drugs causing this allergic syndrome are: *(970)*
   1. trimethroprim/sulfamethoxazole, phenytoin, and carbamazepine.
   2. Bactrim, Dilantin, and Cardizem.
   3. Tegretol, Motrin, and digoxin.
   4. furosemide, Septra, and Cortef.

3. A nursing diagnosis commonly associated with psoriasis is: *(969)*
   1. Risk for injury.
   2. Fluid volume excess.
   3. Disturbed body image.
   4. Ineffective thermoregulation.

4. What is an important teaching point for a patient about self-care for a carbuncle? *(970)*
   1. A clean washcloth and towel should be used for bathing each day.
   2. Use a cold compress for comfort and to promote drainage.
   3. Take sedatives as prescribed for relief of discomfort.
   4. Avoid injury of any kind to surrounding skin.

5. The nurse is caring for several patients on a surgical floor. Which patient needs to be placed in contact isolation? *(966-971)*
   1. Patient with psoriasis with adherent silvery-white scales
   2. Patient has stasis dermatitis with petechiae, and hyperpigmentation
   3. Patient has herpes zoster with small groups of vesicles along nerve pathways
   4. Patient has actinic keratoses with small, scaly, grayish papules

6. Select statements that are true about tinea pedis. It: *(Select all that apply.)* *(973)*
   1. is a fungal disease.
   2. displays with cracks between the toes with peeling and itching.
   3. is often contracted in public showers and spas.
   4. is treated by keeping the foot moisturized and covered.
   5. is treated with antibiotic ointments and systemic drugs.
   6. is a bacterial infection.

7. A high-priority intervention for the patient with serious burns is: *(988)*
   1. cooling the burn areas every 2 hours with running water.
   2. beginning intravenous fluid administration as soon as possible.
   3. cleansing the burn areas thoroughly as quickly as possible.
   4. administering a tetanus immunization within the first hour of treatment.

8. What is the highest priority when caring for the burn patient? *(988-989)*
   1. Preventing contractures from forming
   2. Grafting to cover open burn areas
   3. Preventing infection or controlling it
   4. Providing psychosocial support to the patient

9. The patient arrives by EMS after being rescued from a house fire. The patient sustained minor burns on the hands and forearms and demonstrates a dry hacking cough. She is upset and weeping, but vital signs are currently stable. The physician orders admission for 23-hour observation. What is the priority nursing diagnosis? *(988-993)*
   1. Anxiety related to traumatic life-threatening event
   2. Impaired skin integrity related to burns of hands and forearms
   3. Risk for ineffective breathing pattern related to smoke inhalation
   4. Risk for fluid imbalance related to fluid shifting and edema formation

Copyright © 2013, 2009 by Saunders, an imprint of Elsevier Inc. All rights reserved.

10. Fluid resuscitation is a high priority during the emergent stage of a serious burn. Your patient weighs 182 lbs. His burn percentage is calculated to be 65% of body surface. You are to infuse Ringer's lactate. Using the formula provided in the chapter, within the first 8 hours after the burn, he should receive _____ mL of Ringer's lactate.

CRITICAL THINKING ACTIVITIES

Scenario A: Mr. Marshall is a 27-year-old truck driver who was burned in a vehicular accident. He has been brought to the emergency department of the community hospital. He has burns over the anterior and posterior surface of both arms, chest, and back.

1. According to the rule of nines, what is his total burn percentage? *(982)*

2. One of the burns on his chest is a full-thickness burn. What are the characteristics of a full-thickness burn? *(983)*

3. What are the two major concerns during the first hour after a burn injury? *(984-985)*

4. How would you assess whether Mr. Marshall has a respiratory injury? *(984-985)*

5. What measures would you expect to be carried out to reduce the risk for infection for Mr. Marshall? *(985-986)*

Scenario B: Mr. Marshall has progressed and débridement and grafting on his chest and arms has been carried out. He is undergoing physical therapy; however, he has become progressively withdrawn and less willing to have visitors.

1. When he expresses concern about the scars that are beginning to form, what would you tell him about scar maturation? *(988)*

2. When he resists performing his physical therapy exercises, how would you encourage him to continue them? *(988)*

3. What can you do to help him cope with the psychosocial effects of his injuries? *(993)*

Copyright © 2013, 2009 by Saunders, an imprint of Elsevier Inc. All rights reserved.

Scenario C: Mrs. Ruiz, age 78, is being discharged from the long-term care facility following convalescent care and rehabilitation for a fractured hip. She has a healing stage II pressure ulcer on her left buttock.

1. What equipment would you make certain that the patient has at home to help prevent further pressure ulcer development? *(977-978)*

2. What teaching would you provide as to the care of the skin and of the healing pressure ulcer? *(980-981)*

Scenario D: Mr. Sam Torres is admitted to your unit from the long-term care facility. He is being treated for pneumonia. You discover an area on the right hip that is raw-looking with serous drainage.

1. How would you correctly document this skin problem? *(978-981)*

2. How would you "stage" this ulcer? What stage is it (considering the information above)? *(978, 980)*

3. What skin care measures should be instituted? *(980-982)*

STEPS TOWARD BETTER COMMUNICATION

VOCABULARY BUILDING GLOSSARY

Term	Pronunciation	Definition
proliferation	pro lif' ah ray' shun	rapid increase or multiplication; the reproduction of similar forms, usually meaning cells in medicine
traumatic	traw mat' ik	very emotionally unpleasant

COMPLETION

Directions: Fill in the blanks to complete the statements.

1. Receiving a diagnosis of melanoma would be a _____ experience.

2. A squamous cell skin carcinoma is composed of a _____ of abnormal cells.

Copyright © 2013, 2009 by Saunders, an imprint of Elsevier Inc. All rights reserved.

WORD ATTACK SKILLS

Word Elements

auto-	self
allo-	other (same species)
homo-	same, similar
hetero-	different (individual, tissue)
xeno-	foreign, unlike (different species)
epi-	above, on, upon
derm/a-, dermat/o-	skin
-logy	study or science of
-ist	a person who
-graft	to implant or transplant tissue

Using Word Elements

Directions: What word would mean:

1. Study of the skin: _____

2. On the skin: _____

3. A person who studies the skin: _____

4. Transplant tissue from another person: _____

5. Transplant tissue from oneself: _____

PRONUNCIATION SKILLS

débride'ment (da breed' maw)	removal of dead tissues and foreign material from a wound
xen'ograft (zen'o graft)	graft of tissue between animals of different species

COMMUNICATION EXERCISE

A. If you noticed a skin lesion that looked as if it might be a skin cancer on someone you didn't know well, how would you bring it to the person's attention without offending him or her? Americans normally do not like to have attention called to personal matters, especially any deformities that might be considered negative or personal. However, this is such an important matter that you might want to find a way to approach the person. It would be best to catch the person's attention and speak to him or her in a manner that cannot be overheard by others. Write out what you would say to the person.

_____

_____

_____

_____

Copyright © 2013, 2009 by Saunders, an imprint of Elsevier Inc. All rights reserved.

B. Describe:

1. The attitude you should take with a patient who has a long-term recovery ahead. _____

   _____

2. The diversional and occupational activities you could suggest. _____

   _____

COMMUNICATION EXERCISE

Write a short dialogue explaining to an aging patient why it is important for him to turn or shift his position in bed and in his chair so that he doesn't develop pressure sores. Make some suggestions to help him to remember. (Turn when the TV commercial comes on, when he turns the page in his magazine, when he hears people in the hall, when he returns from a trip to the bathroom.)

_____

_____

_____

_____

_____

Copyright © 2013, 2009 by Saunders, an imprint of Elsevier Inc. All rights reserved.

Care of Patients in Disasters, Bioterrorism Attacks, and Pandemic Infections

chapter

44

Answer Key: Textbook page references are provided as a guide for answering these questions. A complete answer key was provided to your instructor.

COMPLETION

Directions: Fill in the blanks to complete the statements.

1. A disaster exists when the number of _____ exceeds the resource capabilities of the area. *(997)*

2. _____ is a top priority when large groups of people are together in a shelter because the incidence of communicable disease is much greater. *(1003)*

3. Triage for a disaster is based on first saving those with life-threatening conditions and a likelihood of _____. *(999, 1001)*

4. Those exposed to toxic chemicals should be _____ in the field before transport to a medical facility. *(1008)*

5. Exposure to high doses of external radiation that penetrate the body even for a few minutes may result in acute _____. *(1009-1010)*

SHORT ANSWER

Disaster Management Planning

Directions: Read the clinical scenario and answer the questions that follow.

Scenario: You have been asked to sit on a hospital committee to review and update the hospital's disaster management plan. You have been assigned to investigate the roles and responsibilities of the nursing staff and to develop a list of topics that are relevant to disaster nursing.

1. Identify at least five nursing responsibilities in case of a disaster. *(1002-1003)*

    a. _____

    b. _____

    c. _____

    d. _____

    e. _____

Copyright © 2013, 2009 by Saunders, an imprint of Elsevier Inc. All rights reserved.

2. Give four examples of procedures or tasks that you might be expected to perform in the emergency department for patients who may have sustained injury or illness during a disaster. *(1002-1003)*

   a. _____

   b. _____

   c. _____

   d. _____

3. According to the U.S. Department of Health and Human Services, nurses need to be skilled in which three areas if they are providing care during disaster situations? *(1003)*

   a. _____

   b. _____

   c. _____

4. What are the six pathogens that are most likely to be used as bioterrorism agents? *(1011-1015, Table 44-5)*

   a. _____

   b. _____

   c. _____

   d. _____

   e. _____

   f. _____

5. What are four categories of chemical agents that might be used in a terrorist attack? *(1007-1008, Table 44-3)*

   a. _____

   b. _____

   c. _____

   d. _____

   e. _____

6. List four general guidelines for your role in bioterrorism preparedness and response. *(1015)*

   a. _____

   b. _____

   c. _____

   d. _____

Copyright © 2013, 2009 by Saunders, an imprint of Elsevier Inc. All rights reserved.

APPLICATION OF THE NURSING PROCESS

Caring for a Patient with Botulism

Directions: Read the scenario and provide the answers to the following questions.

Scenario: Ms. Kelso is admitted for botulism. She became sick after eating some home-preserved vegetables. Fortunately, she was the only one to eat the vegetables and her family quickly helped her to seek medical attention.

1. What are the early symptoms of botulism? *(1012-1013, Table 44-5)*

    a. _____

    b. _____

    c. _____

2. What is the classic triad of symptoms for this disorder? *(1013)*

    a. _____

    b. _____

    c. _____

3. What is the priority diagnosis for Ms. Kelso? *(1013)*
    a. Risk for ineffective breathing pattern related to flaccid paralysis
    b. Acute confusion related to botulism toxin
    c. Diarrhea related to food poisoning
    d. Impaired physical activity related to decreased strength

4. List at least four interventions (including assessments) to ensure safety for a patient who is having difficulty swallowing. *(1013)*

    a. _____

    b. _____

    c. _____

    d. _____

5. Which statement by the family indicates an understanding of the treatment plan for Ms. Kelso? *(1013)*
    a. "The antitoxin will reverse the muscular paralysis."
    b. "She can be treated with gentamicin (Garamycin)."
    c. "Supportive therapy may be needed for several weeks."
    d. "The drug of choice is ciprofloxacin (Cipro)."

Copyright © 2013, 2009 by Saunders, an imprint of Elsevier Inc. All rights reserved.

PRIORITY SETTING

Disaster Triage

Directions: Read the scenario and correctly tag the disaster victims.

Scenario: You are participating in a disaster drill and have been assigned to assist in the triage area. The drill instructor gives you the following instructions: "An LPN/LVN would not ordinarily be responsible for making initial triage decisions; however, in this scenario, 250 victims have just converged on the hospital and you must do your best to correctly tag patients. You should ask for help in decision-making if you feel that you are unable to accurately assess and appropriately tag the patient. You will have to use your critical thinking skills in each situation." *Correctly tag each patient (RED, YELLOW, GREEN, or BLACK) or refer to RN/ MD. (1001-1002)*

_____ a. Middle-aged man who is having symptoms of myocardial infarction.

_____ b. Child with swollen ankle, decreased ROM, good peripheral pulses.

_____ c. Young woman with vomiting, low-grade fever, and mild abdominal pain.

_____ d. Young man with dislocated shoulder and decreased peripheral pulses.

_____ e. Child with 90% total body burns.

_____ f. Teenager with blunt force abdominal trauma, denies distress, but is diaphoretic.

_____ g. Elderly man with insect bite, reports tightness in throat, has angioedema.

REVIEW QUESTIONS FOR THE NCLEX® EXAMINATION

Directions: Choose the best answer(s) for the following questions.

1. The nurse is assigned to assist in triage. The purpose and goal of triage is to: *(1001)*
    1. sort patients by priority of need for treatment.
    2. ensure that all patients receive treatment.
    3. ensure that medical equipment is available.
    4. identify the need for supplies and support.

2. The nurse is advising a community group about what to do in the event of a natural disaster such as an earthquake or flood. What is appropriate information and advice? *(999-1000)*
    1. Evacuate the area and leave immediately.
    2. Take refuge in the basement during a tornado warning.
    3. During an earthquake, drop to the floor and crawl to an exit.
    4. For flood warnings, push towels into the cracks under the doors.

3. There are multiple victims during a disaster. The majority of these victims will be triaged and identified with which color of tag? *(1001)*
    1. Red tag
    2. Black tag
    3. Yellow tag
    4. Green tag

4. The patient is being treated for radiation exposure. A chelating agent functions to reduce radiation damage by: *(1010)*
    1. binding the radioactive material.
    2. blocking specific isotopes.
    3. mobilizing radioactive material.
    4. reducing concentration of radioactive material.

Copyright © 2013, 2009 by Saunders, an imprint of Elsevier Inc. All rights reserved.

5. What is a simple way to purify water when the supply has been disrupted? *(1003)*
   1. Rolling boil for 3–5 minutes
   2. Adding 16 teaspoons of household liquid bleach
   3. Water that drips from a source into a clean cup
   4. Low-boil the water for 20 minutes

6. Victims who may have residual particulate after radiation or chemical exposure should be decontaminated. Victims should be instructed to: *(1009)*
   1. remove and burn clothing.
   2. wear protective gear and double gloves.
   3. scrub skin with water and soap and rinse well.
   4. brush off and vacuum residual particulate.

7. A patient is admitted with radiation sickness. What would the nurse expect to find documented in the patient's chart? *(1010)*
   1. Cardiac arrhythmias and low blood pressure
   2. Nausea, vomiting, diarrhea, and hair loss
   3. Lethargy, constipation, and blurred vision
   4. Renal failure and electrolyte imbalances

8. The patient is admitted for a diagnosis of anthrax. What is the physician most likely to order to treat this patient? *(1011, 1013, Table 44-5)*
   1. IV fluids and oxygen therapy
   2. Ciprofloxacin (Cipro)
   3. Gentamicin (Garamycin)
   4. Antitoxin type A or B

9. Which task related to disaster management would be appropriate to assign to a nursing assistant? *(1001-1002)*
   1. Assisting victims to shower after exposure to toxin
   2. Debriefing others during a critical incident
   3. Triaging incoming green-tag victims
   4. Moving black-tagged victims to designated areas

10. The nurse is assisting in a temporary housing shelter that has been created for displaced victims of a hurricane. What is the priority diagnosis for this group? *(1003)*
    1. Anticipatory grieving related to loss of property, friends, family, etc.
    2. Ineffective coping related to sudden catastrophic event
    3. High risk for infection related to crowding, poor hygienic conditions
    4. Fatigue related to unfamiliar surroundings and stress

11. The nurse is caring for multiple victims who are rapidly arriving from a nearby disaster site. Which communication strategy is the nurse most likely to use? *(1003)*
    1. Active listening
    2. Short directive statements
    3. Therapeutic touch
    4. Silence and reflection

12. The nursing staff is participating in a discussion about practical measures to prepare for a possible pandemic flu event. Which comment by a staff member indicates an understanding of what should be done? *(1015)*
    1. "The hospital needs to get more ventilators for the intensive care unit."
    2. "None of the nurses with children should have to come under those conditions."
    3. "We need to review respiratory isolation precautions and reinforce handwashing."
    4. "This is not a third-world country; we will be okay if we just use common sense."

Copyright © 2013, 2009 by Saunders, an imprint of Elsevier Inc. All rights reserved.

13. Based on a patient's answers to interview questions, the nurse suspects that the patient may have been exposed to a possible Category A infectious agent. What should the nurse do *first*? *(1011, Table 44-5)*
    1. Notify the supervisor about the possibility of contagion.
    2. Don an N-95 or P-100 respirator mask.
    3. Have the patient and family perform hand hygiene.
    4. Isolate the patient in a negative-pressure room.

14. The nurse is assigned to assist the physician with "reverse" triage during a disaster event. What information is most relevant to this process? *(1000)*
    1. Identifying the patient's blood type and history of transfusions
    2. Knowing the pattern of pain and vital signs over the past few days
    3. Reviewing the past and present medication history
    4. Evaluating the patient's emotional response to the disaster event

15. Which statement by the nurse indicates that the goals of critical incident stress debriefing are being met? *(1016)*
    1. "I still have nightmares about the disaster, but I don't think about it during the day."
    2. "I am surviving, although I guess I am still drinking more than I should."
    3. "I went out with friends the other night and we talked about how we were all doing."
    4. "I am super-prepared now. I check the disaster equipment every day."

CRITICAL THINKING ACTIVITIES

Scenario A: Your supervisor asks you to work some extra shifts. There has been an unexpected influx of patients with flulike symptoms. These patients are rapidly progressing into severe respiratory distress. She tells you that your help is really needed; however, you should be aware that relatively healthy young people with no previous health problems are getting sick and the physicians are not exactly sure what is going on with these patients. *(1002-1003, 1006, 1015-1016)*

1. Discuss how you might feel about being asked to help under these circumstances and/or expose yourself (and your family) to potentially serious communicable disease.

    _____

    _____

    _____

    _____

2. When you are comfortable in your first nursing job, what are some things that you could do (or ask) that would prepare you to face a similar scenario?

    _____

    _____

    _____

    _____

    _____

Copyright © 2013, 2009 by Saunders, an imprint of Elsevier Inc. All rights reserved.

Scenario B: You are working in a downtown walk-in clinic. Typically the clinic services low-income families and the homeless population and provides routine health services such as immunizations for children, treatment for minor illness or accidents, or prescription service for blood pressure medications, etc. *(1010-1016)*

1. Explain in your own words why you would need to have a working knowledge of bioterrorism for this work setting.

_____

_____

_____

_____

_____

_____

2. List seven signs or events that suggest a bioterrorism incident has occurred.

a. _____

b. _____

c. _____

d. _____

e. _____

f. _____

g. _____

Scenario C: You are working in small emergency department in a rural town. There is an explosion in a nearby factory and multiple victims (adult workers) begin to arrive. The physician instructs you to start peripheral IVs (with at least an 18-gauge catheter) on all the patients as they arrive and hang normal saline unless ordered otherwise at 125 mL/hour. The hospital runs out of IV pumps, so you must calculate the flow rate using ordinary IV tubing. Calculate the gtts/min using various tubings.

1. Drop factor 20 gtts/mL _____ gtts/min.

2. Drop factor 15 gtts/mL _____ gtts/min.

3. Drop factor 10 gtts/mL _____ gtts/min.

4. Drop factor 60 gtts/mL _____ gtts/min.

5. The charge nurse tells you not to use mini-drip (60 gtts/mL) tubing unless there is nothing else available. Why would he say this?

_____

_____

_____

_____

_____

Copyright © 2013, 2009 by Saunders, an imprint of Elsevier Inc. All rights reserved.

STEPS TOWARD BETTER COMMUNICATION

VOCABULARY BUILDING GLOSSARY

Term	Pronunciation	Definition
catastrophe	ka tas' tro fee	a terrible event, a disaster
disparity	dis par'itee	difference, inequality
duress	du ress'	forced hardship or difficulty
improvise	im'pro viz	to use whatever is available
triage	tree ahzh'	a system for determining priority of need and order or location of treatment

COMPLETION

Directions: Fill in the blanks with the appropriate words from the Vocabulary Building Glossary to complete the statements.

1. The people who had their homes destroyed in the tornado were experiencing considerable _____.

2. The man's leg was badly fractured, so the nurse had to _____ a splint at the scene of the accident.

3. When Ms. Lyons was admitted, there was evident _____ between the appearance of one leg and the other.

4. Hurricane Katrina was a major _____.

5. The nurse was assigned to _____ for the victims of the tornado.

WORD ATTACK SKILLS

Word Meanings

Directions: For each word on the left, circle the word or phrase with the same meaning on the right.

1. mitigate: reduce   add water   delay

2. acuity: distance   perception   lack of water

3. lethargy: fatal   lack of energy   skin condition

4. aerosolize: spray with a liquid   suspend solid particles in a gas   blow dry

Copyright © 2013, 2009 by Saunders, an imprint of Elsevier Inc. All rights reserved.

ABBREVIATIONS

Directions: Pronounce and give the meaning of each abbreviation.

1. OES:_____

2. FEMA:_____

3. DMAT: _____

4. WMD: _____

5. NOAA: _____

6. CDC: _____

7. CISD (team):_____

8. PTSD: _____

9. VHF: _____

10. EMS: _____

11. HEPA (filter mask): _____

COMMUNICATION EXERCISE

Idioms

Directions: Recall that idioms are usages of language that cannot be translated literally. Idioms are specific to a culture and are often imaginative uses of language. Explain to a partner what the following idioms mean:

1. Telephone tree: _____

   _____

   _____

2. Ground rules:_____

   _____

   _____

Copyright © 2013, 2009 by Saunders, an imprint of Elsevier Inc. All rights reserved.

Student Name_____ Date_____

Care of Patients with Trauma or Shock

Answer Key: Textbook page references are provided as a guide for answering these questions. A complete answer key was provided to your instructor.

TERMINOLOGY

Emergent Conditions

Directions: Match the condition on the left with the description on the right that is most likely to be associated with it.

1. _____ Choking emergency *(1032)*

2. _____ Carbon monoxide poisoning *(1030)*

3. _____ Heatstroke *(1026-1027)*

4. _____ Index of suspicion *(1022)*

5. _____ Hypothermia *(1024)*

6. _____ Mechanism of injury *(1022)*

7. _____ Pneumothorax *(1025)*

8. _____ Triage *(1022)*

9. _____ Penetrating trauma *(1025)*

10. _____ Shock *(1033, 1035)*

a. Labored respirations and decreased breath sounds on one side of the chest

b. Hot, dry skin; victim working outside in summer

c. Vigilance to detect problems that are not obvious

d. Unable to cough or speak, gasping respirations; victim was eating in a restaurant

e. Patient jumped from third-story window

f. Cherry-red skin; victim found unconscious in garage

g. Cool, dry skin; impaired mental ability; elderly victim found at home in winter

h. Presence of knife wound in the abdominal area

i. Decreased perfusion related to depleted blood volume or decreased cardiac output

j. Assessing and sorting to determine order of priority for care

COMPLETION

Directions: Fill in the blanks to complete the statements.

1. _____ laws protect medical personnel from liability when rendering emergency medical care for victims of accidental injury. *(1020)*

2. The purpose of immobilizing the neck of a trauma patient is to keep it as straight as possible, preventing it from _____ or _____. *(1024)*

3. _____ produces paradoxical respirations. *(1024)*

Copyright © 2013, 2009 by Saunders, an imprint of Elsevier Inc. All rights reserved.

4. The amount of _____ and current involved, the length of _____, and the condition of the skin determine how much damage may have occurred as a result of an electric shock. *(1031)*

5. The person who sustains a tick bite in a mountainous area may contract _____ or _____. *(1031)*

6. The heart is extremely sensitive when cold, and the patient must be handled carefully to prevent _____. *(1027)*

CARING FOR A TRAUMA VICTIM IN THE EMERGENCY DEPARTMENT

Directions: Read the clinical scenario and answer the questions that follow.

Scenario: The nurse is working in the ED and several patients have just arrived from the scene of the same accident. All of the victims have been transported by EMS and arrive on stretchers and backboards with C-collars in place. You are asked to help with one of the patients who appears to be less critical than the others at first glance.

1. What are the ABCDEs of assessment? *(1022, 1023, Focused Assessment)*

    A: _____

    B: _____

    C: _____

    D: _____

    E: _____

2. Describe the head-to-toe assessment. *(1023, Focused Assessment)*_____

    _____

    _____

    _____

    _____

    _____

    _____

    _____

    _____

Copyright © 2013, 2009 by Saunders, an imprint of Elsevier Inc. All rights reserved.

3. What kinds of information would you try to get from EMS before they leave the ED? *(1022, 1023)*

_____

_____

_____

_____

4. The patient tells you she has to urinate and asks you to remove the C-collar so that she can get up and go to the bathroom. What should you do? *(1024)*
   a. Tell her that you can't remove the C-collar and obtain an order for an indwelling Foley.
   b. Remove the C-collar and help her to maintain the neck in a straight position.
   c. Ask the physician if spinal injury has been cleared and if it is okay to remove the C-collar.
   d. Instruct the nursing assistant to help the patient use the bedpan.

5. The ED physician tells you that the patient appears to be stable with just a bruise on the lower abdomen, but asks you to check vital signs on the patient every 15 minutes for 1 hour and to repeat the abdominal assessment and to obtain a repeat hematocrit q hour X 3. Why has the physician asked you to do these assessments and what should you be watching for? *(1025-1026)*

_____

_____

_____

_____

_____

SHORT ANSWER

Domestic Violence

Directions: Read the clinical scenario and answer the questions that follow.

Scenario: You are working in an outpatient clinic and Ms. Luten comes in for treatment of a broken wrist. She tells you that she slipped and fell. While you are taking her blood pressure you notice bruises on her upper arms and around her neck. Her medical records show that she has been treated for injuries twice within the past year.

1. You suspect that Ms. Luten may be a victim of domestic abuse. What are five questions that you could ask to assess for abuse? *(1041)*

   a. _____

   b. _____

   c. _____

   d. _____

   e. _____

Copyright © 2013, 2009 by Saunders, an imprint of Elsevier Inc. All rights reserved.

2. List eight physical signs of battering. *(1041)*

   a. _____

   b. _____

   c. _____

   d. _____

   e. _____

   f. _____

   g. _____

   h. _____

3. A clue to the need for an assessment for abuse is _____ in various stages of healing. *(1041)*

4. What are four potential psychological signs of abuse? *(1041)*

   a. _____

   b. _____

   c. _____

   d. _____

5. Which task would be appropriate to assign to the nursing assistant? *(1041)*
   a. Take photos of Ms. Luten's bruises.
   b. Sit with Ms. Luten to provide support.
   c. Collect evidence such as torn clothes.
   d. Obtain an ice pack for her wrist.

APPLICATION OF THE NURSING PROCESS

Allergic Reaction

Directions: Read the scenario and provide answers to the following questions.

Scenario: You are outside with your children and you hear your neighbor, Ms. Andrews, calling for help. She tells you that she was just stung by a bee and "last time I had a really bad reaction to it." Currently, she is anxious, and you can see the sting mark with some redness on her forearm around the immediate area.

1. What is the *first* action you should take? *(1036)*
   a. Call 911 and encourage her to stay calm.
   b. Remove the stinger by gently scraping the skin with a credit card.
   c. Elevate the arm and apply an ice pack.
   d. Assess for hives and general weakness.

Copyright © 2013, 2009 by Saunders, an imprint of Elsevier Inc. All rights reserved.

2. What are eight signs and symptoms of a systemic reaction to a bee sting? *(1036)*

    a. _____

    b. _____

    c. _____

    d. _____

    e. _____

    f. _____

    g. _____

    h. _____

You have assessed Ms. Andrews and she does not appear to be having the signs or symptoms of a systemic reaction to the sting; however, she tells her daughter to run into the house and get the anaphylaxis kit so that you can see it "because you are a nurse and I don't really remember anything about what's in the kit, or how to use it."

3. What is the name, the strength, and the dosage of the emergency drug in the anaphylaxis kit? *(1037)*

    _____

4. What is the name and dose of a typical over-the-counter medication that could be used after the emergency drug is given? _____ *(1037)*

5. Identify four additional self-care measures for bee stings that Ms. Andrews could do at home. *(1036-1037)*

    a. _____

    b. _____

    c. _____

    d. _____

6. Ms. Andrews comes over to your house in the evening to thank you for your help. "I really feel silly about making such a fuss and not knowing anything about that kit." You recognize that while she is not really your patient, she does have some health issues that you can assist her with. What is the priority nursing diagnosis at this point? *(1036-1037)*
    a. Impaired skin integrity related to scratching
    b. Knowledge deficit related to bee sting kit
    c. Risk for ineffective breathing related to throat constriction
    d. Anxiety related to future allergic exposures

Copyright © 2013, 2009 by Saunders, an imprint of Elsevier Inc. All rights reserved.

PRIORITY SETTING

Directions: Read the scenario and prioritize as appropriate.

Scenario: You are at a community swimming pool and there is no lifeguard on duty. Suddenly, one of the women says, "My son is in the water! Please help him! I can't swim!" Prioritize the actions for assisting a drowning victim. *(1019-1020, 1022-1023)*

_____ a. Transport to a medical facility promptly for evaluation and treatment.

_____ b. The rescuer (you) should direct a bystander to call 911.

_____ c. If the child is breathing, place him on his side.

_____ d. Assess for breathing and pulse.

_____ e. Try to reach the victim without going in deep water.

_____ f. Instruct a bystander to assist you in bringing the child out of water.

REVIEW QUESTIONS FOR THE NCLEX® EXAMINATION

Directions: Choose the best answer(s) for the following questions.

1. Implementation of nursing care for the emergency patient who is admitted with frostbite of the foot includes: *(1027-1028)*
   1. applying a heating pad to the frostbitten area.
   2. giving the patient hot fluids to drink.
   3. wrapping the foot in warmed blankets.
   4. immersing the foot in warm water.

2. A toddler is brought to the ED alert and crying; however, EMS reports that the child was pulled from a neighbor's swimming pool and resuscitated at the scene. The toddler is admitted for 23-hour observation. What is most important observation that the nurse is making during the assessment of this child? *(1019-1020, 1022-1023)*
   1. Observing for signs of previous injury that suggest potential child neglect
   2. Monitoring the pulse oximetry readings and auscultating the breath sounds
   3. Assessing the quality of the pulse and rhythm of the heart rate
   4. Assessing the need for education related to child's developmental needs

3. To evaluate the effectiveness of Lasix and morphine for the treatment of pulmonary edema in an emergency patient, the nurse would: *(1033)*
   1. monitor intake and output.
   2. assess respiratory status.
   3. assess for decreased pain.
   4. check the strength of peripheral pulses.

4. The priority goal when planning the care of the emergency patient admitted in shock would be to: *(1033, 1035)*
   1. maintain the patient's body warmth to prevent vasodilation.
   2. decrease the patient's pain to lessen vasoconstriction.
   3. restore the patient's circulating blood volume to promote perfusion.
   4. restore the patient's acid-base balance to aid respiration.

5. A high priority in the immediate treatment of burns of the hands is: *(1032)*
   1. cool burned areas quickly with cool water.
   2. assess ROM to joints and circumferential burns.
   3. cover with blankets or sheets to prevent chilling.
   4. determine the area and degree of the burns.

Copyright © 2013, 2009 by Saunders, an imprint of Elsevier Inc. All rights reserved.

6. The nurse is at a restaurant and observes a person who appears to be choking. He is conscious and partially able to speak. What is the priority action? *(1033)*
   1. Have a bystander call 911 and stay with patient.
   2. Encourage him to cough and breathe as deeply as he can.
   3. Get behind him and perform the Heimlich maneuver.
   4. Strike him sharply between the shoulder blades.

7. There is a multi-car motor vehicle accident and several people stop to assist. Under "Good Samaritan" laws, what applies to voluntary rescuers who assist at the scene? *(1020-1021)*
   1. All rescuers are equally protected against liability.
   2. Rescuers are only protected if they can prove they acted in good faith.
   3. Physicians who stop are held to a higher standard of care than others.
   4. Bad outcomes usually result in liability suits.

8. The patient sustains a venomous snakebite. What is included in the current emergency first-aid treatment? *(1030-1031)*
   1. Wash the wound and lower the extremity.
   2. Apply suction to the area immediately after the bite.
   3. Make an incision over the wound with a sterile tool.
   4. Place a tourniquet above the wound and check the pulses.

9. A group of excited teenagers come to the walk-in clinic; they drag in an adolescent who is unresponsive. There are no obvious signs of injury or bleeding, but his skin is pale and clammy. What questions should the nurse initially ask? *(Select all that apply.)* *(1022-1023)*
   1. "Where are his parents?"
   2. "Does he have any allergies?"
   3. "What is his name?"
   4. "What happened to him?"
   5. "How long has he been like this?"
   6. "Why didn't you call 911?"
   7. "What was the group doing before he passed out?"

10. The nurse is at a community event and a child accidentally sustains a laceration with apparent arterial bleeding. The nurse's immediate action to control the bleeding is to: *(1023-1024)*
    1. apply pressure directly over the wound with the palm of the hand.
    2. place a sterile or clean dressing over the open wound.
    3. elevate the injured part and immobilize the child and the wound.
    4. periodically remove the original dressing to assess for active bleeding.

11. The nurse is making a home health visit to an elderly patient. The temperature in the house is very hot. The elderly patient is responsive, but confused. His skin is hot and dry and he says he feels weak and nauseous. What is the priority action? *(1026)*
    1. Take the patient's temperature and administer an antipyretic.
    2. Notify the physician and update the home health agency.
    3. Remove extra clothing and wipe the skin with cool water.
    4. Start an IV infusion of cool fluids and a cool saline lavage.

12. The patient is in cardiogenic shock secondary to a myocardial infarction. Which emergency treatment will the physician most likely order for this patient? *(1035-1036)*
    1. Fluid bolus and volume expanders
    2. Epinephrine and bronchodilators
    3. Isoproterenol, dopamine, or dobutamine
    4. Fluid bolus and corticosteroids

Copyright © 2013, 2009 by Saunders, an imprint of Elsevier Inc. All rights reserved.

13. An elderly patient is at high risk for septic shock. Which symptom is more frequently associated with shock in elderly patients compared to younger patients? *(1027, 1037-1038)*
    1. Decreased urinary output
    2. Tachycardia
    3. Hypothermia
    4. Slightly elevated temperature

14. The staff is attempting to de-escalate the behavior of a patient who is becoming increasingly upset and frustrated. What is the best approach? *(1041)*
    1. Several staff members should surround the patient.
    2. Allow a family member to privately speak to the patient.
    3. Restrain the patient to give a tranquilizing drug.
    4. Explain the purpose of any planned procedures.

15. The nurse has just completed a community presentation about ways to prevent hypothermia during cold weather outings. Which statement from an audience member demonstrates a need for additional teaching? *(1027-1028)*
    1. "Wearing a hat prevents heat loss through the head."
    2. "I should carry high-energy snacks in case I get lost."
    3. "I should wear or take layers of warm clothing."
    4. "If I get lost I should sit quietly to conserve energy."

CRITICAL THINKING ACTIVITIES

Scenario: You are working in the emergency department. The doctor orders IV fluids for several patients. The RN instructs you to go ahead and hang the fluids and calculate the pump settings.

1. Mrs. Sharon needs a maintenance IV of D$_5$0.45 NS 1000 mL to infuse over 8 hours. What is the pump setting? _____

2. Mr. Swan needs a fluid bolus 300 mL of normal saline over 30 minutes. What is the pump setting? _____

3. Ms. Phillo needs a fluid bolus 100 mL of 5% dextrose to infuse over 20 minutes. What is the pump setting? _____

4. Mr. Damon needs to receive 500 mL before he goes home to infuse at 125 mL/hour. What is the pump setting? _____
   How many hours will it take to complete the infusion? _____

5. When you are using an IV pump, how can you maximize the "volume to be infused" (VTBI) feature to increase the safe delivery of fluids?

_____

_____

_____

_____

Copyright © 2013, 2009 by Saunders, an imprint of Elsevier Inc. All rights reserved.

STEPS TOWARD BETTER COMMUNICATION

VOCABULARY BUILDING GLOSSARY

Term	Pronunciation	Definition
aspirate	as pi rayt'	foreign material becomes lodged in the airway of the respiratory system
battering	bat'ter ing	hitting often and repeatedly
combative	com bat'iv	wanting to fight or argue
corrosive	cor ro'siv	wearing away by chemical action
extremities	eks trem' ah teez	arms and hands, legs and feet
perfusion	per few'shun	passage of fluid through the organs or tissues
triage	tree ahzh'	a system for determining priority of need and order or location of treatment

COMPLETION

Directions: Fill in the blanks with the appropriate words from the Vocabulary Building Glossary to complete the statements.

1. The nurse must _____ patients carefully in order to determine priority and the correct area of treatment.

2. Children frequently _____ hot dogs or hard candy.

3. The patient who had sustained a head injury in the accident became _____ and started to fight with the nurse.

4. The nurse carefully checked all four _____ to see if there were any fractures.

5. There were bruises in various stages and cuts on the woman's body indicating that she was a victim of _____ .

6. The child was brought in by the emergency medical team because he had taken a drink of drain cleaner which is _____ .

7. A warm feeling to the foot, pinkish color, and the presence of a pedal pulse indicated that _____ was occurring in the leg and foot.

WORD ATTACK SKILLS

Word Meanings

Directions: For each word on the left, circle the word or phrase with the same meaning on the right.

1. cessa'tion: a period of time   stopping   hard and fast

2. deter'iorate: increase rapidly   change into bad condition   become smaller

Copyright © 2013, 2009 by Saunders, an imprint of Elsevier Inc. All rights reserved.

Word Elements

circum-   around

oral   mouth

Directions: Write the meaning of the word.

1.   circumoral: _____

PRONUNCIATION SKILLS

Directions: Practice pronouncing the words with a partner

a'queous epineph'rine (ay' kwee us e pin eh' freen)

venomous (VĔN- ō - mŭs)

COMMUNICATION EXERCISE

Directions: Use the information from Box 45-1 and talk to a friend or a family member about how to improve safety in the home. First try using the exact wording in Box 45-1, then try paraphrasing the same information. (Use your own words and style to give the same information.)

Copyright © 2013, 2009 by Saunders, an imprint of Elsevier Inc. All rights reserved.

Care of Patients with Anxiety, Mood, and Eating Disorders

Answer Key: Textbook page references are provided as a guide for answering these questions. A complete answer key was provided to your instructor.

COMPLETION

Directions: Fill in the blanks to complete the statements.

1. A(n) _____ is a recurrent or intrusive thought that the person cannot stop thinking about and these thoughts create anxiety. *(1047)*

2. Persons diagnosed with posttraumatic stress disorder have experienced _____ _____ that produce intense horror and recurrent symptoms of anxiety. *(1047)*

3. Dysthymic individuals feel a sense of _____ and _____ that cannot be alleviated by usual means. *(1051)*

4. The individual who switches from being extremely depressed to becoming manic has a(n) _____ disorder. *(1051)*

5. Two hallmarks of mood disorders are the _____ and _____. *(1058)*

6. The depressed patient may have _____ retardation. *(1055)*

7. A diagnosis of generalized anxiety disorder can only be made when the anxiety is present for at least _____ months. *(1047)*

8. Benzodiazepines are used cautiously for anxiety disorders because they are highly _____ _____. *(1048)*

9. _____ often mimics depressive symptoms. *(1055)*

10. _____ is a speech pattern where the speaker quickly switches from topic to topic and there is little or no connection or linkage of ideas. *(1051)*

Copyright © 2013, 2009 by Saunders, an imprint of Elsevier Inc. All rights reserved.

APPLICATION OF THE NURSING PROCESS

Anxiety

Directions: Read the clinical scenario and answer the questions that follow.

Scenario: A bus full of senior citizens is involved in a minor traffic accident in front of the clinic where you work. The emergency medical personnel have asked to use the clinic as a triage area and have also asked the clinic staff to assist by providing emotional support to the passengers until more help can arrive. One passenger appears to have a broken arm. The others have no obvious physical injuries; however, many of the passengers are very upset.

1. What are six physical signs of severe anxiety that you might expect to find? *(1045-1046, 1048-1049)*

   a. _____

   b. _____

   c. _____

   d. _____

   e. _____

   f. _____

2. List five feelings associated with severe anxiety that these passengers could be experiencing. *(1045-1046, 1048-1049)*

   a. _____

   b. _____

   c. _____

   d. _____

   e. _____

3. In the elderly, signs of severe anxiety are often somatic. What three signs might indicate severe anxiety in an elderly person? *(1050)*

   a. _____

   b. _____

   c. _____

4. What are three medical conditions that should be considered because they can mimic the signs of severe anxiety? *(1050)*

   a. _____

   b. _____

   c. _____

Copyright © 2013, 2009 by Saunders, an imprint of Elsevier Inc. All rights reserved.

5. Write a patient goal with outcome criterion for the following nursing diagnosis: Severe anxiety related to real or perceived threat. *(1050-1051)*

_____

_____

6. List three interventions that could be used to assist a passenger who is experiencing severe anxiety. *(1046-1050)*

    a. _____

    b. _____

    c. _____

7. Which behavior indicates that a passenger is responding to intervention for anxiety? *(1046-1050)*
    a. Passenger cries, but is able to answer questions appropriately.
    b. Passenger cries and repeatedly asks, "What happened to me?"
    c. Passenger is quiet and calm, but will not respond to any questions.
    d. Passenger is wandering around and looking for his car keys.

PRIORITY SETTING

Directions: Read the scenario and prioritize as appropriate.

Scenario: You are caring for several patients in an acute psychiatric admission ward. Mr. Loisi was admitted for major depression and demonstrates marked psychomotor retardation. Ms. Planto has bipolar disorder, and this morning she is very intrusive and loud. Mr. Salest was admitted for a severe episode of generalized anxiety disorder and suicidal ideations. Ms. Tomei has a long history of anorexia nervosa; she denies suicidal thoughts, but she has attempted suicide in the past. Mr. Blanchard was admitted for major depression. Prioritize the order in which the nurse should address the needs of these patients.

_____ a. Mr. Loisi had a bowel movement while sitting in the dayroom, but he will not get up and go to the shower.

_____ b. Ms. Planto is standing at the nurses' station yelling at the unit secretary.

_____ c. Mr. Salest appears secretive as he walks down the hall; he is carrying something large under his shirt.

_____ d. Ms. Tomei is doing jumping jacks and jogging around the unit.

_____ e. Mr. Blanchard is quiet and appears to be on the verge of crying.

REVIEW QUESTIONS FOR THE NCLEX® EXAMINATION

Directions: Choose the best answer(s) for the following questions.

1. When a patient is showing signs of severe anxiety and it is time for him to bathe and dress, it is best if the nurse: *(1046, 1050, Table 46-1)*
    1. leaves the patient alone.
    2. asks the patient why he is feeling so anxious.
    3. explain the rationale for practicing good hygiene.
    4. gives simple directions.

Copyright © 2013, 2009 by Saunders, an imprint of Elsevier Inc. All rights reserved.

2. Which symptoms are most characteristic of depression? *(1055)*
   1. Lack of interest, loss of libido, and flight of ideas
   2. Insomnia, poor hygiene, and grandiose ideas
   3. Overeating, hyperactivity, and rapid speech
   4. Insomnia, anorexia, and lack of energy

3. When communicating with a severely depressed patient, what is the most therapeutic approach? *(1058)*
   1. Be quiet while assisting with activities of daily living.
   2. Interact and talk with the patient and engage him in activities.
   3. Make an extra effort to be cheerful and positive.
   4. Speak in simple, direct sentences when necessary.

4. When planning care for a patient with a mood disorder, what is the highest priority? *(1058)*
   1. Encourage the expression of feelings.
   2. Engage in therapeutic interaction.
   3. Provide a safe environment.
   4. Orient the patient to time and place.

5. The nurse is doing discharge teaching for a manic patient. The patient asks, "Will I have to take lithium forever?" The best answer would be: *(1051)*
   1. "No, only until your symptoms are under control."
   2. "Yes, you will most likely need to take it for your lifetime."
   3. "Possibly your physician will let you discontinue after 4-6 months."
   4. "No, most patients can usually do without it after about a year."

6. Which medication is used to treat anxiety? *(1048)*
   1. Paroxetine (Paxil)
   2. Alprazolam (Xanax)
   3. Phenelzine (Nardil)
   4. Amitryptiline (Elavil)

7. In planning care for the depressed patient, the nurse is aware that the risk for self-harm actually increases when the: *(1058)*
   1. patient is discharged and has to care for himself.
   2. antidepressant medications begin to take effect.
   3. family promises, but fails, to visit him in the hospital.
   4. patient is first admitted and does not trust the staff.

8. An MAO inhibitor such as phenelzine (Nardil) may cause life-threatening: *(1056, Table 46-4)*
   1. respiratory distress.
   2. gastrointestinal bleeding.
   3. cardiac arrhythmias.
   4. hypertensive crisis.

9. The patient is admitted for anorexia nervosa. Which behaviors are most associated with this disorder? *(Select all that apply.) (1060)*
   1. Shifts food around the plate.
   2. Collects recipes.
   3. Makes elaborate meals for others.
   4. Has superstitions about food.
   5. Uses laxatives and vomits in secret.
   6. Practices excessive exercise.

Copyright © 2013, 2009 by Saunders, an imprint of Elsevier Inc. All rights reserved.

10. Which statement by the patient's family indicates the need for more teaching about the treatment of anorexia nervosa? *(1060-1061)*
    1. "If she'll just eat more, we can take her home and she'll be okay."
    2. "She will have to be hospitalized if she has dehydration or electrolyte imbalance."
    3. "Therapy could take between 1–6 years for this disorder."
    4. "Support groups and family therapy are important aspects of treatment."

11. The patient has bulimia nervosa. Which task would be appropriate to assign to the nursing assistant? *(1060-1061)*
    1. Observe for marks on the knuckles during AM hygiene.
    2. Listen outside the bathroom door for sounds of induced vomiting.
    3. Check the patient's belongings for secret caches of snacks and food.
    4. Escort the patient to group therapy or to occupational therapy.

12. A nurse is assessing a patient who has just returned to the unit after receiving electroconvulsive therapy (ECT). Which assessment finding is of greatest concern? *(1057)*
    1. Patient complains of a headache.
    2. Patient does not remember having ECT.
    3. Patient displays a cardiac dysrhythmia.
    4. Patient is disoriented to time.

13. The nurse is talking to an elderly patient who states, "Sometimes I wish that I just would fall asleep and never wake up again." What is the most therapeutic response? *(1060)*
    1. "Oh, don't say things like that, everyone would really miss you."
    2. "Are you thinking about committing suicide?"
    3. "Many people would agree that dying during sleep is the best way to go."
    4. "You seem a little sad today, is there anything I can do to help?"

14. The patient was given an SSRI about 60 minutes ago and is now having change of mental status, a rapid pulse, loss of muscular coordination, and hyperthermia. Which action should the nurse take first to address this life-threatening condition? *(1055-1056, Table 46-4)*
    1. Ensure that there is a patent IV access.
    2. Initiate seizure precautions.
    3. Obtain an order for anxiolytic medication.
    4. Prepare the emergency respiratory equipment.

15. A patient is in the manic phase of bipolar disorder. He is talking very loudly and starting to argue with other patients. Which intervention is the most appropriate to try *first*? *(1052-1053)*
    1. Instruct him to go sit down and watch television.
    2. Talk him for a walk down a quiet corridor.
    3. Invite him to play cards or board games.
    4. Advise him to lower his voice or lose privileges.

16. The nurse is teaching the patient about lithium carbonate. What information is appropriate to include in the teaching? *(Select all that apply.) (1051-1052, Table 46-3)*
    1. It takes 3–4 days to reach therapeutic levels.
    2. It helps to decrease the manic behavior.
    3. There is a small margin of safety between a therapeutic level and a toxic level.
    4. Maintain salt intake and drink adequate fluids; salt depletion may cause toxicity.
    5. Take the medication on an empty stomach.
    6. Do not become dehydrated.

Copyright © 2013, 2009 by Saunders, an imprint of Elsevier Inc. All rights reserved.

CRITICAL THINKING ACTIVITIES

Scenario A: Mr. Dell is brought to the clinic by a friend. He has been awake for 2 days and has ridden over 200 miles on a bicycle. Although he appears exhausted, he continues to pace around the waiting room, talking loudly, with rapid pressured speech and wild gestures.

1. Which nursing diagnosis is a priority for Mr. Dell? *(1051-1053)*
   a. Imbalanced nutrition, less than body requirements, related to shortened attention span while trying to eat
   b. Sleep deprivation related to hyperactivity
   c. Communication, impaired, related to flight of ideas and pressured speech
   d. Risk for injury to self or others related to impulsivity and hyperactivity

2. What are three therapeutic communication interventions that can be used in dealing with a patient in the manic phase? *(1052-1053)*

   a. _____

   b. _____

   c. _____

3. What are two ways you may be able to prevent further escalation of manic behavior in a patient? *(1052-1055)*

   a. _____

   b. _____

4. What strategies can you use to maintain your own patience, understanding and therapeutic efficacy with patients such as Mr. Dell? *(1052-1055)*

   _____

   _____

   _____

   _____

Scenario B: Dixie Jones is 33 years old. She appears to be slightly overweight and suffers from low self-esteem. After lunch, you and other coworkers can frequently hear her vomiting in the bathroom; however, she says she is okay and becomes embarrassed if anybody shows concern. You suspect that she might be bulimic.

1. Write a brief script that could be used to approach Dixie about your concerns. *(1060-1062)* _____

   _____

   _____

   _____

   _____

Copyright © 2013, 2009 by Saunders, an imprint of Elsevier Inc. All rights reserved.

2. What ethical obligations do you have toward a coworker with health problems? _____

_____

_____

_____

_____

_____

STEPS TOWARD BETTER COMMUNICATION

VOCABULARY BUILDING GLOSSARY

Term	Pronunciation	Definition
differentiate	dif er en' shee ate	to see differences
overwhelm'ing	o ver whelm'ing	more than a person can cope with
lethargy	leth'ar jee	extreme tiredness, lack of energy or interest
debilitating	de bil'i tay ting	weakening
elation	ee lay' shun	extreme happiness
recur	re kur'	happen again
somatic	so ma'tik	physical, referring to the body
mimic	mim'ik	act like, imitate
hypervigilant	hy per vij' ah lant	always watchful
escalate	es'ca layt	increase, go to higher levels
frivolity	frih vol' ah tee	light-hearted fun, silliness, gaiety
precipitate	pree sip' ah tayt	to cause to begin
deprivation	dep rah vay' shun	a condition of want and need
conducive	kon doo' siv	helping to cause or produce
lethality	lee thal' ah tee	degree of ability to cause death

COMPLETION

Directions: Fill in the blanks with the correct words from the Vocabulary Building Glossary to complete the statements.

1. Martha was experiencing _____ anxiety after her son was seriously injured and went to surgery.

2. People who are highly anxious may express more _____ complaints than others.

3. Psychotherapy is _____ to resolving moderate depression.

4. During the manic phase, the patient experiences _____.

Copyright © 2013, 2009 by Saunders, an imprint of Elsevier Inc. All rights reserved.

5. The death of her husband seemed to _____ a period of depression.

6. The depressed patient usually shows signs of _____ and is not interested in exercising.

7. Sometimes it is difficult to _____ between moderate and severe anxiety.

8. Side effects of some of the antidepressant drugs can _____ signs of a neurologic disorder such as Parkinson's disease.

9. When interacting with a patient who has expressed a plan for suicide, you must determine the _____ level.

10. Severe anxiety or severe depression can be _____ to a person's life.

11. Episodes of depression may _____.

12. The very anxious person often becomes _____, studying everyone in the immediate environment.

13. In a person with bipolar disorder, the manic phase can _____ quickly.

14. Patients with anxiety disorders may have experienced periods of _____ as children.

15. The patient who can once again engage in _____ is on the way to being well again.

WORD ATTACK SKILLS

Word Elements

The following word elements appear frequently in this chapter:

-thymia   condition of mind, mood
som/a-, somat/o-   body (physical versus mental)

CULTURAL POINT

Attitudes toward suicide vary. Some religions prohibit suicide, while others do not approve of suicide but feel it is an individual's choice, particularly if one is terminally ill and suffering. There is even an organization called the Hemlock Society that provides information and support for those considering suicide. The Hemlock Society's position is that a person has a right to control his or her own life and death. Their concern is "death with dignity." The nurse needs to explore his or her own feelings about suicide. When a patient's views differ from the nurse's views, the nurse must try to be nonjudgmental. It is important to recognize the differences in attitudes and beliefs that are found among various people.

Copyright © 2013, 2009 by Saunders, an imprint of Elsevier Inc. All rights reserved.

COMMUNICATION EERCISE

COMMUNICATION EXERCISE

The following dialogue is an example of one way to interact with a person who is expressing suicidal thoughts.

Patient: "I just can't live like this anymore. I'm going to escape this world and get out of this pain."

Nurse: "It sounds as if you might be planning to take your life. Is that what I am hearing you say?"

Patient: "Yes, I am thinking about it. I'm just not sure yet."

Nurse: "Do you have a plan in mind?"

Patient: "Pills would probably be the easiest way."

Nurse: "Do you have sufficient pills on hand to accomplish your plan? What do you have?"

Patient: "At the moment, I only have a couple of pain pills I and ran out of my antidepressants. I'll have to get some more."

The nurse determines that lethality is not high at the moment.

Nurse: "Have the antidepressants helped you at all?"

Patient: "Not much, and I have been taking them for about 3 weeks."

Nurse: "Antidepressants can take several weeks to work and depression may not resolve for several months. How about talking to your doctor about your medications?"

Patient: "Okay, I'll talk to him today. If I can get even a little pain relief, I'll be okay."

Nurse: "Let's talk tomorrow and you can tell me what the doctor says."

Copyright © 2013, 2009 by Saunders, an imprint of Elsevier Inc. All rights reserved.

Care of Patients with Substance Abuse Disorders

Answer Key: Textbook page references are provided as a guide for answering these questions. A complete answer key was provided to your instructor.

COMPLETION

Directions: Fill in the blanks to complete the statements.

1. It takes the body about _____ hour(s) to metabolize one standard drink. *(1068)*

2. In addition to alcohol, other central nervous system depressants include _____ and _____. *(1071)*

3. The greatest danger related to an opiate overdose is _____. *(1073)*

4. For successful rehabilitation of the heroin addict, in addition to long-term treatment, a change in _____ is essential. *(1073)*

5. Examples of commonly abused inhalants include glue, _____, _____, _____, and other types of solvents. *(1076)*

6. _____ are most frequently abused by teens and children because they are inexpensive and easily accessible. *(1076)*

SHORT ANSWER

Caring for a Patient with Cocaine Abuse

Directions: Read the clinical scenario and answer the questions that follow.

Scenario: Carrie Jacks, a 23-year-old secretary, started using cocaine as a recreational drug on weekends "just for fun." Within a very short time, Carrie started using cocaine after work and spending more time with friends who were also using increasingly larger amounts. On several occasions, Carrie's mother has called in sick for Carrie. Carrie's mother brings her to the clinic for vitamins and information about cocaine abuse "for a friend." You should collect data to determine Carrie's baseline knowledge about cocaine and to assess for signs and effects of substance abuse.

1. What are three effects of cocaine that Carrie could be experiencing? *(1074)*

    a. _____

    b. _____

    c. _____

Copyright © 2013, 2009 by Saunders, an imprint of Elsevier Inc. All rights reserved.

2. You are aware that different methods of using cocaine create different health issues. In what four ways is cocaine used? *(1074)*

   a. _____

   b. _____

   c. _____

   d. _____

3. What are two teaching points to share with Carrie about the risks of using cocaine? *(1074)*

   a. _____

   b. _____

4. What are four common feelings of family members who live with a substance-dependent person? *(1067, 1078)*

   a. _____

   b. _____

   c. _____

   d. _____

5. What two enabling behaviors has Carrie's mother demonstrated? *(1067)*

   a. _____

   b. _____

APPLICATION OF THE NURSING PROCESS

Caring for a Patient with Chronic Alcohol Abuse

Directions: Read the clinical scenario and answer the questions that follow.

Scenario: Mr. Briganti is a 56-year-old homeless man who frequently comes to the walk-in clinic for health care, and sometimes for food or a place to rest. He admits to chronic alcohol abuse and has expressed some thoughts of quitting, but has never followed up on referrals. Today, he is admitted to the hospital for severe malnutrition and electrolyte imbalances. He admits to drinking heavily just before going to the clinic.

1. The diagnosis of alcohol dependence is based on what criteria? *(1068)*

   a. _____

   b. _____

   c. _____

   d. _____

   e. _____

Copyright © 2013, 2009 by Saunders, an imprint of Elsevier Inc. All rights reserved.

2. When assessing Mr. Briganti for a substance abuse problem, what are three things you should ask about substance abuse during history-taking? *(1076)*

   a. _____

   b. _____

   c. _____

3. Name three goals of care for a patient with a substance abuse disorder. *(1077, 1079-1081, Nursing Care Plan 47-1)*

   a. _____

   b. _____

   c. _____

4. What is the priority diagnosis for Mr. Briganti? *(1077, 1079-1081, Nursing Care Plan 47-1)*
   a. Noncompliance related to abstinence from substance
   b. Injury, risk for, related to alcohol consumption/withdrawal
   c. Home maintenance management, impaired, related to homelessness
   d. Imbalanced nutrition, less than body requirements, related to excessive alcohol consumption and self-neglect

5. Early symptoms of alcohol withdrawal (anxiety, irritability, and agitation) may manifest as early as: *(1068)*
   a. 1–2 hours after the last drink.
   b. 6–12 hours after the last drink.
   c. 24–48 hours after the last drink.
   d. 2–3 days after the last drink.

6. Write a sample outcome statement for Risk for injury related to complications of withdrawal from alcohol. *(1077, 1079-1081, Nursing Care Plan 47-1)*

   _____

   _____

7. Give three nursing interventions to prevent injuries related to complications of withdrawal from alcohol. *(1077-1078)*

   a. _____

   b. _____

   c. _____

8. The doctor orders a 500 mL fluid bolus of dextrose 5% with normal saline to infuse over 90 minutes for Mr. Briganti. What is the pump setting? _____ mL

9. Which task would be appropriate to assign to the nursing student in providing the care for Mr. Briganti? *(1078)*
   a. IV insertion with your supervision.
   b. Telephoning the doctor to give lab results.
   c. Assessing Mr. Briganti for Risk for injury.
   d. Talking to Mr. Briganti about the alcohol abuse.

Copyright © 2013, 2009 by Saunders, an imprint of Elsevier Inc. All rights reserved.

PRIORITY SETTING

Prioritizing for a Patient with Alcohol Withdrawal

Directions: Read the clinical scenario and prioritize as appropriate.

Scenario: You are caring for a patient who has a history of chronic alcohol abuse. It has been approximately 8 hours since the patient last had a drink. You are vigilant for the signs of withdrawal. The patient currently has a blood pressure of 160/85, pulse 110. Place the interventions in the order of priority. *(1068, 1077-1078)*

_____ a. Orient the patient to person, place, and time.

_____ b. IV fluids are administered to correct dehydration as ordered.

_____ c. Encourage a balanced diet high in proteins and multivitamins.

_____ d. Give chlordiazepoxide HCl (Librium) as ordered.

_____ e. Establish IV access.

REVIEW QUESTIONS FOR THE NCLEX® EXAMINATION

Directions: Choose the best answer(s) for the following questions.

1. What are the two main defense mechanisms used by substance abusers? *(1066-1067)*
   1. Repression and regression
   2. Sublimation and splitting
   3. Denial and rationalization
   4. Displacement and identification

2. The patient is taking lorazepam (Ativan) for anxiety. The nurse advises him not to drink alcohol while taking this drug for which reason? *(1069)*
   1. There is an increase in blood pressure caused by frequent use.
   2. There is an additive effect on the nervous system.
   3. There is a decrease in therapeutic response caused by frequent use.
   4. There is increased risk for insomnia and gastrointestinal distress.

3. The nurse is caring for an elderly patient who is prescribed triazolam (Halcion) for insomnia. Benzodiazepines must be used cautiously in the elderly because: *(1072)*
   1. they have a long half-life and are not excreted readily.
   2. they are toxic to the aging endocrine system.
   3. tolerance causes use of increasing doses.
   4. they may be used along with alcohol.

4. The nurse is caring for a patient with a history of substance abuse. What is the most important intervention in the initial treatment of the substance-abuse patient? *(1077-1078)*
   1. Careful detoxification procedures
   2. Sympathetic care by all health professionals
   3. Medical diagnosis of dependence on the substance
   4. Regular participation in a 12-step program

5. Which assessment should the nurse perform in order to prevent a life-threatening complication of CNS stimulant withdrawal? *(1074, 1078)*
   1. Observe frequently for respiratory depression.
   2. Monitor for cardiac dysrhythmias.
   3. Monitor urinary output.
   4. Watch for bleeding signs.

Copyright © 2013, 2009 by Saunders, an imprint of Elsevier Inc. All rights reserved.

6. During the physical assessment, the nurse notices bruises and needle marks on the patient's antecubital space. What is the best response? *(1076-1077)*
   1. "What are these marks? Are you injecting IV drugs?"
   2. "I am going to ask the doctor to look at your arms."
   3. "I see you have some bruises. Can you tell me what happened?"
   4. "Let me clean and bandage your arm to prevent infection."

7. The nurse is talking to the patient's mother about enabling. Which statement by the mother indicates that additional intervention is needed for the enabling behavior? *(1067)*
   1. "I am going to let her take responsibility for her decisions."
   2. "I'm her mother, I'll always be there for her no matter what."
   3. "We have all been denying the problem for a long time."
   4. "I will support her recovery by attending Al-Anon."

8. A patient with CNS stimulant abuse displays agitation and aggression. Which medication is the physician most likely to prescribe to address these symptoms? *(1069)*
   1. Methylphenidate (Ritalin)
   2. Lorazepam (Ativan)
   3. Ondansetron (Zofran)
   4. Naloxone (Narcan)

9. The doctor has ordered large doses of thiamine for the patient. This treatment is appropriate for which of condition? *(1071)*
   1. Wernicke's encephalopathy
   2. Korsakoff's syndrome
   3. Opiate overdose
   4. Methamphetamine abuse

10. The nurse is assisting the alcohol abuse patient to plan activities that will help him to maintain a healthy lifestyle after he is discharged from the hospital. *(Select all that apply.) (1070-1071, 1081-1082)*
    1. Remind the patient that the physical symptoms of withdrawal will not last forever.
    2. Help him to make a list of activities that would distract him from the cravings.
    3. Ask him to contact old drinking buddies to tell them that he has stopped using.
    4. Encourage him to socialize with an old drinking buddy and talk about happier times.
    5. Participate actively and frequently in a 12-step program.

11. The nurse believes that another nurse is "stealing" narcotic doses from the patients and self-injecting the medication. What should the nurse do *first*? *(1067)*
    1. Follow the nurse around to verify suspicions.
    2. Confront the nurse and ask for an explanation.
    3. Ask the patients if they are getting pain relief.
    4. Ask a supervisor to give advice about the situation.

12. A patient with a chronic substance abuse problem has a nursing diagnosis of Ineffective denial related to psychological dependence. Which outcome statement is most appropriate? *(1079-1080)*
    1. Patient will stop denying dependence on substances.
    2. Patient will list three negative effects that substances have on his life.
    3. Patient will decrease substance use in 2 weeks.
    4. Patient will talk to wife about reasons for substance abuse.

13. Which social situation most strongly indicates that a recovering alcoholic needs to be advised to call his Alcoholics Anonymous sponsor? *(1071)*
    1. There is an after work get-together where alcohol will be served.
    2. A friend is getting married and the toasting will be done with champagne.
    3. A weekend hunting trip with friends will include beer and other liquors.
    4. A niece is having a birthday party and her father always drinks.

Copyright © 2013, 2009 by Saunders, an imprint of Elsevier Inc. All rights reserved.

14. The nurse is caring for a patient on a medical-surgical unit. The patient admits to being a heavy drinker. What is an early symptom of alcohol withdrawal? *(1068)*
    1. Slurred speech
    2. Anxiety
    3. Diaphoresis
    4. Hallucinations

15. The nurse is talking to a teenager who says, "Marijuana is not that big of a deal. It should be legalized." What is the best response? *(1075-1077)*
    1. "Actually marijuana is a gateway substance that can lead to more serious drug use."
    2. "Well, marijuana does help control nausea for chemotherapy patients."
    3. "You should really talk to your parents about this and get their opinions."
    4. "So, it sounds like you have some first-hand experience with marijuana."

CRITICAL THINKING ACTIVITIES

Scenario: You are asked to help develop a community presentation about smoking cessation. One of your tasks is to collect some accurate information that can be used in the presentation.

1. Two serious long-term results of smoking nicotine that may occur are: *(1075)*
   a. addiction to nicotine and impaired coordination.
   b. low blood pressure and cardiac arrhythmias.
   c. stained teeth and bad breath.
   d. lung cancer and emphysema.

2. What are three physical changes that nicotine causes? *(1075)* _____

   _____

   _____

   _____

3. What are the withdrawal symptoms? *(1075)* _____

   _____

   _____

   _____

4. What treatments are available for nicotine addiction? *(1075)* _____

   _____

   _____

   _____

Copyright © 2013, 2009 by Saunders, an imprint of Elsevier Inc. All rights reserved.

STEPS TOWARD BETTER COMMUNICATION

VOCABULARY BUILDING GLOSSARY

Term	Pronunciation	Definition
alleviate	ah lee' vee ayt	make easier or less severe
arousal level	ah row' zel lev' el	ease with which a person can be awakened
denial	dee ny' al	a defense mechanism in which a person will not admit unpleasant or painful realities
diminish	di min' ish	become less, get smaller
eradicate	eh rad'i cayt	get rid of; remove
foster	fos'ter	encourage and help
withdrawal	with drawl'	a group of symptoms that are present when a person stops using a drug
enabling	en ayb'ling	making something easier; doing something for someone that he could do for himself; acting so that one person supports another person's behavior
self-righteous	self ry' chus	very sure that oneself is right and has the correct answers
stigma	stig'ma	a mark of shame

WORD ATTACK SKILLS

Word Meanings

Directions: Underline the correct word in each pair to complete the sentence with the correct meaning.

1. Buying alcohol for an alcoholic spouse who has drunk too much is an example of (self-righteous / enabling) behavior.

2. Extreme jumpiness and nervousness can be a symptom of (denial / withdrawal) from alcohol in the hospitalized patient.

3. Joining a 12-step group such as Alcoholics Anonymous will help (foster / eradicate) a person's decision to stop drinking.

Number Words in Order

Directions: Number these words in order, with the strongest word first.

_____ a. alleviate

_____ b. diminish

_____ c. eradicate

Copyright © 2013, 2009 by Saunders, an imprint of Elsevier Inc. All rights reserved.

Word Elements

Directions: The following words from Chapter 47 end in the word element -tion. This ending usually indicates the result of an action. In each word defined below, identify the base word, define the base word, and give the whole word's part of speech.

1. Predisposi'tion—being more vulnerable or likely to attain something:

    _____

    _____

2. Rationaliza'tion—an unconscious defense mechanism in which a person finds logical reasons for his actions while ignoring the real:

    _____

    _____

3. Valida'tion—showing approval, agreeing to the correctness or appropriateness of an action:

    _____

    _____

PRONUNCIATION SKILLS

Directions: Beneath each "s" in the following words write "s" or "z" to show how the letter "s" should be pronounced.

1. predisposition

2. arousal

COMMUNICATION EXERCISE

With a partner, practice asking and answering the questions in Focused Assessment on p. 1076 in the textbook. Ask for clarification if you do not understand the pronunciation or meaning of what your partner is saying.

Copyright © 2013, 2009 by Saunders, an imprint of Elsevier Inc. All rights reserved.

Student Name_____ Date_____

Care of Patients with Cognitive Disorders

chapter

48

Answer Key: Textbook page references are provided as a guide for answering these questions. A complete answer key was provided to your instructor.

TERMINOLOGY

Directions: Match the term on the right with the meaning on the left.

1. _____ Delirium *(1085)*

2. _____ Cognition *(1085)*

3. _____ Dementia *(1085)*

4. _____ Confabulation *(1086)*

5. _____ Global amnesia *(1097)*

6. _____ Delusion *(1086)*

7. _____ Wandering *(1098)*

8. _____ Sundowning *(1094)*

a. Becoming confused and disoriented only at night

b. Making up conversation to fill gaps in memory

c. Acute confusion

d. Deficit in memory and other cognitive areas

e. Leaving a place or moving with no plan

f. Unable to recall events, or remember friends and family

g. Belief in a false idea

h. Mental processes of perception, memory, judgment, and reasoning

COMPLETION

Delirium and Dementia

Directions: Fill in the blanks to complete the statements.

1. The patient experiencing delirium may demonstrate disorganized and distorted thinking and incoherent _____. *(1086)*

2. One of the first things you should assess in a patient who is exhibiting signs of delirium is what _____ the patient is receiving. *(1086)*

3. A difference between delirium and dementia is that dementia occurs over a(n) _____ _____. *(1085-1086)*

4. The most common degenerative disease of the brain is _____. *(1087)*

5. For elders, medications should be given in the _____ amounts possible and increased when the symptoms indicate. *(1086)*

Copyright © 2013, 2009 by Saunders, an imprint of Elsevier Inc. All rights reserved.

SHORT ANSWER

Caring for a Patient with Acute Confusion

Directions: Read the clinical scenario and answer the questions that follow.

Scenario: Mr. James is an elderly man who resides at an assisted-living facility. Although he is occasionally forgetful, he is usually alert and cheerful and enjoys telling stories about his family and his career in the military. He is able to function with minimal assistance. The nursing assistant tells you that today Mr. James seems drowsy, disoriented, and extremely irritable.

1. Name four types of medications that could be causing Mr. James' change in behavior. *(1086)*

   a. _____

   b. _____

   c. _____

   d. _____

2. What five areas are involved in a quick assessment for delirium and dementia? *(1093-1094)*

   a. _____

   b. _____

   c. _____

   d. _____

   e. _____

3. What are five possible causes of acute confusion? *(1085)*

   a. _____

   b. _____

   c. _____

   d. _____

   e. _____

4. List five things you can do to help decrease Mr. James' confusion using reality orientation. *(1096)*

   a. _____

   b. _____

   c. _____

   d. _____

   e. _____

Copyright © 2013, 2009 by Saunders, an imprint of Elsevier Inc. All rights reserved.

APPLICATION OF THE NURSING PROCESS

Caring for a Patient with Alzheimer's Disease

Directions: Provide the answers to the following questions.

Scenario: Mr. Thompson, age 85, lives with his daughter Jane. He was diagnosed with Alzheimer's disease several years ago. Jane is concerned because her father left the house last week and he was missing for several hours before the neighbor helped him back to the house. Jane also reports that her father has not recognized her on several occasions.

1. The doctor has told Jane that her father may begin to have signs of moderate Alzheimer's. List four of the behaviors associated with moderate Alzheimer's. *(1087, Box 48-1)*

   a. _____

   b. _____

   c. _____

   d. _____

2. Jane reports that her father has been losing weight and that she has to remind him to eat and sometimes she even has to feed him. She tells you that, "When Dad was younger, he used to weigh over 250 lbs. and now he is down to about 145 lbs. Convert Mr. Thompson's current weight to kg. _____

3. Which nursing diagnosis would be a priority for Mr. Thompson? *(1089)*
   a. Confusion, chronic, related to slow progressive memory loss
   b. Confusion, acute, related to biochemical changes in the brain
   c. Social interaction, impaired, related to inability to recognize friends and family
   d. Injury, risk for, related to faulty judgment
   e. Wandering related to disorientation to time and place
   f. Risk for caregiver role strain related to prolonged 24-hour responsibility to give care

4. List three ways in which you can help Jane to reduce her own stress. *(1098)*

   a. _____

   b. _____

   c. _____

5. For a patient who is confused or tends to wander, list five teaching points to share with the caregiver to ensure the patient's safety. *(1092, Nursing Care Plan 48-1)*

   a. _____

   b. _____

   c. _____

   d. _____

   e. _____

Copyright © 2013, 2009 by Saunders, an imprint of Elsevier Inc. All rights reserved.

6. Which statement indicates that Jane understands how to manage Mr. Thompson's confusion? *(1095)*
   a. "If I repeat time, date, and year every morning, he will become oriented to time."
   b. "I'll use several different caregivers; he will be stimulated by other faces."
   c. "I'll provide general orientation to the year by using holiday decorations."
   d. "We'll have big family parties every weekend, just like we used to."

PRIORITY SETTING

Directions: Read the scenario and prioritize as appropriate.

Scenario: You are working in an extended-care facility. You have just received shift report on your six patients. Indicate the order in which you would attend to the needs of these patients.

_____ a. It is the scheduled time for Mr. Jeandron's AM insulin.

_____ b. Mrs. Slipik is more confused today than she usually is.

_____ c. Mr. Motton has a complaint about the night-shift nurse.

_____ d. Mr. Tize has a low-grade fever.

_____ e. Mrs. Palabo has fallen in the bathroom.

_____ f. Mr. Newton is asking for his scheduled pain medication.

REVIEW QUESTIONS FOR THE NCLEX® EXAMINATION

Directions: Choose the best answer(s) for the following questions.

1. The nurse is caring for a patient with Alzheimer's. Which signs and symptoms are associated with mild Alzheimer's? *(1087, Box 48-1)*
   1. Slow, progressive loss of intellectual ability and difficulty learning new things
   2. Unable to speak or ambulate and profound memory loss
   3. Social withdrawal and decreased in ability to perform usual activities of daily living
   4. Outbursts of anger, hostility, paranoia, and wandering

2. What factors cause elderly patients to be at risk for substance-induced delirium? *(1086)*
   1. Increased metabolism and reduction in cardiac and liver function
   2. Decreased metabolism and reduction in cardiac and respiratory function
   3. Decreased metabolism and reduction in kidney and liver function
   4. Increased metabolism and reduction in neurologic and immune function

3. During data collection, the patient's son tells the nurse, "Mom can remember her name, but she doesn't seem to know where she is." Based on this information, which question should the nurse ask *first*? *(1088-1089)*
   1. "How does she like to be addressed?"
   2. "When did you first notice this?"
   3. "What kind of medications does she take?"
   4. "When did she last see the doctor?"

4. The patient is suffering acute delirium related to a systemic infection. During the evening, the patient appears to be very frightened by the IV tubing. The nurse recognizes that the patient might be experiencing which disturbance? *(1086)*
   1. Hallucination
   2. Illusion
   3. Delusion
   4. Confabulation

Copyright © 2013, 2009 by Saunders, an imprint of Elsevier Inc. All rights reserved.

5. A 25-year-old patient is brought to the emergency department by the police. He is a poor historian, but the police tell the nurse that they were called because he was wandering down the middle of the freeway. He appears confused, disheveled, and malnourished. Which nursing diagnosis on the care plan would be of highest priority for this patient? *(1089, 1093)*
    1. Bathing/hygiene/feeding self-care deficit
    2. Wandering related to disorientation to time and place
    3. Injury, risk for, related to impaired decision-making
    4. Imbalanced nutrition, less than body requirements

6. The nurse is caring for a patient in the moderate Alzheimer's. In planning care, the nurse should anticipate the need for which intervention? *(1087, 1093)*
    1. Repeat the date and time frequently.
    2. Restrain the patient to protect from falls and wandering.
    3. Vary routine and provide unstructured environment.
    4. Allot extra time for grooming and toileting.

7. The nurse is working on a busy medical-surgical unit. An elderly patient has fallen out of bed twice, despite repeated verbal instructions to call for assistance. What are appropriate interventions to ensure safety? *(Select all that apply.)* *(1095-1097)*
    1. Encourage family members and friends to stay with the patient.
    2. Obtain an order for an anxiolytic medication.
    3. Keep patient close to the nurse's station.
    4. Check on patient frequently to offer nutrition, fluids, pain relief, and toileting.
    5. Place the bed in the lowest position with three side rails up.
    6. Temporarily place restraints and secure knots to the bedrails.
    7. Advise the patient that the hospital is not liable if he refuses to cooperate.

8. The doctor has ordered that the patient be restrained for 24 hours because he is a danger to self or others. Which task is appropriate to assign to the nursing assistant? *(1096)*
    1. Selecting the type of restraint.
    2. Checking the circulation in the area distal to the restraint.
    3. Performing 1:1 observation.
    4. Obtaining consent from the patient's family to use restraints.

9. The nursing student is assisting the nurse to apply restraints to a patient. Which action by the student indicates that she understands the procedure? *(1097, Box 48-4)*
    1. She checks the circulation and then applies the restraints.
    2. She ties the knot so that it is not readily visible to the patient, family, or staff.
    3. She states that she will check on the patient every 2–4 hours.
    4. She documents the care that was given while the patient was in restraints.

10. The patient is prescribed donepezil (Aricept). Which statement by the patient's wife indicates that she understands the information about the drug? *(1089, Table 48-1)*
    1. "It slows progression of symptoms, but is not a cure."
    2. "If he takes the medication, the symptoms will resolve."
    3. "This medicine may improve memory, but it is experimental."
    4. "The side effects include headaches and blurred vision."

11. The nurse is planning care for a patient with a cognitive disorder. Which task can be assigned to the nursing assistant? *(1093, 1096)*
    1. Determine which patients need assistance with hygienic care.
    2. Evaluate the patients' responses to reality orientation therapy.
    3. Assist patients to ambulate in hall or enclosed courtyard.
    4. Observe patients for changes in mental status during the shift.

Copyright © 2013, 2009 by Saunders, an imprint of Elsevier Inc. All rights reserved.

12. A patient is experiencing acute delirium with confusion related to medication side effects. What is the best environmental intervention to use with this patient? *(1089, 1093, 1095)*
    1. Turn on a favorite television program to provide a familiar distraction.
    2. Ask several family members to come and talk about everyday topics.
    3. Put the patient close to the nurse's station with the door open.
    4. Assign a nursing assistant to observe 1-to-1 in a quiet room.

13. The nurse is making a home visit to an elderly patient with Alzheimer's. The patient's wife says, "Jim is more confused compared to usual." What is the best response? *(1098)*
    1. "It's hard to see someone that you love deteriorate."
    2. "What kind of changes are you seeing?"
    3. "When was the last time your husband saw a doctor?"
    4. "With Alzheimer's, the symptoms do worsen."

14. The nurse hears in report that a patient has global amnesia. The nurse will allot extra time for which intervention? *(1097)*
    1. Talking about family members and their recent visits
    2. Reminiscing about family holidays and past events
    3. Reorienting to person, place, and time
    4. Placing signs and arrows to the bathroom and dining room

15. An elderly patient with mild dementia has demonstrated ability to feed himself, perform toileting independently, and dress himself; however, he frequently says, "You do it for me." What should the nurse do to encourage independence? *(1090-1091, Nursing Care Plan 48-1)*
    1. Instruct him to try and then come back later to see what he has accomplished.
    2. Verbally coach him through the task and observe his performance.
    3. Point out to him that he needs to be independent for as long as possible.
    4. Ask him why he frequently does not want to do things for himself.

CRITICAL THINKING ACTIVITIES

Scenario: You are working at an extended-care facility. In report, you hear that Mr. Kuapoo was restrained during the night for "inappropriate behavior." When you check the chart, you cannot find any order for restraints and the documentation does not include any details about the behavior, the type of restraints, or the care given while the patient was in the restraints.

1. What is your first action? *(1096-1097)*
   a. Call the doctor and obtain an order for restraints.
   b. Call the nurse at home and ask for details.
   c. Report the incident to the nursing supervisor.
   d. Assess the patient and remove the restraints.

2. During the report, what information should be clarified with the nurse before he or she leaves? *(1096-1097)*

_____

_____

_____

_____

Copyright © 2013, 2009 by Saunders, an imprint of Elsevier Inc. All rights reserved.

3. What are your ethical obligations in this situation? What are the ramifications of following through? *(1096-1097)*

_____

_____

_____

_____

_____

_____

STEPS TOWARD BETTER COMMUNICATION

VOCABULARY BUILDING GLOSSARY

Term	Pronunciation	Definition
cognition	kog ni' shun	the mental process of thinking, perceiving, and remembering
confabulation	kon fab u la' shun	inventing or making up untrue or exaggerated stories and answers to questions
abstract	ab strakt'	not concrete, not material, or not physical; (noun) ideas or theories with no specific application
respite care	res'pit care	short-term care to give relief to the family caregiver for an afternoon or weekend
insight	in' site	ability to see and understand the truth about something
blunted	blun'ted	not sharp; not perceptive; plain and flat
remote memory	ree mot' memory	distant in time, long ago
advance directives	ad vans' di rek' tivz	instructions about what to do in case of medical emergencies, incapacity, and death; may include power of attorney
confront	kon front	to talk face to face about difficult problems, sometimes argumentatively

COMPLETION

Directions: Fill in the blanks with the appropriate words from the Vocabulary Building Glossary to complete the statements.

1. A patient suffering from advanced Alzheimer's disease generally has a(n) _____ affect.

2. When dementia is present, the patient has difficulty comprehending _____ ideas.

Copyright © 2013, 2009 by Saunders, an imprint of Elsevier Inc. All rights reserved.

3. When patients begin to have great difficulty with memory, they tend to make things up in order to fill gaps; this is called _____.

4. As dementia worsens, _____ decreases, although long-term memory may remain intact.

5. The family caregiver of an Alzheimer's patient badly needs occasional _____ _____ for the patient.

6. A patient who frequently loses his way does not usually have any _____ as to why this is happening to him, and is frightened.

7. The dementia patient often has difficulty with recent memory but can remember things from childhood that reside in _____.

8. All adults should have _____ in place, in case an accident or illness incapacitates them.

SHORT ANSWER

Memory Examples

Directions: Give two examples each of immediate memory, recent memory, and remote memory.

1. Immediate memory:

   e.g., I just drank a cup of coffee.

   a. _____

   b. _____

2. Recent memory:

   a. _____

   b. _____

3. Remote memory:

   a. _____

   b. _____

Copyright © 2013, 2009 by Saunders, an imprint of Elsevier Inc. All rights reserved.

WORD ATTACK SKILLS

Word Meanings

Directions: Match the adjectives on the left with their correct meanings on the right.

1. _____ Impaired
2. _____ Fragmented
3. _____ Incoherent
4. _____ Disturbed
5. _____ Disoriented
6. _____ Distorted
7. _____ Disorganized
8. _____ Diminished

a. Changed from its true nature or shape
b. Damaged
c. Divided in pieces
d. Less, smaller
e. Not certain of time, place, or identity
f. Not making sense
g. Upset, worried; not normal
h. Without an order or system

PRONUNCIATION SKILLS

Directions: Put the following words in the correct column depending on whether the pronunciation of "-ed" in the word is -id, -d, or -t.

blunted, diminished, disorganized, disoriented, distorted, disturbed, fragmented, impaired

-id	-d	-t

Copyright © 2013, 2009 by Saunders, an imprint of Elsevier Inc. All rights reserved.

COMMUNICATION EXERCISE

Scenario: Mr. Jones is trying to leave the unit. He repeatedly walks towards the door, saying that he has to go to work. The nursing assistant has called you to intervene because Mr. Jones is becoming increasingly agitated and will not move away from the door.

Distraction is the first method to be used, then negotiation.

Nurse:	"Mr. Jones, I'm Sandra, the charge nurse on this unit. Did you enjoy your breakfast this morning?"
Mr. Jones:	"Well, I guess it was OK."
Nurse:	"Let's talk a walk together down to the common room. There is a group activity going on."
Mr. Jones:	"That would be nice, but I have to go to work now.
"**Nurse:**	"Well, there are some people here that really need your help and advice. They would like to see you now."
Mr. Jones:	"Okay, I guess I could see them now. "
"**Nurse:**	"I know they will appreciate seeing you."

CULTURAL POINT

The elderly often have difficulty with recent memory but like to talk about pleasant memories from the past. Conversation with them might be directed at childhood memories of holidays and special vacations or events. Various foods, smells, and pieces of music may remind them of such times. The nurse's own life can be enriched by sharing of memories.

Copyright © 2013, 2009 by Saunders, an imprint of Elsevier Inc. All rights reserved.

Care of Patients with Thought and Personality Disorders

chapter
49

Answer Key: Textbook page references are provided as a guide for answering these questions. A complete answer key was provided to your instructor.

TERMINOLOGY

Thought Disorders

Directions: Match the term on the left with the correct definition or statement on the right.

1. _____ Psychotic features *(1102)*
2. _____ Delusions of grandeur *(1104)*
3. _____ Hallucination *(1102)*
4. _____ Word salad *(1109)*
5. _____ Ideas of reference *(1104)*
6. _____ Neologisms *(1109)*
7. _____ Illusion *(1104)*
8. _____ Flat affect *(1104)*
9. _____ Delusion *(1102)*
10. _____ Alogia *(1104)*

a. Person has an inflated notion of self-importance despite logical reasoning
b. Absence or near-absence of emotional expression
c. Misinterpretation of reality
d. Sensory perception without a corresponding stimulus
e. The person feels that objects, events, or people in his environment have an unusual significance only for him
f. Disorganized mix of words, phrases, and fragments that do not make sense
g. Hallucinations, delusions, and disorganized speech or behavior
h. Made-up new words for expressing confused thoughts
i. False fixed belief
j. Poverty of thoughts

COMPLETION

Schizophrenia

Directions: Fill in the blanks to complete the sentences.

1. When assessing thought disorders, the interview must be _____ because it is difficult for the individual to _____ for very long. *(1108)*

2. Schizophrenia usually develops in _____ or in the early _____. *(1103)*

3. A schizophrenic's behavior can cause vulnerability to psychosocial problems. These include _____, _____, _____, and _____. *(1106)*

4. Examples of atypical antipsychotic medications which are used to treat schizophrenia include _____, _____, and _____. *(1105, Box 49-1)*

Copyright © 2013, 2009 by Saunders, an imprint of Elsevier Inc. All rights reserved.

5. Because of the negative symptoms of _____ and _____, elderly schizophrenics are not as likely to seek help. *(1104, 1116)*

SHORT ANSWERS

Thought Disorders

Directions: Read the clinical scenario and answer the questions that follow.

Scenario: Ms. Lalani, age 45, was diagnosed with schizophrenia at age 21. She is frequently admitted to the psychiatric unit for relapse. Currently, she is delusional and verbally hostile. Her appearance is disheveled and she wears layers of clothes inside out and backward. She has a flat affect and sits by herself, talking and gesturing to the air. In the past, she has been prescribed the conventional antipsychotic medication thioridazine (Mellaril). The doctor is trying to give her ziprasidone (Geodon) to see if her symptoms can be controlled by one of the newer medications.

1. List six desirable outcomes for the negative symptoms of schizophrenia. *(1104)*

   a. _____

   b. _____

   c. _____

   d. _____

   e. _____

   f. _____

2. What are four assessment findings for Ms. Lalani that suggest that she has a thought disorder? *(1102)*

   a. _____

   b. _____

   c. _____

   d. _____

3. Which nursing diagnoses would be appropriate for Ms. Lalani and are likely to be included in her plan of care? *(Select all that apply.) (1108)*
   a. Communication, impaired
   b. Sensory perceptions, altered
   c. Activity intolerance
   d. Social isolation
   e. Bathing/hygiene/feeding self-care deficit
   f. Risk for other-directed or self-directed violence
   g. Dysfunctional grieving

4. What are three nursing interventions for patients with Altered thought processes related to delusional thinking? *(1109-1112, Nursing Care Plan 49-1)*

   a. _____

   b. _____

   c. _____

Copyright © 2013, 2009 by Saunders, an imprint of Elsevier Inc. All rights reserved.

5. What signs and symptoms should you look for when assessing for extrapyramidal or neuromuscular side effects that are associated with antipsychotic medications? *(1105-1108, Table 49-2)*

a. Pseudoparkinsonism: _____

_____

b. Dystonic reaction: _____

_____

c. Akathisia: _____

_____

d. Tardive dyskinesia: _____

_____

_____

_____

6. List six common anticholinergic side effects that are seen with the use of antipsychotic medications. *(1105-1108, Table 49-2)*

a. _____

b. _____

c. _____

d. _____

e. _____

f. _____

7. The doctor orders a maximum fluid intake of 2500 mL of water/24 hours, because Ms. Lalani is known to drink excessive water and this puts her at risk for hyponatremia. Convert 2500 mL into the total number of 8-ounce glasses of water that Ms. Lalani is allowed to drink. _____ glasses

APPLICATION OF THE NURSING PROCESS

Caring for a Patient with Schizophrenia

Directions: Read the scenario and choose the best answer(s) for the following questions.

Scenario: Mr. Hinton is a 25-year-old patient who was recently admitted with the diagnosis of schizophrenia. The police were called to a local restaurant because Mr. Hinton had barricaded himself in the men's room and was yelling about terrorists. He is disheveled and appears suspicious and distrustful.

1. In report, the nurse states that Mr. Hinton displays positive symptoms of schizophrenia. Which symptoms are considered positive symptoms? *(1103-1104)*
   a. Delusions and hallucinations
   b. Self-care deficits and lack of motivation
   c. Blunted affect and poverty of speech
   d. Social withdrawal and manipulative behavior

Copyright © 2013, 2009 by Saunders, an imprint of Elsevier Inc. All rights reserved.

2. You observe Mr. Hinton. He is standing in a corner by himself and suddenly he puts his hands over his ears and begins to sway back and forth. You hear him say "Shut up, just stop it, shut up!" What does this behavior suggest? *(1103)*
   a. Mr. Hinton is seeking attention.
   b. Mr. Hinton is displaying echolalia.
   c. Mr. Hinton is experiencing a drug side-effect.
   d. Mr. Hinton is having an auditory hallucination.

3. Mr. Hinton insists that terrorists once kidnapped him. He is afraid that they will return to "finish the job." What is the best response? *(1109-1113, Nursing Care Plan 49-1, Box 49-2)*
   a. "Tell me more about why you think terrorists are after you."
   b. "I can see that you are afraid, but I believe that we are safe here."
   c. "You seem very afraid, but we will protect you from those people."
   d. "Your story about this kidnapping is frightening, but it's illogical."

4. In the acute phase, which is the priority diagnosis for Mr. Hinton? *(1108)*
   a. Acute confusion related to a chemical imbalance
   b. Social isolation related to fear and feelings of persecution
   c. Other-directed or self-directed violence, risk for, related to delusional thinking
   d. Self-care deficit related to cognitive impairment

5. Mr. Hinton loudly argues with the medication nurse and refuses to take his morning medications. "She is a terrorist and is trying to poison all the patients!" What is your first action? *(1109-1110, 1113, Box 49-2)*
   a. Point out to Mr. Hinton that other patients are taking the medicines without ill effects.
   b. Call the physician and ask for a temporary emergency order to administer medications.
   c. Support the authority of the medication nurse by gathering 4 or 5 other staff members.
   d. Distract Mr. Hinton and then later see if he will accept the medication from another nurse.

6. Which activity would be most appropriate for Mr. Hinton in the early acute phase of hospitalization? *(1109-1112, Nursing Care Plan 49-1)*
   a. Attending a music therapy class
   b. Walking in an enclosed patio garden
   c. Playing cards or checkers in the day room
   d. Sleeping in his room undisturbed

SHORT ANSWER

Borderline Personality Disorder

Directions: Read the clinical scenario and answer the questions that follow.

Scenario: You are working on a medical-surgical unit. You hear in report that all of the nurses are having trouble dealing with Ms. Aunders, who was admitted several days ago. One of the RNs suggests a psychiatric consult be obtained because the patient is extremely manipulative, demanding, and "unlikely to follow the treatment plan." Old medical records show that Ms. Aunders has been previously diagnosed with a borderline personality disorder.

1. What are the four characteristics of personality disorders? *(1113)*

   a. _____

   b. _____

   c. _____

   d. _____

Copyright © 2013, 2009 by Saunders, an imprint of Elsevier Inc. All rights reserved.

2. What are four things to assess for in a patient whom you think might have a personality disorder? *(1115, Box 49-4)*

   a. _____

   b. _____

   c. _____

   d. _____

3. Write an outcome for the nursing diagnosis: Self-esteem, chronic low, related to past failures and negative responses from significant others. *(1115-1116)*

   _____

   _____

   _____

4. What are two nursing interventions used to deal with manipulative behavior of patients who have personality disorders? *(1113, Box 49-2)*

   a. _____

   b. _____

PRIORITY SETTING AND ASSIGNMENT

Directions: Read the scenario and prioritize as appropriate.

Scenario: You are caring for Mr. Radcheck. He has been rocking and fidgeting and refuses to interact with the staff or other patients. You have observed him talking to himself and you suspect that he may be having command hallucinations.

1. What is the priority nursing diagnosis? *(1106)*
   a. Acute confusion with delusions
   b. Sensory perceptions, disturbed (hallucinations)
   c. Social interaction, impaired
   d. Risk for other-directed or self-directed violence

Mr. Radcheck is now pacing. He yells at one of the other patients and then comes to you and says, "That blearsoning boop is rounding, rounding! Get her down! Stick her with a knife and glass and dead her head!"

2. What is the priority intervention? *(1109)*
   a. Try to figure out what he is saying and empathize.
   b. Firmly instruct him to calm down and go sit down.
   c. Gently tell him his behavior is inappropriate.
   d. Redirect him to a quiet and isolated area.

3. Mr. Radcheck is unable to follow your verbal instructions. His pacing increases and he begins to wildly gesture. What is the priority action? *(1109-1113)*
   a. Remove the other patients and allow him to pace.
   b. Gather several staff members to stand behind you.
   c. Call the doctor for an order for chemical restraints.
   d. Repeat your verbal instructions and state the consequences.

Copyright © 2013, 2009 by Saunders, an imprint of Elsevier Inc. All rights reserved.

4. The nursing assistant is available to help you with Mr. Radcheck. What task would be appropriate to assign to the assistant? *(1109-1113)*
   a. Ask the assistant to try to calm him down.
   b. Ask the assistant to go call the doctor.
   c. Have the assistant do 1:1 as ordered by the doctor.
   d. Assign the assistant to put the patient in four-point restraint.

5. The next day, Mr. Radcheck is calm and quiet. Which task would be appropriate to assign to the nursing assistant? *(1109-1113)*
   a. Sit with Mr. Radcheck and ask him how he is feeling.
   b. Encourage Mr. Radcheck to take a shower.
   c. Talk with Mr. Radcheck about his future plans.
   d. Observe Mr. Radcheck for any agitated behavior.

REVIEW QUESTIONS FOR THE NCLEX® EXAMINATION

Directions: Choose the best answer(s) for the following questions.

1. A nurse is caring for a patient with paranoid schizophrenia. Which behavior indicates that the patient is having delusions of persecution? *(1104)*
   1. Tilts head and appears to be listening.
   2. Paces around the dayroom with arms folded.
   3. Refuses to eat food unless it is packaged.
   4. Strikes out at a curtain that is waving in the breeze.

2. The patient is taking an antipsychotic medication, fluphenazine (Prolixin). Which side effect, if noted, should the nurse identify as most significant, requiring immediate intervention? *(1105)*
   1. A fixed upward gaze
   2. A shuffling gait
   3. Tapping of the foot
   4. Irritability

3. The patient was admitted yesterday following an episode of violence at a library. He is currently quiet, but displays psychotic behaviors. When planning care for the patient, the nurse plans to avoid which action? *(1109, 1113, Box 49-2)*
   1. Address the patient by name and establish rapport.
   2. Use therapeutic touch to communicate caring.
   3. Control environmental stimuli such as loud music.
   4. Allow the patient to move about in an enclosed area.

4. The patient tells the nurse that there are a several men in dark coats that are watching her and planning to steal her belongings. The best response from the nurse is: *(1113, Box 49-2)*
   1. "There are no men watching you."
   2. "Tell me more about these men."
   3. "I did not see any men."
   4. "They won't hurt you."

5. The nurse is working in an acute admission ward in a psychiatric facility. Which safety precautions should the nurse take when caring for these acutely ill patients? *(Select all that apply.)* *(1109-1110)*
   1. Avoid wearing flashing or dangling jewelry.
   2. Avoid wearing a white coat or white uniform.
   3. Avoid wearing a stethoscope, scarf, or tie around the neck.
   4. Avoid casual touching without asking permission.
   5. Avoid doorways and exits.
   6. Avoid any patients who appear sullen or depressed.

Copyright © 2013, 2009 by Saunders, an imprint of Elsevier Inc. All rights reserved.

6. The patient is taking olanzapine (Zyprexa) as prescribed. Which patient comment suggests that the medication is successfully treating the patient's positive symptoms? *(1113)*
   1. "I can leave the hospital whenever I want to."
   2. "Nurse, I am ready to go home. Would you call my mother?"
   3. "I can still hear the voices, but they are very distant."
   4. "The angel stopped talking; now she just sits and waves."

7. The patient is ready to be discharged. The nurse teaches him about his antipsychotic medication and he asks, "What will happen if I stop taking my medication when I go home?" Which is the best reply? *(1104-1105, 1108, 1113)*
   1. "You should never stop taking your medication."
   2. "Someday you may be able to do without the medication."
   3. "If you can get organized and reduce stress, perhaps you can get along without it."
   4. "If you stop taking your medication, the symptoms will probably return."

8. The patient will be discharged within a day or two. Which statement by the patient's family indicates a need for further discussion about the diagnosis of schizophrenia? *(1105, 1108)*
   1. "A stable home environment will help to prevent relapse."
   2. "He might always hear voices, but the medications will help."
   3. "Medication will eliminate his blunted affect and social isolation."
   4. "If he fails to take his medication, it will probably lead to readmission."

9. A patient with schizophrenia comes to the nurse and says, "Here we go, got flacks and sacks and jibbogny tomorrow. Would you like some?" What is the best response? *(1109)*
   1. "Say that again. I couldn't understand what you are saying."
   2. "Sure thing, flacks and sacks and jibbogny sounds great to me."
   3. "I don't quite understand, but I do appreciate you including me."
   4. "You are not making any sense. Try to speak clearly."

10. The nurse is assessing a new patient who was just admitted for schizophrenia. The patient is easily distracted and is rocking back and forth. What strategy should the nurse try *first*? *(1109, 1113, Box 49-2)*
    1. Get as much information from the chart as possible.
    2. Attempt to get a phone number for a family member.
    3. Use short sentences that can be answered with a yes or no.
    4. Delay the assessment until the patient is more coherent.

11. What is a potential complication of residual negative symptoms that do not respond to medication? *(1104, 1113)*
    1. Apathy results in failure to adhere to medication regimen.
    2. Bizarre behavior such as public nudity results in social stigma.
    3. Tardive dykinesia is permanent and debilitating.
    4. Auditory hallucinations continue, but are less problematic.

12. A patient is admitted to the unit with a diagnosis of borderline personality disorder. Which behavior most typifies this disorder? *(1114)*
    1. Can decide what to eat for breakfast without help
    2. Eyes are cast downwards when speaking to others
    3. Suddenly gives her favorite blouse to another patient
    4. Glares at strangers when they enter the room

Copyright © 2013, 2009 by Saunders, an imprint of Elsevier Inc. All rights reserved.

13. The nurse is talking with a patient who has a borderline personality disorder. The patient says, "I'll tell you a secret, because you are the best nurse here." Which comment should the nurse identify as most significant, requiring immediate notification of the registered nurse? *(1114-1116)*
    1. "I lied to get in here, because I was sick of living with my mother."
    2. "The charge nurse is a lesbian. I've seen her in the lesbo clubs."
    3. "I am going to give myself a little superficial cut, so that the doctor will see me."
    4. "I stole some money from my father and he might hurt me when I get out."

14. The nursing diagnosis for a patient is Chronic low self-esteem. The nurse instructs the patient to do which activity to promote self-esteem? *(Select all that apply.)* *(1109-1110)*
    1. Make a list of things that she is good at.
    2. Give and receive positive feedback.
    3. Set small, realistic goals.
    4. Describe personal failures in detail to a friend.
    5. Critique personal performance for errors.
    6. Keep a journal of success stories.

CRITICAL THINKING ACTIVITIES

Scenario: You have talked to Christy Smith and feel that rapport has been established. Ms. Smith has shared personal information with you. She states, "I really like talking to you." You leave Ms. Smith to admit a new patient. Later, when you return, Ms. Smith hits you and tries to run out the door.

1. What are your initial thoughts about this scenario? _____

_____

_____

_____

2. What factors may have triggered Ms. Smith's aggressive behavior? *(1108-1109, 1113, Box 49-2)*

_____

_____

_____

_____

3. What types of things should you do to protect yourself, patients, and others? *(1108-1109, 1113, Box 49-2)*

_____

_____

_____

_____

Copyright © 2013, 2009 by Saunders, an imprint of Elsevier Inc. All rights reserved.

STEP TOWARD BETTER COMMUNICATION

VOCABULARY BUILDING GLOSSARY

Term	Pronunciation	Definition
trigger	trig′ger	start a reaction, cause to begin
de-escalation	dee esk ah lay′ shun	process of coming back down, as in the calming of a nervous, hyperactive patient
extrapyramidal	eks′ trah pir ram′ i dal	symptoms outside the pyramidal tracts of the nervous system
erratic	eh rat′ik	inconsistent, not performing normally; irregular
odd	awd	something or someone different, strange, unusual, or surprising
eccentric	ek sen′ trik	showing unusual behavior; unconventional, peculiar
impulsive	im puhl′ siv	acting on sudden urges or desires without thinking of the consequences
boundaries	bown′dreez	limits to behavior or movement
recur	ree ker′	happen again
rationale	rah shun al′	the reason for doing something; the thoughts about why to do something
acting out	ak′ ting owt	expressing feelings through nonverbal behavior
borderline	bor′ der lyn	on the edge or boundary; precarious
"get under the skin"		causing a reaction, such as irritation or attraction
traits	trayts	characteristic actions or behaviors
subsequent	sub′ see kwent	later, following, after a previous event

CHOOSING THE CORRECT WORD

Directions: Underline the word in parentheses that correctly completes the thought.

1. The patient would often take things from stores; this is an example of (eccentric/impulsive) behavior.

2. The patient was removing her clothes in the dayroom after her husband came to visit; this is an example of (subsequent/acting out) behavior.

3. The patient demonstrated (erratic/odd) behavior by weaving pieces of Styrofoam and old milk cartons into her hair.

4. The nurse was firm with the borderline personality disorder patient, setting (boundaries/rationale) for acceptable behavior.

5. The family did not know what would (trigger/recur) manic behavior in the patient.

6. Lying and manipulative behaviors are characteristic (traits/de-escalation) of people with borderline personality disorders.

Copyright © 2013, 2009 by Saunders, an imprint of Elsevier Inc. All rights reserved.

COMMUNICATION

The following is a sample dialogue showing how a nurse can intervene when a patient is becoming agitated. The patient, Anna, is speaking in a loud voice and waving her hands in her daughter's face.

Anna: "You must accept Jesus as your savior or you won't go to heaven. Why haven't you been going to church? You'll be damned forever. I'm saved. Why can't you save yourself?"

Nurse (to patient): "Anna, I see your daughter is here to visit. I like the dress you have on, Anna. You have on your new shoes too!

Nurse (to daughter): "Anna chose this outfit, because she knew you were coming today"

Daughter: "You look really nice, Mom."

Nurse: "Yes, she is all ready to have lunch with you in the garden room. Anna, are you hungry? Let's go down to lunch."

The nurse has used distraction to de-escalate Anna's behavior. At the same time, the attention to Anna and the sincere compliments help increase Anna's self-esteem and establish that the nurse is caring and empathetic.

DESCRIPTIVE TERMS

Directions: Place the characteristic behaviors listed below with the correct type of disorder in Cluster A, B, or C as listed in Box 49-3 on p. 1114 in the textbook.

clinging	impulsive	perfectionist	socially inhibited
attention-seeking	submissiveness	suspicious	eccentric
distrustful	need for admiration	fears rejection	feels inadequate
lacks empathy	odd	need for control	needy
grandiosity	disregards rights of others	extremely emotional	distorted feelings
lability of emotions	distorted thinking		

Cluster A (Odd/Eccentric)	Cluster B (Dramatic/Erratic)	Cluster C (Anxious/Fearful)
1.	1.	1.
2.	2.	2.
3.	3.	3.
4.	4.	4.
5.	5.	5.
6.	6.	6.
	7.	7.
	8.	8.

Copyright © 2013, 2009 by Saunders, an imprint of Elsevier Inc. All rights reserved.